Cambridge History of Medicine

EDITORS: CHARLES WEBSTER and CHARLES ROSENBERG

Public health in British India

After years of neglect the last decade has witnessed a surge of interest in the medical history of India under colonial rule. This is the first major study of preventative medicine in British India. The author considers the purposes, nature and political significance of colonial medical intervention. Familiar themes such as medicine's role in the consolidation of colonial rule are examined in a new and more critical light, exposing the gap between the rhetoric and the reality of colonial medical policy. The book also explores many previously unresearched areas such as European attitudes towards India and its inhabitants, and the way in which these were reflected in medical literature and medical policy; the fate of public health at local level under Indian control; and the effects of quarantine on colonial trade and the pilgrimage to Mecca. The book places medicine within the context of debates about the government of India, and relations between rulers and ruled. In emphasising the active role of the indigenous population, and in its range of material, it differs significantly from most other work conducted in this subject area.

Cambridge History of Medicine

EDITED BY
CHARLES WEBSTER
Reader in the History of Medicine, University of Oxford,
and Fellow of All Souls College

CHARLES ROSENBERG
Professor of History and Sociology of Science,
University of Pennsylvania

For a list of titles in the series, see end of book

Public health in British India: Anglo-Indian preventive medicine 1859–1914

MARK HARRISON

Wellcome Institute for the History of Medicine, London

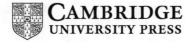

CAMBRIDGE
UNIVERSITY PRESS

Published by the Press Syndicate of the University of Cambridge
The Pitt Building, Trumpington Street, Cambridge CB2 1RP
40 West 20th Street, New York, NY 10011–4211, USA
10 Stamford Road, Oakleigh, Melbourne 3166, Australia

© Cambridge University Press 1994

First published 1994

Printed in Great Britain at the University Press, Cambridge

A catalogue record for this book is available from the British Library

Library of Congress cataloguing in publication data
Harrison, Mark.
Publis health and preventive medicine in British India, 1859–1914
/ Mark Harrison.
p.   cm. – (Cambridge history of medicine)
Includes bibliographical references and index.
ISBN 0-521-44127-7 (hc)
1. Medicine, Preventive – Government policy – India. 2. Public
health – India – History – 19th century. 3. Public health – India –
History – 20th century. 4. Medical policy – India – History – 19th
century. 5. Medical policy – India – History – 20th century.
6. India – History – British occupation, 1765–1947. I. Title.
II. Series.
[DNLM: 1. Public health – History – India. 2. Preventive Health
Services – History – India. 3. Health policy – History – India.
WA 11 J14 H3p 1994]
RA395.I5H38   1994
362.1'0954 – dc20
DNLM/DLC
for Library of Congress   93– 15646   CIP

ISBN 0 521 44127 7 hardback
ISBN 0 521 46688 1 paperback

To my parents

Contents

Illustrations

Plates

All illustrations are reproduced by courtesy of the Trustees of the Wellcome Trust, London

Figures

Tables

Preface

When I first began research for the doctoral thesis, of which this book is an extended and revised version, the history of medicine in British India was a neglected field of historical enquiry. There existed only a few articles – several of which were exploratory in nature – in contrast to a voluminous literature on public health in Britain, and a rapidly expanding body of scholarship on medicine in colonial Africa. Today this is happily no longer the case. Recent years have seen a growing interest in the subject, and a number of scholars are currently engaged in research on various aspects of medicine in colonial India. However, there is, as yet, no book-length account of public health in British India, and it is that historiographical gap that this volume attempts to fill.

This is a thematic rather than a narrative account, and its subject matter – given British India's diversity – is necessarily selective. Key dimensions of preventive medicine – professional, cultural, and administrative – have been chosen to illustrate the range of factors affecting the development of public health in India. I have done my best to place these firmly within the broader socio-political context of the subcontinent under British rule. The place of preventive medicine in colonial India is analysed with respect to its role in consolidating British dominion, its place in disputes over how best to govern India, and its significance for relations between rulers and ruled. It is hoped that this volume will make a contribution to current debates over the 'impact' of British rule in India, as well as to the history of colonial medicine.

In the course of my research I have incurred many debts, intellectual and otherwise. My supervisors, Margaret Pelling and Paul Weindling, deserve special thanks for guiding me through the troubled waters of post-graduate research. Drs Brian Harrison and Ian Catanach provided help at a formative stage in my research; while, in its final stages, this volume has benefited greatly from the comments and suggestions made by the examiners of my thesis – Professor David Arnold and Dr John Darwin. I have also to thank fellow students and colleagues at Corpus Christi and Green Colleges, and at the Wellcome Unit for the History of Medicine, Oxford; at NISTADS, New Delhi; and most recently at the Wellcome Institute for the History of Medicine, London. In particular, I would like to thank Humaira Ahmed for her advice on preparing earlier drafts of my manuscript; Gillian Maude for copy editing the typescript; Paul Gladding for assistance with graphics; and Helen Power and Molly Sutphen for sharing their knowledge of Leonard Rogers and William Simpson respectively.

I am indebted, too, to the staff of the following libraries for their patience and helpful advice: the India Office Library, London; the National Archives of India, New Delhi; the Wellcome Institute Library, London; the London School of Tropical Medicine; the Public Record Office, London; and the Indian Institute, Bodleian, and Radcliffe Science libraries, Oxford. Invaluable financial assistance was also provided by the Economic and Social Science Research Council; the Wellcome Trust; Corpus Christi and Green Colleges, the Arnold, Bryce and Reed Fund, and the trustees of the Curzon Memorial Prize, at Oxford University; and the trustees of the Singer Prize, awarded by the British Society for the History of Science.

I would also like to thank the editors of the *British Journal for the History of Science* and the *Indian Economic and Social History Review* for their permission to re-print articles from their journals, see chapters 2 and 5 respectively.

Lastly, and most importantly, I am indebted to my parents and family, and most recently to Emma Harrison, for their constant support and encouragement.

Select abbreviations

AMD	Army Medical Department
AMS	Army Medical Service
ASC	Army Sanitary Commission
BHO	Bombay Health Officers Quarterly Reports
BMA	British Medical Association
BMJ	*British Medical Journal*
Capt.	Captain
CCS	Certificate of the Corporation of Surgeons
Col.	Colonel
Comm.	Commissioner
Conf.	Conference
CP	Central Provinces
Dep.	Deputy
DGIMS	Director-General, Indian Medical Service
FKQCP	Fellow, Kings and Queens College of Physicians, Ireland
FRCP	Fellow of the Royal College of Physicians
FRCS	Fellow of the Royal College of Surgeons
Gen.	General (military)
Genl.	General
GOBe	Government of Bengal
GOBo	Government of Bombay
GOI	Government of India
GOM	Government of Madras
ICS	Indian Civil Service
IJMR	*Indian Journal of Medical Research*
IMG	*Indian Medical Gazette*
IPHMJ	*Indian Public Health and Municipal Journal*

IMS	Indian Medical Service
IOR	India Office Records
IPC	*Reports of the Indian Plague Commission*
IPS	Indian Police Service
IRFA	Indian Research Fund Association
JTM	*Journal of Tropical Medicine*
LAH	Licentiate of the Apothecaries' Hall (Dublin)
LFPSG	Licentiate of the Faculty of Physicians and Surgeons, Glasgow
LKQCP	Licentiate of Kings and Queens College of Physicians, Ireland
LMS	Licentiate in Medicine and Surgery, India
LRCP	Licentiate of the Royal College of Physicians
LRCS	Licentiate of the Royal College of Surgeons
LSA	Licentiate of the Society of Apothecaries
Lt.	Lieutenant
Maj.	Major
MB	Bachelor of medicine
Medl.	Medical
MD	Doctor of medicine
MFPSG	Member of the Faculty of Physicians and Surgeons, Glasgow
MKQCP	Member of the Kings and Queens College of Physicians
MOH	Medical Officer of Health
MRCP	Member of the Royal College of Physicians
MRCS	Member of the Royal College of Surgeons
NAI	National Archives of India
NMS	Navy Medical Service
NWP (and O)	North West Provinces (and Oudh)
Physl.	Physical
Procs.	Proceedings
RAMC	Royal Army Medical Service
San.	Sanitary
SCA	*Report of the Sanitary Commissioner for Assam*
SCBe	*Report of the Sanitary Commissioner for Bengal*
SCBo	*Report of the Sanitary Commissioner for Bombay*
SCCP	*Report of the Sanitary Commissioner for the Central Provinces*
SCGI	*Report of the Sanitary Commissioner with the Government of India*
SCM	*Report of the Sanitary Commissioner for Madras*
SCNWP	*Report of the Sanitary Commissioner for the North West Provinces and Oudh*

SCP	*Report of the Sanitary Commissioner for the Punjab*
Sci. Mems.	*Scientific Memoirs of Medical Officers of the Army of India*
Sec.	Secretary
Surg.	Surgeon
Trans.	Transactions
VR	Vaccination records
WIHM	Wellcome Institute for the History of Medicine

Glossary

Anglo-Indian	Briton living in India
ayurveda	Hindu medicine
babu	western-educated Indian
bhadralok	'respectable folk' in Bengal
Brahmin	priestly caste
busti	slum dwelling
Eurasian	person of mixed European and Indian parentage
hakim	practitioner of Islamic medicine
halacore	street sweeping and night-soil collection
lakh	100,000
mofussil	hinterland of provincial capital
octroi	trades tax
panchayat	village union
ryot	peasant
tahsil	sub-division of a district
taluka	as above, in NWP and O
unani	Islamic medicine
vaid	practitioner of Hindu medicine
zemindar	landowner

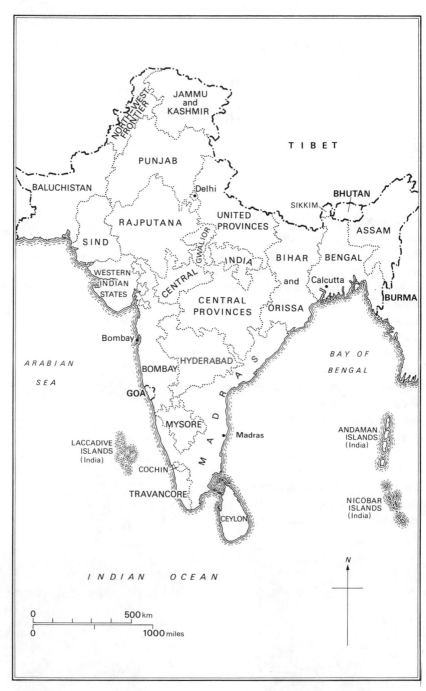

British India in the first half of the twentieth century

Introduction

My main aim in writing this book has not been simply to provide an account of the development of public health in British India, but to explore its broader social and political significance. In so doing, I have ventured into largely uncharted territory, and I am acutely conscious of the fact that I have left many areas of public health in India uncovered. However, it is probably impossible to give a comprehensive account of public health in India within the confines of a single volume and, in any case, undesirable, given India's ethnic, epidemiological, and administrative diversity. What follows is a thematic study of several key areas of preventive medicine and public health, illustrating the theoretical, professional, and administrative aspects of its development. The latter dimension is examined at local, national, and international levels.

Although the subject of this book is a relatively new one, it was not conceived in a historiographical wilderness. The last decade, especially, has witnessed a surge of interest in the medical history of British India, and of the European colonies more generally. Much of this literature has been of an exceptionally high quality, and I owe a great debt to its authors for the insights they have given me. In this volume I do my best to address many of the questions and issues raised in this literature, while offering many explanations and interpretations for which I, alone, am responsible. I have found it necessary to take issue with some of the claims made by certain scholars, and to qualify or modify the arguments of others, but this book does not represent a fundamental historiographical revision. Indeed, it is probably unwise at the present time to speak of a scholarly consensus with respect to medicine in India, for much of the literature has been of an exploratory nature. Moreover, the only universal theme in this literature – the limited scope and effectiveness of colonial medical intervention – is one which I endorse.

This book differs from most existing scholarship chiefly in the weight it gives to certain factors in explaining these limitations and, in particular, the importance of political relationships with sections of the indigenous population.

1

It also stresses to a much greater extent the active role of Indians as policy makers at local and municipal level; the varied and often conflicting viewpoints of colonial administrators and medical officers; and the importance of practical constraints, such as local revenues. Another important difference lies in the conclusions which are drawn about medicine's role in the consolidation of imperial rule in India. Preventive medicine, I argue, was less central to this process than is sometimes imagined.

Medicine's role as a 'tool of empire' is probably the most familiar theme in the historiography of colonial medicine to date, and has its origins in the writings of colonial medical officers and imperial politicians. Their principal concern was with the health of Europeans in the tropics, and especially of troops – the ultimate guarantors of imperial rule. The vulnerability of Europeans in the tropics has also formed the subject of several more recent studies, most notably Philip Curtin's 'The White Man's Grave' and *The Image of Africa*, which were published in the early 1960s.[1] Curtin's latest book – *Death by Migration* – returns to the same theme, with a study of 'relocation costs' among European soldiers in the tropics between 1815 and 1914. Here, Curtin emphasises the human costs of empire, but argues that improvements in hygiene and medicine began to make a significant impact on mortality among European troops from the middle of the century.[2] In a similar vein, Daniel Headrick, in his influential *Tools of Empire*, lists medicine among several technologies which proved crucial to the success of European expansion and dominion over large parts of the globe.[3]

These studies have done much to illuminate an important and neglected dimension of imperial history, although they perhaps raise as many questions as they answer. As David Arnold has pointed out, Headrick's reading of the evidence is rather selective, and he certainly exaggerates the effectiveness of medical intervention in the form of quinine prophylaxis against malaria.[4] More serious is Headrick's emphasis on means rather than motive. Was it, perhaps, imperial expansion which provided the stimulus to technological innovation, rather than the inverse relationship which Headrick describes? Certainly, the absence of effective medical intervention did not prevent the development of plantation agriculture in the West Indies, the British conquest of India, French dominion in Algeria,[5] or the Dutch presence in the East Indies.[6] Equally, Curtin's analysis of relocation costs does not address the effects of high mortality on European *perceptions* of the tropics or its implications for the colonial enterprise. His exclusive emphasis on mortality rates also gives the impression that the threat posed to European colonialism by disease declined considerably from the middle of the century. But, as I attempt to show in chapters 2 and 3, especially, morbidity rates present a very different picture, and were a major cause of anxiety well into the twentieth century. It was not mortality from diseases such as cholera, but the persistent incapacitating effects of malaria, typhoid, and venereal disease which most concerned colonial authorities.

It was not only in the military sphere that medicine came to be viewed as a 'tool of empire'. In the early eighteenth century, medicine entered the discourse of economic efficiency, with inoculation against smallpox introduced on slaving vessels, and limited medical provisions being made for slaves in plantations in the West Indies and the Americas.[7] But medicine did not become prominent in the rhetoric of empire until the late nineteenth century, following concerns over colonial indebtedness, and with the growing political importance of imperial themes. For the colonial secretary Joseph Chamberlain, medical progress seemed to offer the prospect of improved labour efficiency, and the opening-up of hitherto impenetrable areas of the tropics.[8] One manifestation of this 'constructive imperialism' was the establishment of the London School of Tropical Medicine in 1899, while the Liverpool School, founded the previous year, was promoted by mercantile interests as an investment in colonial trade.[9] These notions persisted into the interwar period, although economic adversity made governments more reluctant to intervene. Such texts as Balfour and Scott's *Health Problems of the Empire* – published in 1924 – were written largely to convince British and colonial administrations of the economic utility of medical intervention.[10] How far such considerations shaped public health policy in India is, as yet, little understood. I argue here that the gap between rhetoric and reality was considerable.

Medicine has also been viewed as an instrument of 'social control' in the colonies, providing means of 'knowing' the indigenous population, and rationales for social segregation. In an influential article of 1977 Maynard Swanson described how the presence of bubonic plague in the Cape Colony provided a pretext for racial segregation, with public health officials at the forefront of such demands.[11] Indeed, fear of infection from the indigenous population served to reinforce segregated residential patterns throughout colonial Africa,[12] and to some extent in India.[13] More generally, public health measures have been viewed as powerful tools for the domination of indigenous peoples. These took the form of selective and degrading medical intervention,[14] detention and isolation,[15] controls on population movement,[16] and demonstrations of colonial benevolence intended to reduce resistance to imperial rule.[17] It is also claimed that medicine played an important role in the creation of the colonial subject, although how far the negative images portrayed in colonial medical texts affected indigenous peoples' understanding of themselves is still largely unknown.[18] The role of medicine as a 'colonising discourse' is considered in chapter 2 of this book, while the subsequent chapters assess the extent to which public health measures were conceived in terms of 'social control', and their effectiveness in performing this function. I argue that medicine both shaped and reflected an increasingly negative view of India and its people, but that the desire to control and contain the indigenous population was checked by the political and economic imperatives of colonial rule.

Another major theme of this book concerns contradictions and rivalries within the imperial order itself, and the way in which these were illustrated or exposed by debates on public health. I argue that the relationship between colonial priorities and medical policies was much less straightforward than has generally been suggested.[19] The formulation of public health policy is, perhaps, best understood as a contest between two different conceptions of empire. The one, authoritarian and paternalistic, emphasising Europe's 'civilising' mission in the tropics. The other, liberal and decentralist, stressing the constraints imposed upon government action by shortages of revenue, indigenous resistance, and competing claims on the resources of local and central government.[20] I aim to show how these different conceptions of empire manifested themselves in the administration of public health from central government down to district and municipal commissions.

Although the development of public health in British India reflected the relative dominance of these competing imperial ideologies, it was affected also by prevailing attitudes and events outside the subcontinent. The importance of medical issues in relations between the imperial 'metropole' and the colonial 'periphery' was a theme which I first began to explore in an analysis of the international sanitary conferences and their effects on colonial trade, and the annual pilgrimage of Indian Muslims to Mecca and Medina. I argued that international pressures to restrict the passage of Indian vessels through the Suez Canal exposed a cleavage between the British and Indian governments. The former taking a stance diametrically opposed to the wishes of the Indian government, compelling it to pursue a sanitary policy which threatened to jeopardise its relations with the Muslim community.[21] Here, I elaborate upon this theme using additional evidence concerning the role of Muslim élites in the pilgrimage controversy, and with reference to imperial interference in other spheres of public health.

In addition to the imperial determinants of sanitary policy it is necessary to consider the attitudes and responses of indigenous peoples themselves. At present very little is known about Indian responses to colonial medical initiatives, although excellent work has been done on the political dimensions of the Indian plague epidemics of 1896 onwards.[22] However, the fate of indigenous medicine under colonial rule has attracted more attention, and demonstrates both competition and accommodation between western and traditional systems; though with the displacement of certain specialisms such as bone setting and lithotomy.[23] Together, these studies suggest the importance of medicine as an index of convergence and divergence between eastern and western cultures; a theme which is developed in the present study through an examination of Indian responses to public health measures, and the role of Indians in the policy-making process at municipal and district level.

It is argued that the dominance of indigenous élites in municipal adminis-tration from the 1870s, and European fears of provoking the Indian masses after the mutiny/rebellion of 1857, were two of the most important factors shaping the development of sanitary policy in India. The need to co-opt indigenous élites into the governance of India, and to avoid civil unrest, acted as a brake upon authoritarian elements within the British administration, and fostered an official approach to public health based on co-operation rather than confrontation. However, frustration with the slow pace of reform in many cases served to increase tension between the Anglo-Indian and indigenous populations. Many Europeans (and Indian Muslims) resented moves towards self-government which resulted in the dominance of local administration by the majority Hindu community, and demanded a reversal of these reforms in the name of sanitary progress. Hindu municipal commissioners were, themselves, divided over the question of sanitary reform. The rhetoric of reform was appropriated by modernising nationalists, but contested by more orthodox sections of the community, and by the landed interests who had most to lose from increases in local taxation, or regulations concerning rented properties. These themes are considered in chapter 7, together with other factors affecting the development of sanitation under local self-government, and in a more detailed way in chapter 8 – a case study of Calcutta. In the latter, I argue that the economic interests of the city's Indian *rentier* class constituted the single greatest obstacle to sanitary reform.

1

The Indian medical service

Science and reason is not enough. A man must also have a heart and be capable of understanding the beauties of art and literature. (J. G. Farrell, *The Siege of Krishnapur*)

The role of medical officers in shaping public health policy in British India can only be fully understood in the light of their aspirations, priorities, and grievances. This chapter attempts to place the Indian Medical Service (IMS) in its political and social context: to assess its standing in colonial society and in relation to the medical profession in Britain. It is argued that medical officers in India were unable to achieve the same degree of occupational control and influence over society which was achieved by the medical profession in nineteenth-century Britain, and that this was due principally to the conflicting priorities of the colonial regime. The 'imperial' designs of the medical profession only rarely coincided with those of the Indian government, which was wary of interfering with indigenous medical practices and which generally subordinated medicine to the military and political imperatives of colonial rule.[1] As a result, the IMS was far less attractive to potential recruits than either the Indian Civil Service (ICS) or the British and Indian armies, and suffered in extreme form from the conservatism and internal tensions which afflicted all colonial services to varying extents. The inertia and status anxiety which gripped the IMS had important implications for the development of public health in British India. Innovation in medical theory and practice was often positively discouraged by senior officers in the service, while the military orientation of the IMS, and its lack of internal dynamism, fostered fatalism about the plight of the Indian people.

The question of professional status has been explored in several historical studies of the British medical community,[2] but there have been few systematic or detailed studies of the social composition of the uniformed medical services – colonial or military. Existing work in this area has been confined largely to

6

official, and generally uncritical, participant histories; though some, like Crawford's *History of the Indian Medical Service*, are remarkably comprehensive and rich in social data.[3] There are, however, several good accounts of the development of the state medical services in Britain, and of other Indian services, which provide valuable comparative material for this study of the IMS.[4]

The medical services: their origins and structure

The British medical presence in India dates from 1600, when a small number of ship's surgeons arrived on board the East India Company's first fleet. The number of British surgeons in India increased steadily as the Company extended its trading operations, but there was no regular medical establishment until 1763, when the Bengal Medical Service was formed.[5] The Bengal service set fixed grades or ranks, and definite rules for promotion; it comprised 4 head surgeons, 8 surgeons, and 28 surgeon's mates. Medical services were soon formed on similar lines in the other two presidencies of Bombay and Madras. In 1775 the medical services were expanded, and medical boards set up in each presidency to administer European hospitals.

The major stimulus to reorganisation was the Company's expansionist policy in the mid-eighteenth century, which drew it into wars against the French and with Indian rulers. Hitherto, the Company had employed no regular forces except small garrisons at the more important 'factories', including Calcutta and Madras, but open warfare between the English and French companies during 1750–4 and the Seven Years War against France (1756–63) made necessary the establishment of a larger and more permanent military presence in India, and a corresponding expansion of military medical services. Under rules issued by Governor-General Lord Cornwallis in 1788, surgeons were not permitted to enter civil employment until they had performed almost 2 years' military service. A century later, the situation had changed little, with surgeons being required to undergo at least 2 years in the military wing of the Indian Medical Service (formally separated from its civil wing in 1858), before being eligible for a civil-surgeoncy, and they remained liable to be recalled for military service in the event of an emergency. The Indian medical services, then, were predominantly military in orientation – inescapably so, given the Company's reliance on military power as the ultimate guarantee of its dominance in India.

The wars of the eighteenth century also highlighted the need for assistants and orderlies in European hospitals in India.[6] From very early times, the Company employed Indians, and occasionally European soldiers, as compounders, dressers, and apothecaries. In Bengal, in the 1760s, these assistants were organised into a Military Subordinate Medical Service (SMS), and similar measures were taken in the other presidencies in the early nineteenth century.[7] By 1833, a comparable civil establishment had come into being in Bengal, and

2 years later, with the founding of Calcutta Medical College, military and civil assistant surgeons and hospital assistants (as they were now termed) were required to undergo a 2-year course of instruction, and an apprenticeship at a recognised medical institution. The strength of the SMS grew steadily from 20 to 40 men per presidency in 1848, to over 500 throughout India by 1914.[8]

The expansion of the SMS and the superior service in the first half of the nineteenth century paralleled British territorial expansion in India. Since Clive's assumption of the *diwani* (the right to collect land revenues) in Bengal in 1765, the Company was increasingly involved in administrative matters and, by 1833, after successive alterations to its charter, it ceased to have any trading interests. At the same time, with the passage of Lord North's Regulating Act in 1773, and Pitt's India Act of 1784, the British government began its long involvement in the administration of India; initially through the Board of Commissioners for Indian affairs. The consolidation, and continued expansion, of British rule from the late eighteenth century, brought a rapid growth in the number of Europeans serving there, and a commensurate increase in the demand for civil medical services.

By 1857 the British were in possession of much of northern and southern India (with the exception of Mysore), and of western and lower Burma. But, with the abolition of its trading charter in 1833, the position of the East India Company became increasingly untenable. The Indian mutiny/rebellion of 1857 sounded the death-knell of the Company rule and, in the following year, the administration of India was transferred to the Crown. Henceforth, the Indian medical services became the responsibility of the British government. Surgeons in the Indian medical services became commissioned officers, although the Indian military medical service remained distinct from that of the British Army, which had its own medical service – the Army Medical Department (after 1898, the Royal Army Medical Corps). In 1896 the three presidency medical services were amalgamated into a single Indian medical service.

The history of public health administration in India also dates from the assumption of Crown rule. In 1859, in the wake of the mutiny, a special commission was set up to inquire into the sanitary state of the British Army in India. Epidemic disease had seriously depleted the fighting capacity of British troops in 1857, and, in the light of the public outcry over preventable deaths in the Crimea, there was increasing concern in Britain over military hygiene in India. In 1863 the commission reported that an average of 69 out of every 1,000 British troops in India died annually of disease. These findings caused an uproar in Britain and created a climate favourable to the reform of military hygiene in India. The commission also resulted in the establishment of sanitary commissions to monitor conditions in and around military cantonments.[9]

Hygiene within military stations was now regulated by the 1864 Military Cantonments Act, which established a system of sanitary police under the overall charge of military medical officers, and a scheme for the registration of deaths.[10] The provisions of the act, which covered the Indian as well as the European population of cantonments, was an indication of the growing conviction that the health of Europeans could not be considered in isolation. Though Europeans inhabited barracks or 'civil lines' usually at some remove from indigenous dwellings, they had frequent contact with Indian servants, and troops moved under few restrictions among the bazaars and the entourage surrounding military cantonments. It was this increasing concern with sanitary conditions immediately outside of European quarters that led to the reorganisation of colonial public health administration in 1868.

In that year the joint military/civilian presidency sanitary commissions were abolished. Military hygiene became the preserve of military medical officers, and civilian health of 'Sanitary Commissioners' attached to provincial governments, and the Government of India. The sanitary commission with the Indian government was aided by a statistical officer, and, from 1874, by two special scientific assistants. This central establishment was merged with the Vaccination Department in 1870 to form a central Sanitary Department. At provincial level, sanitary commissions were merged with the vaccination service at different times between 1870 and 1879. The sanitary commissioners served in an advisory capacity to government, having no executive powers: they were expected to 'ascertain as exactly as possible the existing sanitary condition of the country, and to suggest measures for its improvement'. This entailed making regular sanitary tours of each province, and the collection of vital and meteorological statistics.[11]

At local level, public health work was conducted by civil surgeons or, occasionally, by 'Executive Officers of Health' (modelled on British medical officers of health), employed by municipal authorities rather than by government, as in the case of sanitary commissioners. Any member of the civil IMS was eligible for employment as a sanitary commissioner or a health officer, though the latter, being a municipal appointment, was open to practitioners outside the IMS. Health officers worked under a patchwork of sanitary legislation, again modelled on British legislation, but adapted to Indian conditions. Usually, municipal sanitary regulations provided for the sweeping of streets and the collection and disposal of night soil ('conservancy'), and placed restrictions on 'noxious trades'. A 'small army' of Indian subordinate staff – including some supervisors and sanitary inspectors – was employed in connection with these duties, under the executive charge of the health officer.

Conditions of service

Officers of the IMS laboured under a double handicap. The low esteem in which the medical profession was held in mid-Victorian Britain was compounded in

India by the seeming indifference of the colonial administration. The social standing of the British profession was uncertain, even after the Medical Registration Act of 1858. Jeane Peterson reminds us that 'Victorian society in 1858 had limited confidence in the power of medical science and serious reservations about medical men's social authority and prestige.' Surgery had still not shaken off its status as a craft, and incomes from medical practice were barely sufficient to enable medical men to attain the status of 'gentleman'.[12] There were also marked variations in status within the medical profession. The old tripartite division between physicians, surgeons, and apothecaries (in descending order) was being replaced by new divisions, between general practitioners and consultants, and between those with lucrative private practices and those employed by local authorities as Poor Law medical officers or medical officers of health.[13]

Local authority appointments were often unpopular with medical graduates because the work was badly paid and lacked the autonomy associated with private practice. This was less true of the medical services in India, but there was still considerable dissatisfaction with levels of remuneration, and with other conditions of employment. Throughout the 1870s and 80s, the root cause of much discontent in the IMS was over-staffing, which meant that many new recruits were placed on lower rates of pay ('unemployed pay') until suitable posts were found for them. This arrangement often lasted for several years. Grievances about 'unemployed pay' had an important effect upon recruitment, and attracted a good deal of attention at the time. The mood of the 1880s is captured in this mischievous piece of doggerel written by a young surgeon, who had been on unemployed pay for some years:

> Sure of his creed, he longs to strive,
> Knowing the fittest will survive.
> Behold him then, in India's land,
> Anxiously waiting to turn his hand
> To the well-loved task, but he waits in vain
> Till dull grows the mind and torpid the brain;
> For the field's over-stocked and the work's too small;
> There's not enough work for the hands of all.[14]

But this situation did not last for long. Severe famines and the plague epidemics of the late 1890s stretched the medical services to their limit; personnel shortages and overwork became common causes of complaint. The *Indian Medical Gazette* warned in 1897 that 'much dissatisfaction is being felt in the Indian Medical Service owing to the continued stoppage of leave', due to the occurrence of plague, famine, and frontier disturbances.[15] These complaints were echoed in evidence given to the Indian Plague Commission in 1898–9. Major Grayfoot of Bombay insisted that his staff was not large enough to cope with plague, and that emergency measures like bringing assistant-surgeons out of retirement had failed to solve the problem. His subordinates had been unable to take leave for 3 years.[16]

Such conditions almost certainly deterred many medical graduates from joining the IMS. This was also true of the IMS's sister service, the Army Medical Service, which ministered to the British Army in India. Overwork and cancellations of leave in the 1890s exacerbated recruitment problems which had afflicted the AMS for much of the nineteenth century. As the *Indian Medical Gazette* put it, 'nearly every man who has been induced to enter the service of late years, and finds how he has been treated, personally warns his brothers, cousins and friends not to submit themselves to the treatment which unfortunately he has had to endure'.[17] The effects on recruitment were readily apparent: 'at the last examination . . . thirty-three men were obtained to fill fifty vacancies. Since then, a very large number of retirements has taken place . . . The service must be on its last legs as regards members.'[18]

But, if conditions in the medical services left much to be desired, they did at least offer financial stability. As the *Indian Medical Gazette* pointed out, the Indian Government offered the new recruit to the IMS Rs 420 per month; nearly double his market value at home. The service did not 'offer the great prizes, professional and pecuniary, which fall to the most successful men in the European capitals, but the on the other hand it has no blanks'.[19] This statement is in accord with Peterson's assertion that the IMS could provide a serviceable, if not brilliant, career.[20]

Much the same could be said for other Indian services. The IPS recruit started on Rs 250 per month, rising to a maximum in the case of presidency commissioners of Rs 1,500.[21] Yet, the IMS recruit fared substantially better than his equivalent in the IPS: the basic pay of a surgeon-captain in 1903 starting at Rs 450 per month, rising to a maximum of Rs 550 after 10 years. Higher ranks also earned more than senior IPS officers, but slightly less than their counterparts in the ICS.[22] Sanitary commissioners received a higher basic salary than ordinary IMS officers in compensation for the exclusion from private practice. Deputy sanitary commissioners (equivalent to the rank of surgeon captain) commanded a minimum monthly salary of Rs 500, rising to Rs 700 after ten years.[23]

This small increase in salary may seem like inadequate compensation for exclusion from private practice, but the rewards of private practice in India were uncertain and varied enormously from region to region. Those Indians who looked favourably upon western medicine tended to prefer treatment by their countrymen, especially as the fees charged by IMS men were so high. Indeed, complaints about the exorbitant fees charged to wealthy Indians were acted upon by government, which, anxious not to offend indigenous élites, placed a ceiling on charges for private practice by IMS men. Rising to the defence of the service, the *Journal of Tropical Medicine* denied that there had

been anything in the conduct of the members of the Service as a body to justify any
restriction of their constitutional rights whatsoever, and we challenge the Government of India to publish any sufficient number of cases of extortion to justify their
inflicting the gratuitous insults implied in these orders on a highly charitable and
honourable body of gentlemen.[24]

However, the record of the IMS does not stand up to scrutiny. While fees may
not have been excessive by Harley Street standards, they were far higher than
those charged to Europeans in India, and for some time these discriminatory
practices were sanctioned by government officials. Writing in defence of Major
Lane, an IMS officer who had attended the raja of Mandi and his family, the
commissioner of Jullunder Division, Punjab, maintained that 'Rs 10,000 [£666]
is a reasonable fee . . . Most London specialists would have charged at least
50 guineas a day . . . The traditional fee in India [for attendance on non-official
families] is Rs 300 a day for a Civil Surgeon and Rs 500 for a consultant from a
Presidency town.'[25]

These fees were far in excess of those charged to European civilians, for
whom IMS officers usually imposed a ceiling of Rs 160 a month. IMS officers
knew that western medicine was popular with the Indian aristocracy, for whom
it was a mark of high social status. The raja of Farid Kot, for instance, offered
the truly kingly sum of Rs 50,000 for successful treatment of his family.[26] But,
at the other end of the scale, the civil surgeon was finding it increasingly hard to
make a living from private practice. He had to compete with large numbers of
graduates from the Indian medical schools, and with unqualified persons
claiming to be 'doctors of medicine'. The value of the rupee relative to that of
sterling was another important consideration. In the 1870s and 80s the value of
the rupee fluctuated wildly, as the price of silver rose and fell in relation to that
of gold. After 1898 India was on a gold exchange standard, but the medical
profession in India was still lamenting the depressed state of the rupee in 1913.[27]

The position of the Subordinate Medical Service was much less satisfactory.
Indian hospital assistants (first class) received a starting salary of Rs 25 per
month, rising to a maximum of Rs 55 – equivalent to £20–40 per annum.[28] This
compared unfavourably with the pay of *tahsildars* (village headmen) who were
on a scale of Rs 50–250 per month. 'It can hardly be denied', commented the
Journal of Tropical Medicine in 1906, 'that the class is wretchedly paid in
proportion to the amount and the responsibility of the work expected of it, and
the scale of remuneration . . . compares ill with that accorded to public servants,
drawn from a similar class of Indian society, belonging to other departments'.[29]

Indian students taking the 4-year course qualifying them for entrance into the
subordinate service demanded a minimum of Rs 50 and an increase in their
maximum salary to Rs 150. There was also discontent over the English test
which was an essential requirement for entry into the service, and over their
professional designation. 'Assistant surgeon' or 'extra assistant surgeon' were

thought more appropriate for an individual who had completed a lengthy period of training, than 'hospital assistant'. The hospital assistants received the unwavering support of the *Journal of Tropical Medicine*[30] and the senior service in their demands.[31] But during the period under examination only one of their grievances was satisfactorily redressed – the designation 'hospital assistant' being changed to that of 'sub-assistant surgeon' in 1910.[32]

Another cause of discontent in the superior service was the slowness of promotion. Up to the rank of lieutenant-colonel, promotion was made primarily on the basis of seniority, and the lack of meritocracy within the service was a constant source of discontent among more ambitious medical officers.[33] In 1872 the *Indian Medical Gazette* protested that 'Assistant-Surgeons of eleven and twelve years standing have two hundred officers before them, to be promoted or otherwise disposed of, before they can gain the rank and pay of a Surgeon. They may have to wait for as much as twenty-one years before promotion.'[34]

Promotion to senior administrative ranks was even more difficult to achieve:

> twenty-six years was then [in 1880] considered the normal time at which an officer of the IMS might expect promotion to the administrative rank. Even then, this was far from being the case . . . Nowadays, with the rate at which promotion in the IMS has run for many years past, the idea sounds Utopian. For a long time past, an officer has been exceptionally fortunate if he had attained administrative rank with less than thirty years service.[35]

In 1909 there were 60 officers of more than 26 years service in the IMS who had not reached the rank of full colonel and, in 1911, the block in promotion was apparently 'as firm as ever'. Three years later, the government finally took steps to remedy the situation: a scheme of 'accelerated promotion' being introduced, whereby men of 16 years service became eligible for promotion to the rank of major 6 months earlier than usual. But it was a case of too little too late, and these measures did nothing to stem the rising unpopularity of the service.[36] Intense competition for promotion had a strong negative influence upon the service's willingness to innovate, and to assimilate new scientific ideas and medical practices. 'While in former times', wrote the editor of the *Madras Times* in 1880, 'medical officers . . . often set to work vigorously in India, they now scarcely, if ever, think of any but the work actually required of them'.[37] To 'get on', a recruit had to toe the line; as the *Journal of Tropical Medicine* put it in 1906, 'Once in the service stick to routine work, preferably on the military side, as the civil branch no longer presents any particular pecuniary advantages . . . Above all, avoid suspicion of originality or special ability in any direction.'[38]

Few recruits to the IMS appeared to question this advice. Even some of its most distinguished members, such as Ronald Ross (discoverer of the malaria vector), entered the service with few ambitions, and with little predilection for medicine. Ross had joined the service principally because his father (an Indian

Army general) had urged him to do so, and because it afforded excellent sporting opportunities – especially fishing, polo, and pig-sticking. It was only late in his Indian career that Ross acquired an interest in scientific research and in public health.[39] The recreational activities which attracted him to the IMS also loom large in the diaries of other medical officers stationed in India; often to the exclusion of any detailed description of medical practice.[40] The same is true of an article in *Dollar Magazine* entitled 'The Indian Medical Services as a career', which left any mention of medical practice until last, concentrating on the opportunities presented to the new recruit 'not only in the field of athletics, but in the wider field of sport such as he is unlikely to get in this country'. An officer in the military wing of the service apparently had a good deal of free time, which he generally devoted to games 'in a way which is unknown to anything like the same extent at home', while the 2 months annual leave available to even the most junior officer were commonly spent on hunting and fishing expeditions.[41]

Yet, as the writer of this article was well aware, there was much about service in India that was unattractive; not least the perceived dangers of the Indian climate.[42] Medical men were not immune to the diseases which took a heavy toll among the personnel of other services, and high mortality amongst them acted as a deterrent to potential recruits. In 1839–60, 207 of the 558 who were due to retire from the Bengal Medical Service died at their posts from illness, and 24 were killed in action. In 1865–85, the number fell significantly (probably due to improved sanitary arrangements and fewer military campaigns) to 77 out of 841, but increased again in 1886–96 to 44 out of 199.[43]

High rates of sickness among medical officers also adversely effected the provision of medical care. In 1853 the inspector-general of hospitals for India – Sir John Hall – regretted that medical provisions in military cantonments in the Bombay Presidency had been seriously undermined by the invaliding of almost one quarter of the medical officers.[44] Some years later in his personal diary Surgeon-Major Thomas Wood complained of being left alone in attendance of the British garrison at Poona, 'the surgeon sick, and the second assistant surgeon declaring himself unfit for duty' – a state of affairs which was apparently 'too often the case in this climate'.[45] Captain William Morrison, serving with the Army Hospital Corps in Ceylon, also complained that he and many of his colleagues suffered perpetually from diseases of the digestive tract, and from the 'listlessness' thought to be generated by the tropical climate.[46]

The high incidence of sickness among the European medical profession led practitioners to set up medical funds in each of the presidencies in the early nineteenth century. The Madras Medical Fund, for example, was established in 1807 to provide subsistence to the widows and children of medical men who subscribed to the scheme in times of bereavement or illness. The fund also provided assistance to those medical officers who were obliged to go to Europe because of ill health, and for those who had been forced to retire.[47] Such organisations provided affordable life assurance at a time when premiums in Britain were rising steeply for those venturing to the tropics.[48] In 1911 James Cantlie, editor of the *Journal of Tropical Medicine* called upon the insurance companies of Britain 'to realize their duty to the State by ceasing to hinder the unity of the Empire by callousness in their business'.[49] But such warnings went unheeded, and insurance companies continued, with good reason, to discriminate against those who chose imperial service.

The education of a profession

Gentlemen and scholars

In nineteenth-century British society a liberal education was one of the essential hallmarks of a gentleman. If that education was received at public school and consolidated with an MA from Oxford or Cambridge, then so much the better. Though public school education was rare among members of the British medical profession, it materially increased an individual's prospects of a lucrative appointment in the metropolis, or of a fellowship of one of the royal colleges. The British Medical Association was very much aware of the link between education and status, and licensing bodies instituted preliminary 'arts' examinations in an attempt to improve the social standing of licentiates.[50]

This preoccupation with 'gentility' was also a feature of the medical profession in India. In 1868 the *Indian Medical Gazette* declared that 'we have not the slightest objection to the sons of men of "low birth" being admitted into our profession, but we do insist that the sons themselves shall be, not only professionally, but liberally well educated, and that they shall have some notion of the laws of good society'.[51]

But, while the *Gazette* was largely satisfied with the standard of professional education attained by British recruits to the IMS, it was less happy with the quality of medical graduates from Indian universities and medical schools:

> we have reason to believe that the Asiatic Society of Bengal are endeavouring to move government to provide facilities for the teaching of natural and physical science in the schools and colleges set apart for general education in this country. This movement must, if successful, result in raising the qualifications and status of the native alumni of Indian medical schools.[52]

After the introduction of competitive examinations in 1855, the IMS had been opened up to Indians, though, as the examinations were held in Britain, very few Indians actually joined the service until the turn of the century. Yet the presence of Indians, however few, was sufficient to lower the status of the IMS in European eyes, and this was compounded by the fact that Indians allegedly received an inferior professional training. The Subordinate Medical Service, which was composed entirely of Indian assistant surgeons and hospital assistants, posed a slightly different problem. It was feared that inadequately trained subordinate personnel might tarnish the reputation of western medicine. Equally, it was expected that the qualifications held by 'native assistants' should be of sufficient standard to maintain morale in the service, and to ensure a steady supply of new recruits. In 1869 the *Gazette* called for the standardisation of examinations to the subordinate service, in order to ensure that the 'dignity of their diploma' would be enhanced.[53] For the same reason, in 1909, the *Indian Public Health and Municipal Journal* supported Bombay University Senate in its opposition to the provincial government's proposals to substitute a licence for the medical degree of the university. The government's rationale was that more Indians would be prepared to take a shorter course. But, according to the editor of the *Municipal Journal*, quackery was 'rampant' and the only way of suppressing it to ensure 'that the licensed practitioner shall be many times removed from the level of a man who is a hereditary hakim'.[54]

Medical registration

The journal's pronouncement drew attention to the precarious position of Anglo-Indian medical practitioners. Since the passing of the Medical Registration Act of 1858, the British medical profession had been effectively closed to unlicensed practitioners, though this had not, of course, put an end to 'unofficial' practice outside the profession. The act legally defined a 'medical practitioner' and established a register of all those so qualified. A General Medical Council was also established to adjudicate on professional matters.[55] The profession in India had no such safeguard, and had the additional problem of establishing itself in the face of deep-rooted indigenous medical traditions.

Agitation for medical registration in India began just a few years after the act was passed in Britain, but, by 1865, it was clear to all concerned that the Government of India had no intention of following suit. Its failure to enact similar legislation, according to the *Indian Medical Gazette*, was yet 'another instance of the indifference with which all matters affecting state medicine are regarded'.[56] The government's reluctance to consider such a move reflects the comparatively low priority attached to medical matters by the colonial administration, but also, and more importantly, the cultural and political limits of state intervention in the Indian context.

Though such an act would not have made illegal the practice of indigenous systems of medicine, like *unani* (Islamic medicine) and *ayurveda* (Hindu medicine) it drew an implicit distinction between legitimate and illegitimate medical practice. In the wake of the mutiny, the government was reluctant to tread heavily on the cultural sensibilities of its Indian subjects and, in the case of *vaids* and *hakims* (practitioners of *ayurvedic* and *unani* medicine respectively), these sensibilities were particularly acute, as their position had already deteriorated under British rule, with growing numbers of western-educated Indians consulting western instead of traditional practitioners.[57] Many Indian practitioners of western medicine were, however, in favour of registration. The Bengal surgeon Gopaul Chunder Roy, for instance, demanded action to curb the activities of the 'band of lawless resolutes' (quacks and empirics) which 'infest the country like locusts, and cause more devastation amongst humanity than the diseases which they pretend to combat'.[58]

The campaign for medical registration revived in Bombay in 1880 and culminated in a proposal by Dr Van Dyke Carter, principal of Grant Medical College, to restrict the practice of unqualified practitioners. His chief concern was the large number of 'quacks' and persons posing as qualified practitioners of western medicine in the city. Failed medical students and tradesmen seeking to supplement their income were thought to constitute the bulk of those claiming to be 'doctors'. A similar campaign was conducted in Calcutta in 1887, with the backing of certain Hindu notables, but neither met with any success.[59] Reflecting on the situation in 1899, the *Journal of Tropical Medicine* noted that

> medical graduates of the Universities and licentiates of the Colleges, who had settled in the large towns, had only too much reason for complaint. They were surrounded by barbers, carpenters, washermen, milksellers, cooks, painters, masons, etc., who, having failed at their calling, had betaken themselves to the practice of medicine.[60]

After being raised at the Indian Medical Congress of 1894, the issue lay dormant until 1912, when it was pressed once more by the Hon. R. A. Lamb, a member of the Bombay Legislative Council. Lamb appears to have largely accepted medical arguments that registration was in the public interest: 'While the exclusion from practice of the native *hakim* and *vaid* remains both undesirable and impracticable, it has become necessary to protect the public as well as the medical profession from the irregularly qualified doctor who has received a training in medical science at an unrecognized medical institution.'[61]

In its reluctance to exclude practitioners of indigenous medicine, Lamb's proposal acknowledged the cultural limits of state intervention rather than any respect for traditional systems. As already suggested, the state's relationship with indigenous medicine was an ambivalent one, characterised more by political expediency than by any balanced assessment of its medical value. The administration never officially recognised *unani*, *ayurveda*, or the increasingly popular strain of homeopathic medicine that had taken root in Bengal, as 'scientific systems' on a par with western medicine.[62] In March 1900, the viceroy Lord Curzon was advised not to consent to a request made by an

Indian homeopathic practitioner that the latter's latest treatise on plague be dedicated to him. 'Such encouragement', warned the lieutenant-governor of Bengal, 'must tend to lower the regular system – which is supported by Government as the correct one – in the eyes of the people of this country'.[63] Likewise, while the Indian government had no objection to the opening of a *unani* medical college in the Punjab in 1912, it refused to grant it official recognition.[64]

The justification for British rule in India was that it ordered Indian society in a rational and humanitarian way; 'rationality', too, was what allegedly distinguished western from indigenous medicine. Medical and political authority, therefore, intersected, but reservations about interference with traditional practices meant that the two did not always march hand in hand. Indeed, at times of crisis, such as during the plague epidemics of 1896 onwards, traditional practitioners were engaged in order to make custodial measures more acceptable to the indigenous population, or where staff shortages made medical administration impracticable without indigenous support. In both cases, the employment of traditional practitioners proved unpopular with European medical officers, who put up a dogged and ultimately successful resistance.[65]

After the turn of the century, however, colonial administrators were more sympathetic to the demands of medical officers. Medicine and medical science had become part of the rhetoric of 'colonial efficiency', and doctors' objectives were now more closely identified with those of the Indian administration. More importantly, there were now more Indian practitioners of western medicine, in whose own interests it was to support moves to restrict unlicensed practice. For these reasons, Lamb's proposal was successful, and resulted in the passage of India's first Medical Registration Act in 1912. The act established a Medical Council for Bombay which was empowered to judge the standard of instruction at universities and medical colleges in the presidency. Henceforth no one except a registered practitioner was allowed to hold posts in hospitals or in government service (this had, in any case, been the convention prior to 1912), and persons masquerading as registered practitioners were subject to a fine of up to Rs 300. In 1914 identical legislation was enacted in Bengal and Madras.

The reaction of Indian practitioners to the acts was predictable. Opinion was divided between those schooled in western medicine, and practitioners of traditional systems. Though the legislation did not interfere directly with the practice of traditional medicine, its practitioners felt that the government was 'expressly putting its stamp of approval on western systems and of disapproval on other systems of medicine'. In Bombay, the legislation was 'opposed in the interests of *vaids*, by almost all the elected representatives of the Hindus in the Council', while the Hon. M. N. Ahmed took up the cudgels on behalf of the *hakims*, and expressed regret at the action of the government in introducing a measure that 'tended to discourage the indigenous medical systems of the country'. However, in Madras, the Hon. K. P. Raman Menon – a practitioner of western medicine – maintained that opponents of the bill had been motivated by 'a false sense of patriotism', and that government had long bestowed its stamp of approval upon western medicine. In response to the argument that indigenous medical systems would die out if only the western system was granted official recognition, Menon argued that 'it is not the fault of the Government if these systems die out, but . . . the fault of the practitioners, who do not care and have no idea whatsoever how the system should be worked on scientific lines'.[66]

Education and recruitment

Though the relationship between professional qualifications and professional status is by no means straightforward or unproblematic, the level of education attained by members of a profession does provide some indication of its standing in society and of its ability to compete in the recruitment stakes with other professions. From 1863, all prospective entrants to the IMS had to undertake a one-year course of study at the Royal Army Medical College at Netley, and pass a qualifying examination common to those wishing to enter the AMS and the Navy Medical Service. IMS recruits compared favourably with entrants to the other two services in respect of scores obtained in this examination, and on only five occasions between 1879 and 1901 did IMS recruits score a lower aggregate mark than their fellow AMS students. The examination covered surgery, medicine (including diseases of women and children), pharmacy, hygiene, anatomy, physiology, botany and zoology.[67] However, comparison with the British medical profession requires a closer analysis of the qualifications held by individual recruits to the IMS.[68] Figure 1.1 shows the qualifications held by recruits to the IMS between 1851 and 1914 – figures in brackets represent the percentage of recruits holding a particular qualification. Prior to 1896 the data relate to the Bombay Medical Service only, but after 1896 to the united IMS. Details of educational qualifications are available for virtually all recruits.[69]

The dramatic fall, shown in figure 1.1, in the number of IMS recruits holding only a single licence such as the Licence of the Society of Apothecaries (LSA) as their highest qualification compares favourably with similar trends in England. Likewise, the percentage of IMS recruits holding the more prestigious double licences was only marginally behind provincial practitioners in England, and on a par with MOsH. The percentage of IMS recruits educated to degree level also increased significantly between 1851 and 1871, being higher than for the provincial medical profession as studied by Hilary Marland.[70] In the 1880s, competition for entry into the IMS was particularly acute: the service still offered reasonable prospects for lucrative civil employment, if not rapid promotion.[71]

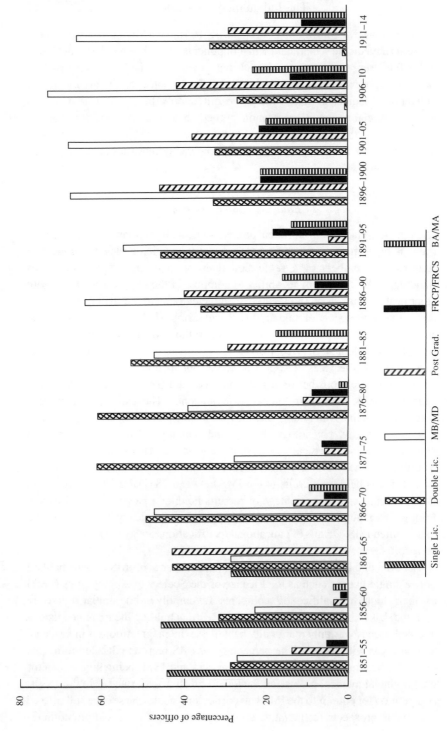

Figure 1.1 Qualifications held by IMS officers

However, the percentage of IMS recruits between 1857–87 who held medical degrees was somewhat lower than among British MOsH (35.4 per cent as against 39.7 per cent). But by 1886–90 the majority of IMS men held medical degrees, and between 1896 and 1914 this rose to 68 per cent.[72] Fellowships of the Royal Colleges of surgeons and physicians were relatively uncommon among the ranks of the IMS, but were more common than among British MOsH and the provincial medical profession.[73]

Analysis of the educational composition of the IMS in the last quarter of the nineteenth century also reveals a marked rise in the number of officers who had achieved a high level of proficiency in arts subjects before going on to study medicine. Equally striking is the sharp rise in specialist post-graduate qualifications obtained by IMS men after 1886. In this respect the IMS followed closely the pattern of British MOsH, for whom the Diploma of Public Health became compulsory in 1888. The DPH was also the specialist qualification most commonly held by IMS men, reflecting the creation in India of specialist sanitary posts. The first IMS officer to hold a DPH was Ronald Ross, who obtained the qualification while on furlough in London in 1886. After 1898, with the founding of the London and Liverpool Schools of Tropical Medicine, an increasing number of IMS men came to hold the Diploma of Tropical Medicine, or the Diploma of Tropical Medicine and Hygiene. In 1912, the DPH also became a requirement for employment in India as a sanitary officer or a first- or second-class health officer.[74]

Though these figures indicate favourable trends in the recruitment of well-qualified medical men to the IMS, and their subsequent achievements, there occurred in the 1870s a decline in the standard of recruits, perhaps reflecting widespread discontent about the place of the IMS in the 'table of precedence' issued by the Home Department of the Indian government. The 'table' set down the relative social rank of all the public services (civil and military) in India, and the IMS did not fare particularly well: 'while certain classes of the military are unduly exalted, the medical profession in India gains not at all . . . We have military officers, by virtue of holding a civil position, promoted to a status, two or three steps above their bona fide standing.'[75]

The 1870s was a period of discontent with promotion prospects and of rivalry between the civil IMS, and the newly formed Sanitary Department. In the early 1870s, guarded enthusiasm for the new service among senior IMS men gave way to bitter resentment. This resentment stemmed from the rapid promotion of relatively junior officers to positions of influence within the new department. 'It has come to pass', protested the *Indian Medical Gazette*, that 'Government find it necessary to appoint a junior officer from the Indian Medical Service to advise them upon [sanitary] matters . . . which the head of the [Medical] Department is incapable of doing, – the minor fulfilling the functions of the major.'[76] A subsequent *Gazette* editorial continued in the same vein:

The interests of the medical profession in India . . . demand that its members should work in union . . . under one leader in whom they have confidence . . . and it appears to us that the newly created sanitary service as at present constituted tends to weaken the medical department, creating schism amongst the executives which is highly desirable to avoid.[77]

Thus, it was feared that the ordinary civil IMS would become a 'second-class' service.

A noteworthy aspect of this rivalry with the Sanitary Department was an attack on the alleged specialist status of its members. 'Every Assistant-Surgeon who has had the privilege of attending Netley, or . . . who possesses a copy of Parkes's *Practical Hygiene*', argued the *Indian Medical Gazette*,

is just as capable of faithfully and satisfactorily carrying out such an investigation [of drinking water] as the Examiner of Potable Waters and it is only because the Government will not encourage such an example of zeal, and assist the department to use its scientific knowledge by the supply of ordinary apparatus and material, that the lights are thus hidden under a bushel.[78]

It would appear, therefore, that resentment of new specialist appointments was bound up with existing grievances about under-funding of the IMS. A *Gazette* editorial of 1908 entitled 'A forgotten service grievance' firmly equated hostility towards the Sanitary Department with frustration at the slowness of promotion in the IMS. This was particularly true of brigade-surgeons (equivalent to the military rank of lieutenant-colonel) who had been denied promotion to administrative appointments due to economies in the service, and the preference given to relatively junior members of the Sanitary Department: 'When they saw that these reductions had deprived them of their promotion, which they might otherwise have reasonably expected, it was small consolation to them that several of their juniors in the Sanitary Department had, by piece of unexpected good fortune, been pitchforked over their heads.'[79] It would seem from this editorial that these conflicts were a thing of the past, yet W. G. King, sanitary commissioner for Madras, claimed that important sanitary schemes were still curtailed by senior IMS officers, jealous of their juniors in the Sanitary Department, who were in a position to advise the government.[80]

The years immediately before the First World War were, indeed, worrying times for many officers of the IMS. From 1910 there was a fall in the percentage of recruits educated to degree level, of those holding postgraduate qualifications, and of those who went on to become fellows of a royal college. At the same time there occurred an increase in the percentage of recruits whose highest qualifications were only double or single licences. This is the period cited by Roger Jeffery as the beginning of the 'terminal decline' of the IMS. As further evidence of its growing unpopularity, he states that, in 1907, there were only 25 applicants for 23 posts.[81] From 1905 the IMS was undergoing rapid changes in its ethnic composition, and the vast majority of those recruits holding only the single LMS (a qualification in medicine and surgery unique to India) were of Indian origin.

The decline in the educational standards of recruits in the IMS both reflected and compounded the inferior status of the medical services in India. In 1913 the *Indian Medical Gazette* concluded that:

> the cause [of the fall in the quality of recruits] can only be a general dislike and mistrust of the conditions of service in India at the present time. This disinclination to accept service in India affects all the Indian services more or less . . . The unrest in India, the treatment of that unrest by the authorities and the political develop-ments of the present day, have made men hesitate before embarking on an Indian career.

But conditions inside the service were also to blame: 'civil practice is not what it was, little money can be made in many stations; mofussil life is less attractive than it used to be; and . . . the pay with the present raised prices all over the world is not attractive'.[82]

Sanitary and presidency services

Thus far, this chapter has analysed recruitment patterns for the IMS as a whole, but it is also illuminating to consider variations in the educational status between different branches of the service. Figure 1.2 presents data relating to sanitary specialists within the service. Since there is no one reliable record of those officers employed as full-time preventive practitioners, data have been gathered from a variety of sources and may not, admittedly, represent the full strength of the sanitary service in India.[83]

As befits their specialist status, the percentage of sanitary officers holding post-graduate qualifications (usually the DPH) was much higher than for the IMS as a whole. However, a more telling indicator of educational status was the percentage of sanitary officers who held medical degrees. With the exception of the 1890s and 1911–14, the proportion of sanitary officers who held medical degrees was significantly higher than was the case in the general IMS. In addition the percentage of sanitary officers who held only a single or double licence as their highest qualification was lower than for the IMS as a whole. The percentage of sanitary officers who went on to become fellows of one of the royal colleges was also significantly higher. The greater opportunities and the more rapid promotion afforded by a career in the Sanitary Department may help to explain why so many of the best qualified recruits entered the department.

As table 1.1 shows, there were also significant differences in the qualifications obtained by recruits to the medical services of the three presidencies.

What emerges most clearly from this table is the dominant position of the Bengal Medical Service. The Bengal service generally contained a higher

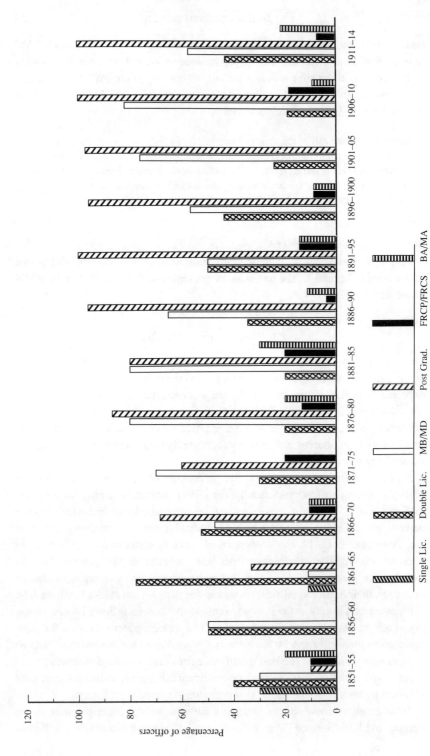

Figure 1.2 Qualifications held by IMS officers appointed to full-time sanitary posts

Table 1.1. *Qualifications held by officers of the presidency medical services*[84]

Qual.	Bengal		Madras		Bombay	
	1839–60	1865–96	1839–60	1865–96	1839–60	1865–96
LSA/LAH	122	79	38	46	46	30
	(21.9)	(1.4)	(13.1)	(17.2)	(17.0)	(15.9)
MRCS	369	225	158	82	168	74
	(66.1)	(41.7)	(54.5)	(28.3)	(62.0)	(39.1)
LRCS	94	97	32	54	38	53
	(16.8)	(18.0)	(11.0)	(20.2)	(22.2)	(28.0)
FRCS	83	95	30	54	25	16
	(14.9)	(18.0)	(10.3)	(20.2)	(9.2)	(8.5)
MD/MB	274	256	118	126	81	107
	(49.1)	(47.5)	(40.7)	(47.2)	(29.9)	(56.6)
MKQCP/MRCP	28	23	9	33	4	11
	(5.0)	(4.3)	(3.1)	(12.4)	(1.4)	(5.8)
LKQCP/LRCP	17	209	7	115	79	92
	(3.0)	(38.8)	(2.4)	(43.1)	(29.1)	(48.7)
FRCP	0	2	4	3	1	1
LFPSG	4	15	1	16	1	0
MFPSG	0	0	5	11	1	6
CCS	1	0	0	0	0	0
LMS	0	13	0	12	1	11
		(2.4)		(4.5)		(5.8)
No. of men	558	539	290	267	271	189

Figures in parentheses indicate percentages.

percentage of recruits who held medical degrees and who were fellows of one of the royal colleges than either the Madras or Bombay services, though it lost ground, and was in some cases overtaken by the other two services in 1865–96. This pattern reflects more general trends concerning the popularity of the three presidencies. As in the ICS, performance in the competitive examination and personal preference determined where a recruit was stationed, although it was sometimes possible to move to another presidency at a later stage in one's career. Bengal was generally the preferred appointment since, until 1911, it was the home of the Indian capital (Calcutta), and the hub of European culture.

Bengal, with its preponderance of European stations, also offered the most lucrative opportunities for private practice and the best prospects for advancement to a prestigious post with the Indian government. Appendix A shows that, without exception, those who went on to become sanitary commissioners with the Government of India and/or DGIMS between 1860 and 1914 were initially recruited to the Bengal service. As Spangenberg notes in his study of the ICS, 'provincial affiliation was one of the chief determinants of one's relative

Table 1.2. *Medical schools, teaching hospitals, and universities attended by IMS recruits*[85]

Institution	1839–60	1865–96	1897–1914
Edinburgh	205 (38.6)	173 (16.7)	163 (19.0)
Other Scottish	78 (14.7)	125 (12.1)	69 (8.0)
London	151 (28.4)	324 (31.3)	327 (38.2)
Other English	15 (2.8)	44 (4.3)	49 (5.7)
Irish	45 (8.5)	194 (18.7)	91 (10.6)
Indian	14 (2.6)	74 (7.2)	78 (7.8)
European	19 (3.6)	33 (3.2)	9
Other colonies	2	2	5
Oxbridge	2	21 (2.0)	66 (7.7)
Total known	531	1034	857
Total no. of recruits	1119	995	655

Figures in parentheses indicate percentages.

prestige and status', and preoccupation with status itself served to sharpen provincial antagonisms, providing an obstacle to administrative efficiency.[86]

Any assessment of the bearing of education upon professional status would not be complete without some consideration of the institutions at which IMS recruits received their education.

Though graduates from the London medical schools comprised the largest single element of the IMS between 1839 and 1914, the proportion of IMS officers drawn from Irish and especially Scottish schools was highly significant. Edinburgh, in particular, occupied a dominant position in 1839–60, and this is reflected in the number of senior positions taken by Edinburgh graduates between 1860 and 1880.[87] Medical training in the Scottish schools was generally respected for its rigour, but the London schools were increasingly popular after mid-century, and attendance there seemed to offer the best prospects for the development of a practitioner's career. Family ties also appear to have been important factors affecting choice, as was the expense of living in a particular locality. The majority of IMS recruits, then, had gained their medical education at institutions widely respected by members of the British profession, and increasingly by the lay public. However, qualifications obtained from Irish universities – of which there were a substantial number in the IMS – were looked upon with less favour.[88]

Of greater concern to senior IMS men was the increasing number of recruits educated at Indian universities. Qualifications from Indian medical schools were recognised by the British General Medical Council (GMC) after 1892, but in 1907 the council expressed its concern over the standard of education received at these institutions, particularly in midwifery. In 1930 the GMC actually withdrew recognition from qualifications obtained at the Indian schools, though it was reintroduced in 1936. Part of the problem was the lack of a regulating body like the GMC. The issue was raised in 1910 by the DGIMS Pardey Lukis, but the proposal had to be shelved because of the allegedly high expenditure involved in creating a system of regulation. It was not until 1933 that an Indian Medical Council was established.[89]

Professional status, as Eliot Freidson reminds us, is essentially a historical construction.[90] The status of a particular profession can only be determined with any accuracy if we take into account the views of historical actors themselves, of how the members of an occupational group saw themselves and how they were perceived by others. In this respect it is illuminating to make comparisons between the IMS and other Indian professions on the basis of their social composition, training, and conditions of service, since these became the criteria by which 'professional status' was judged.

For most of the nineteenth century, senior Indian civil servants were dissatisfied with the standard of entrants into the ICS. The vast majority of ICS men (unlike their British counterparts) did not possess an Oxford or Cambridge education (18.7% were educated at these institutions), and many had not attended any university (some 43%). Spangenberg attributes the inability of the ICS to attract a higher standard of recruits to the declining value of the rupee (relative to the pound and to prices in India), lack of promotion prospects, the inferiority of the civil to the military establishment, and dislike of service in India among the higher classes of British society.[91]

Yet, while the IMS compared more favourably with the British medical profession than did the ICS with its British counterpart, the ICS was ranked above the medical service in the table of precedence, and was able to boast more socially prestigious Oxford and Cambridge MAs than the IMS. ICS men also appeared to get the upper hand in situations where civil servants and medical men competed for administrative posts. 'It will hardly have surprised our readers', wrote the editor of the *Indian Medical Gazette* in 1871, 'that the Lieutenant-Governor of Bengal has, on the earliest opportunity, substituted a civilian for a medical officer as Superintendent of Jails. Mr Campbell, as is generally believed, entertaining no exaggerated notions regarding the value of the medical profession.'[92]

Compared to the Indian Police Service, however, the IMS appears especially well qualified, both in terms of professional qualifications and education in the liberal arts. Like the IMS and the ICS, the IPS held competitive examinations for entrance into its 'superior ranks' (the subordinate service being comprised entirely of Indians and Eurasians), but expected to attract candidates with, at best, a public school education and 'possibly a year or two at university'. It was acknowledged that the IPS was unlikely to attract candidates as well qualified as those entering the ICS. The police recruit's basic course of instruction, unlike that of the IMS and ICS, took place at colleges set up within India, lacking the

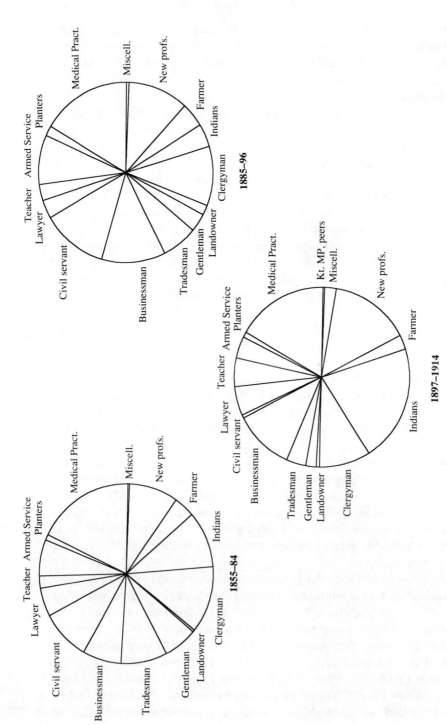

Figure 1.3 IMS recruits 1837–1914: occupation of father

prestige of institutions like Haileybury (the ICS college) and Netley. Training for police recruits was also constituted on a provincial basis, making local forces even more insular than branches of the ICS or the IMS.[93]

Class and professional status

Peterson's study of the medical profession in mid-Victorian London illustrates the importance of social class in determining professional status. The small proportion of medical men of genteel parentage which appears in Peterson's sample was both a consequence and a cause of the profession's low standing in metropolitan society.[94] Evidence for the social composition of the IMS (i.e. occupation of father) is provided by the birth certificates which were often appended to recruitment files. For those years in which such data is available, an average of over 70 per cent of recruitment records carry details relating to circumstances of birth, compared to an average of only 57 per cent in Peterson's sample.[95]

Figure 1.3 shows that recruits to the IMS were more likely to come from a medical family than any other, mirroring the pattern of 'internal recruitment' observed by Peterson and Marland in the English profession. Other similarities include the preponderance of clergymen and the relative significance of military men among the fathers of IMS recruits, as has been found with medical men in London, and in the English provinces.

This figure shows that the most important difference between the social composition of the IMS and the English profession – as described by Peterson and Marland – was the higher percentage of recruits drawn from the 'lower middle class', the 'new professions', the business and manufacturing communities, and later from the teaching profession. The reverse side of this trend is to be found in the comparatively small proportion of IMS men whose fathers ranked among the gentry. In terms of social composition, therefore, the IMS ranked lower than the provincial medical profession as studied by Marland, and significantly lower than the fellows of the royal colleges of London who form part of Peterson's sample. In some respects the IMS was on a par with the London apprentice apothecaries – the other base for Peterson's study. However, the social composition of the apothecaries is more varied than the IMS, drawing a substantial proportion of recruits from the sons of gentlemen and of tradesmen. The IMS was more uniformly – and increasingly – lower middle class; a factor to which we may perhaps attribute some of the status anxiety and conservatism characteristic of medical officers in this period.[96]

The lower percentage of tradesmen's sons among IMS officers reflects the fact that a substantial number of IMS recruits had family ties with India. This trend of recruitment from families who had served in India became more marked around the turn of the century, as service in India became less popular due to growing political unrest and the depressed state of the rupee. European civilians in India were almost exclusively 'professional people', doctors, police super-intendents, and civil servants. There were comparatively few European tradesmen in India outside of the armed forces.

The absence of detailed information on the social composition of other Indian services makes difficult any assessment of the relative social status of IMS officers. The only figures available relate to officers of the Indian Army. Of nineteenth-century Indian Army officers, 44.1% were sons of British army officers, 24.1% of Indian army officers, 6.9% of ICS men, 3.8% of surgeons, 3.1% of gentleman farmers, 3.1% of clergymen. 1.5% of civil engineers, 1.5% of physicians, and 6.2% from other unspecified backgrounds.[97] A number of important points arise from this comparison. Firstly, the Indian Army followed a pattern of 'internal recruitment' far more significant than the IMS, with between one quarter and one half of its recruits drawn from military families, as opposed to an average of 17.2% from medical families in the case of the IMS, between 1855 and 1914. Second, comparatively few Indian army recruits came from commercial or 'new professional' families, with a larger proportion of officers than the IMS drawn from the landed gentry. In sum, the officer class of the Indian army appears to approximate more closely than the IMS to the gentlemanly status so prized by aspiring Victorian professions. The social composition of the two services reflects their standing in Anglo-Indian society, the military ranking above the medical profession in the Home Department's 'table of precedence'.

Ethnicity and professional status

The two most noteworthy features of the ethnic origin of IMS recruits are the high percentage of recruits drawn from Scotland and Ireland, and the increasing number of Indians entering the service after the turn of the century. It has been possible to provide a relatively complete picture of the birthplace of recruits only for the period 1837–96, and a comprehensive set of data regarding the recruit-ment of Indians is available for the period 1896–1914.

Table 1.3 below illustrates the high proportion of IMS recruits of Scottish and Irish origin.

Although England was generally the single most important source of IMS recruitment, men of Scottish and Irish birth constituted a percentage of the service out of proportion to the populations of these two countries. Indeed, in 1855–84, the number of recruits from Ireland even exceeded those from England. A sizeable proportion of IMS recruits was also born in India, often to parents of Irish or Scottish descent. The pattern of recruitment to the IMS resembles closely that of the AMS, which, from 1859 to 1864, drew 230 men from Ireland, 115 from England, and 85 from Scotland. Thus the proportion of

Table 1.3. *Birthplace of IMS recruits 1837–1896*[98]

Birthplace	1837–54	1855–84	1885–96
England	377 (43.4)	181 (25.5)	114 (34.4)
Scotland	197 (22.7)	141 (19.1)	40 (8.3)
Ireland	91 (10.5)	186 (26.2)	42 (12.6)
Wales	13 (1.3)	11 (1.5)	3
Isle of Man	1	1	1
Channel Islands	4	2	3
Mediterranean	5	1	1
India (European)	141 (16.2)	110 (15.9)	100 (30.1)
India (indigenous)	2	50 (7.0)	11 (3.3)
Indian Ocean Islands	4	5	3
Australia	1	3	1
New Zealand	0	0	2
Canada	4	10 (1.4)	1
West Indies	11 (1.3)	7	5
South Africa	3	3	3
West Africa	1	0	0
At sea	3	1	0
Europe	11 (1.3)	3	1
Other Asian	1	1	1
Unknown	37	231	16
Total no. of recruits	906	941	348

Figures in parentheses indicate percentages.

AMS recruits from the so-called 'celtic fringe' was even higher in this period than for the IMS. Recruitment from Scotland, and more especially from Ireland, was important in terms of professional status since it reflected the popularity of the service among British medical graduates.

It is clear that medical men considered employment in one of the uniformed medical services as a last resort, comparable with employment in the Poor Law Medical Service in Britain. There were fewer prospects of making a reasonable living from private practice in Scotland and Ireland, and the IMS – with its clearly defined salary scales – provided an opportunity to earn a steady and serviceable income.[99] In respect of the preponderance of Irish and Scottish officers, the IMS was similar to the IPS, another low-status colonial service (at least in the period prior to 1914).[100] It is also interesting to note that the peak period of recruitment from Ireland – 1855–84 – coincided with a period in which professional grievances over promotion and status in the IMS were particularly acute.

Equally significant in determining the character and status of the IMS was the recruitment of indigenous Indians. Though the service had been opened up to competitive examination in 1855, the number of Indians entering the service until the turn of the century was low. In 1905 only 5% of IMS were of Indian origin.[101] From 1905, following Secretary of State Morley's decision to limit the

Table 1.4. *Recruitment of Indians to the IMS 1896–1914*[102]

	Total number of recruits	Number of Indian recruits	% of total number of recruits
1896–1900	147	3	3.4
1901–5	229	8	3.5
1906–10	183	25	13.7
1911–14	111	29	26.1

number of places open to European recruits, the numbers of Indians joining the service increased substantially to around one quarter of the intake between 1911 and 1914.

Morley's decision reflected the Liberal government's desire to speed up the process of 'Indianisation' in executive and legislative councils, and in other branches of the administration. Opening up the professions was a sop to 'moderate' Indian opinion at a time when the British and Indian governments were concerned at violent protests against British rule and the growth of 'extremist' influence in the Indian National Congress.[103]

It has been argued that the slowness of Indianisation prior to 1905 was a reflection of Indian unease at the military character of the service, since new recruits were posted first to a military station, being eligible for transfer to civil duties only after 5 years' military service.[104] However, the martial character of the service was, probably, not in itself a deterrent to the recruitment of Indians,[105] and indigenous traditions of medicine and public service also meant that medical work was not an entirely alien concept. The expansion of medical education in India from the mid-nineteenth century, and the lack of official support for traditional systems of medicine, encouraged many Indians to train in western instead of Indian medicine. The recognition of Indian degrees by the GMC in 1892 also presented opportunities for practice throughout the British Empire, and the IMS provided a useful springboard for such a career.

One additional factor needs to be considered: until the assumption of direct rule by the Crown in 1858, the Brahmin caste had possessed a monopoly of intellectual life, with the Indian landowning class dominant in the political and economic spheres. By taking advantage of new openings in medicine, and more particularly law, Indians could break through these monopolies and achieve an unprecedented degree of social mobility.[106] The most significant obstacle facing medically trained Indians considering a career in the IMS was the fact that the entrance examination took place in England, and that post-graduate training took place at the Army Medical School at Netley. Besides the financial difficulties of embarking upon such a course, travel outside of India was considered by many Hindus to be ritually polluting, entailing loss of caste. Well into the 1880s,

Indian newspapers such as the *Hindoo Patriot* continued to discourage travel abroad, although those representing the new professional classes, such as the *Bengalee*, welcomed the provision of scholarships to enable Indians to gain an education in Britain.[107]

Racial discrimination within the IMS was probably the other most important factor deterring Indians from joining the service. The entry of Indians into the IMS was viewed with concern by British medical officers because of its consequences for the standing of the service in Anglo-Indian society, and its implications for recruitment in Britain. In order to understand this reaction it is necessary to place the service within the wider social context of British India. The mutiny of 1857 had been a major factor in the racial alienation of the British in India. It had hardened prejudices against the Indian population and produced a 'fortress mentality' among Europeans, which provided a formidable obstacle to the formation of constructive relationships with Indian leaders.[108] European attitudes towards Indians were strongly coloured by the conviction that Indians were incapable of internalising western values and behaviour patterns, contrasting sharply with the optimistic and virulently westernising utilitarian doctrines that had shaped official policy in the 1830s.[109]

These attitudes were typified by the widespread conviction among British medical men that Indians and Eurasians (those of mixed Indian and European parentage) were unsuitable for public health work, because of the alleged absence of any such tradition among indigenous peoples. Public demonstrations of racism among IMS officers, as in other colonial services, were, however, rare.[110] The profession appears to have been concerned primarily with the educational standard of Indian recruits and its effects upon status, but the underlying social tensions created by Indianisation could not always be suppressed. In his *Race, Sex and Class Under the Raj*, Kenneth Ballhatchet highlights the case of a Eurasian IMS officer, Josiah Dashwood Gilles. Gilles was an outstanding student, gaining the MRCP and the MD degree, and acceptance into the IMS as an assistant surgeon despite – at 29 – exceeding the age limit for the service. But Gilles was accused of incompetence and of inappropriate conduct while attending a European woman. Though these claims were later dismissed by the DGIMS, he was still of the opinion that it was a mistake to make Eurasians commissioned officers; appointment at warrant officer level being considered more suitable: 'this course would not have withdrawn them from their own class, or placed them in a false position, one in which though equals in virtue of holding Her Majesty's Commission, they are . . . not looked upon by the other officers of the service as on an equality in a social sense'.[111] The appointment of well-qualified Indians and Eurasians troubled many of the older medical officers, discontented with their promotion prospects and aware of suspicions of incompetence.

If Indian and Eurasian officers did actually feel alienated from the IMS establishment one would expect there to have been a large proportion who retired early from the service. This appears to have been the case, with many Indians retiring comparatively early, after only 17 years' service.[112] By 1914 only ten officers of Indian origin had completed the full service term of 30 years, and only ten had risen to the rank of lieutenant-colonel. Before 1914 only one Indian had risen above this rank to take an administrative position: H. M. Banatlava, who was promoted colonel in 1914. Banatlava held the double licence common among Indian recruits, but had the distinction of an MD from Brussels university.[113]

One other Indian who went on to distinguish himself in the IMS was S. G. Chakravarty. Chakravarty joined the service in 1855, after gaining a medical degree from University College London. After rising through the ranks of the IMS, he became professor of clinical medicine at Calcutta Medical College and held the coveted and lucrative position of first physician at the college hospital. It is noteworthy that Chakravarty was more 'westernised' than most Indian recruits to the IMS, and hence more acceptable to the IMS establishment. Although born a Brahmin, Chakravarty converted to Christianity whilst in London, and endeared himself to an influential medical circle in the metropolis. He also played an active part in advancing the interests of the medical profession in India by taking a leading role in the formation of the Bengal Medical Association, which eventually became a branch of the BMA.[114]

By the 1910s, concern over Indianisation of the medical service was compounded by talk of opening up state medical positions to medical men from outside the IMS. These proposals, which stemmed from governmental concerns about the lack of well qualified recruits then entering the IMS, eventually became law in 1912.[115] The new arrangements met with a good deal of hostility from the medical profession in India and its champions in the British medical press. The *Journal of Tropical Medicine* declared that

> while we entirely agree that there is a wide opening for the extension of the employment of Indian medical men, we would most emphatically protest against the principle of 'filling appointments from the outside'.[116]

But these protests fared ill against Secretary of State Morley's determination to lay the foundations of an independent medical profession in India; a process which continued apace after the first world war.[117]

Conclusion

The educational standard of IMS recruits compared favourably with other Indian services and with the medical profession in Britain, yet medical officers continued to occupy a marginal position in Anglo-Indian society, above officers of the IPS, but below those of the ICS and the British and Indian armies. The position of IMS men in India's table of social precedence was mirrored by their predominantly lower to middle-class origins, contrasting with the more genteel parentage of many of those who held army commissions or senior positions in the ICS. But, like most Indian services, the IMS recruited disproportionately from the 'celtic fringe' and from European families already living in India. It was also subject to the same internal tensions and contradictions: those created by Indianisation, the slowness of promotion, manic fixation with status, and discontent with remuneration and conditions of service.

The legal status of the Indian medical profession was equally problematic. IMS officers found themselves in a position similar to that of British medical men prior to the Medical Registration Act of 1858: as registered practitioners, they enjoyed legal status in Britain, but in India, where there was no registration act until 1912, they faced competition from practitioners of indigenous medicine, and from numerous unqualified persons posing without fear of conviction as doctors of western medicine. Attempts to introduce legislation similar to that passed in Britain, brought medical men into conflict with the Indian administration, which was more sensitive than the colonial medical profession to the likely political implications of any interference in traditional practices. Only when a significant number of Indians began to qualify in western medicine, and themselves demand restrictions on unlicensed practice, was the government prepared to contemplate legislation on British lines.

The slowness of promotion within the IMS, the pervasive anti-intellectualism, and bitter internal conflicts, fostered a climate in which innovation in theory and practice was positively discouraged. Equally, the military orientation of the service and the narrow outlook of many of its officers encouraged fatalism and indifference to the plight of the Indian people. The effects of this institutional inertia will become increasingly apparent in the following chapters, in which medical theory and medical policy are examined more closely. It will be seen that the IMS was slow to respond to, and actively resisted, medical trends emanating from the metropole, while the minority of active reform-minded medical officers within the IMS was marginalised and unable to exercise much influence on sanitary policy.

2

Tropical hygiene: disease theory and prevention in nineteenth-century India[1]

It seems agreeable to Reason and Experience that the Air operates sensibly in forming the Constitutions of Mankind, the Specialities of Features, Complexion, Temper, and consequently the Manners of Mankind which are found to vary much in different Countries and Climates./(John Arbuthnot, *An Essay Concerning the Effects of Air on Human Bodies*, London, 1731, p. 146)

Tropical hygiene before 1858

European attitudes towards India and its inhabitants were varied and often ambivalent, yet there was one basic assumption underlying all colonial medical texts from 1770 until at least 1858. That is, a belief in the uniqueness of the Indian environment and its maladies, and the need for a fundamental reappraisal of European medical knowledge in the light of these new circumstances. 'It required no long time', wrote the naval surgeon Charles Curtis in 1807, 'to convince [the author] that European nosology and definitions would, in India, prove but uncertain or fallacious guides'. Curtis' work at the naval hospital at Madras in 1782–3 engendered in him the belief that there was 'scarce a single production, whether of the animal or vegetable kingdom . . . to be met with [in India] bearing a true resemblance to its prototype in Europe'.[2] This use of the word 'prototype' is puzzling, seemingly implying that natural phenomena in India had in some way deviated from archetypal forms in Europe. But whatever Curtis' views on the priority of tropical and temperate species, there can be no mistaking his conviction of the uniqueness of the tropical disease environment. The 'illusive and varying forms' under which the symptoms of known diseases presented themselves in India led Curtis to the conclusion that nosology and etiology were local phenomena, and that diseases there accordingly required different forms of treatment than in Britain. In his defence, Curtis cited another Madras surgeon John Paisley, on cholera:

In Europe cholera is produced by an increased acrimony, and increased secretion of bile . . . but it seldom there brings on sudden weakness at the first onset. On the contrary, bleeding is often unnecessary in the beginning. But when it is epidemic here, it is totally a disease of highly putrid bile, which . . . brings on sudden prostration of strength, and spasms over the whole surface of the body.[3]

Curtis' other chief concern was hepatitis, which seemed to him to prevail in India much more than in other countries of a similar latitude. Again, there was much to distinguish 'Indian' hepatitis from its European counterpart. 'All the inflammatory affections of [the liver] are dominated here, as well as in Europe, by the general name of Hepatitis', he observed, 'But Indian Hepatitis includes a variety of affections of this bowel, different in their nature, extent, and termination.'[4] Similar opinions were expressed by the army surgeon, George Ballingall, stationed in India for 7 years at the beginning of the nineteenth century. Ballingall, who went on to become the first professor of military surgery at Edinburgh, was preoccupied with dysentery – one of the principal causes of sickness and admissions to hospital among British troops in India. He was especially concerned that medical men new to India might misunderstand the disease, as it appeared there, and saw it as his duty to 'warn young men how little they will find the Dysentery of India corresponding with the description given of it in Europe; and to prevent them from automatically employing treatments which might not be fitted to the disease in India'. 'Instead of the *pyrexia contagiosa* which . . . is the first characteristic described by Dr. Cullen', he continued, 'the dysentery in India often makes considerable progress and has very severely, perhaps irreparably, injured the intestinal canal, before any urgent symptoms or pyrexia became either distressing to the patient, or conspicuous to his medical attendant'.[5] In opposition to most European authorities, Ballingall maintained that there were two types of dysentery: one confined to the large intestine; the other, a more chronic form, which extended its influence to the liver. He insisted that mercury, then favoured by doctors in Europe as a treatment for dysentery, was valuable only in the hepatic form of the disease, and preferred to prescribe purgatives in most cases.[6]

Acclimatisation

Belief in the distinctiveness of the tropical disease environment raised two fundamental questions: whether or not it was possible for Europeans to acclimatise their bodies to their new surroundings; and whether, and in what ways, their cultural practices could be adapted to suit their new environment. The first of these – the 'acclimatisation question' – was of great political significance because, potentially, it cast doubt on the long-term presence of Europeans in the tropics. The second – the question of cultural practices – drew Europeans to consider the utility of indigenous medical knowledge, and to assess their own lifestyle in relation to that of their subjects. In neither case were European responses uniform, or necessarily consistent.

The fecundity of the tropical environment elicited a variety of responses from Europeans, inducing visions both of paradise and of hell. In the tropics, wrote the naval surgeon James Lind in 1768,

> all nature seemed to be at enmity with man. [Men] were prevented from walking in the wood by tygers . . . and if by going armed or in small parties, they should escape these, . . . they exposed themselves to the views of venomous serpents . . . The river swarmed with crocodiles: the earth had its white ants, the air its wild bees, its sand-flies its mosquittoes [sic].[7]

But attitudes towards tropical environments were rarely uniformly hostile. The overwhelming tendency, as in Europe, was to distinguish between healthy and unhealthy localities. Writing in 1773, the East India Company surgeon John Clark found the coast of Malabar 'temperate and healthy' and had been reliably informed by another English gentleman that the Carnatic region was 'remarkably pleasant and fertile', with the air, even in the warmest months, causing no great inconvenience to health.[8] Women, too, flourished in the salubrious climate of India's south-eastern coast, and, according to Clark, enjoyed 'a remarkable immunity from the endemic and popular diseases of a warm climate'. But, in the port of Madras, women seemed especially susceptible to the intense heat: 'The lovely bloom and ruddy complexion they bring from Europe are soon converted into a languid paleness: they become supine, and enervated; and suffer many circumstances of ill health peculiar to their sex, from mere heat of climate and relaxation of system.'[9]

Most medical men in India shared Clark's view that Europeans thrived best in climates that most resembled those at home. But, underlying this differentiation of the Indian climate into 'healthy' and 'unhealthy' zones, there was a general belief that, over time, Europeans might gain immunity to the vicissitudes of climate and disease in the tropics. Such ideas were convenient in the sense that they boosted Europeans' confidence in their ability to rule parts of the globe with climates very different from their own. This was particularly important in eighteenth-century India, where the British territorial expansion was encountering military resistance from Indian rulers and their imperial rivals, the French. Yet, this belief in the adaptability of physical constitutions was more fundamental in that it was derived from popular and Hippocratic notions of environmental influence,[10] which reached a high stage of sophistication in the eighteenth century in the writings of Montesquieu, Buffon, and others. According to these doctrines, climate in particular exerted a powerful effect upon human health and physical characteristics, and in the writings of Montesquieu, even on the nature of political institutions.[11] Doctrines of climatic influence were also prominent in Indian writings in the eighteenth and nineteenth centuries, and may have served to reinforce those which emanated from Europe.[12]

This conviction in the adaptability of European bodies fostered guarded optimism about the prospect for European settlement in the tropics, as is shown in James Lind's *Essay on the Diseases Incidental to Europeans in Hot Climates*. Lind, as we have seen, was by no means enthralled by every aspect of the tropical environment, but still felt that Europeans could soon become acclimatised to their new surroundings:

> By length of time, the constitution of Europeans becomes seasoned to the East and West Indian climates, if it is not injured by repeated attacks of sickness, upon their first arrival. Europeans, when thus habituated, are generally subject to as few diseases abroad, as those who reside at home.[13]

Nor were such views peculiar to Anglo-Indians. The army surgeon John Hunter, writing of his experience in Jamaica, was convinced that 'the human frame acquires by habit a power of resisting noxious causes'. Hence Europeans, after remaining some time in the West Indies, were less likely to be affected by fever on their first arrival. Indeed, Hunter believed that Europeans would become blacker over generations, their constitutions adapting to their new environment. That they had not done so already, was primarily a consequence of their reluctance to adopt indigenous life styles, which would have rendered them liable to the full effects of climate.[14] Man's capacity to adapt to new environments was a mark of his rationality – a reflection of eighteenth-century optimism about human progress. As the English physician William Falconer put it in 1781, 'he was intended by nature to inhabit every part of the world'.[15]

Preventive medicine

Most medical men in India believed that there was nothing inevitable about sickness in the tropics, and that much could be done to prevent it. The fact that one ship which docked at an Indian port might be visited by disease and another be exempt was, for Clark, 'the strongest proof that sickness is not an inevitable evil, but, in general, the consequence of inattention and mis-management'.[16] The Indian climate was not necessarily harmful to Europeans provided they were disciplined and attentive to excess. But indiscipline was endemic among young British troops new to India; a consideration which led the army surgeon George Ballingall to propose that only those soldiers who had reached 25 years of age should be stationed there; older troops being thought less likely to pick up intemperate habits from those already garrisoned in India.[17]

The naval surgeon Charles Curtis drew attention instead to the inappropriate diet of Europeans: he believed that over-consumption of meat was the root of many of their ills. 'They cannot too soon . . . accustom themselves to what are called the native dishes', he maintained, 'which consist for the most part of boiled rice, and fruits, highly seasoned with hot aromatics, along with meat items and sauces, but with a small proportion of animal matter'. Alas, the majority of Europeans injured themselves 'from a kind of false bravado, and the exhibition of a generous contempt for what they reckon the luxurious and effeminate practices of the country'.[18]

Curtis' sentiments were echoed by the Calcutta surgeon Adam Burt. According to Burt, human beings, 'no less than vegetables' were 'materially changed by transition from their native to a different soil', and must, in order to survive, adapt their life styles in ways appropriate to that climate. 'The too liberal use of wine', he warned, 'combines with the climate to render Europeans ill-qualified for digesting the great quantity of animal food which most of them continue to devour as freely as before they left their native country'. Although he did not think it advisable to emulate Indian dietaries in every respect, they seemed to him to suggest 'very useful hints' for survival in hot climates.[19]

Europeans also borrowed extensively from indigenous medical practices. From the early seventeenth century, European medical men made extensive use of indigenous medical knowledge, using local medicinal plants and consulting practitioners of Indian systems of medicine. By the end of the seventeenth century, Europeans had grown more confident, and, having assimilated a good deal of local knowledge, began to distance themselves from Indian practitioners. But consultation did not cease altogether, and by the end of the eighteenth century Indian medical systems had become the subject of a more penetrating and systematic investigation.[20] These developments were a consequence of a more general awakening of interest in Indian culture stimulated by orientalist scholars like William Jones.[21] Jones attempted, with mixed success, to bring traditional texts to the notice of European practitioners. Though not uncritical of ancient medical texts, he felt they still contained much that was of value. The East India Company took heed of Jones' advice and urged its own surgeons to become better acquainted with local medicines and Indian medical texts, then slowly becoming available in translation. Although 'orientalism' needs to be placed within the wider context of European political domination, it was not simply a 'conquest of knowledge' for the purposes of command.[22] It represented equally the lure of the 'exotic', and, for writers such as Voltaire, the Orient provided models of government and rational religion which western societies would do well to emulate.[23] Yet, Indian culture was respected for its former greatness: it was to a supposed 'Golden Age' rather than its 'degenerate' eighteenth-century forms which most Europeans looked for inspiration.

The willingness of Europeans to learn from indigenous medicine reflected epistemological similarities between European and Indian medical systems. Until the mid-nineteenth century, western medicine, *ayurvedic* or Hindu medicine, and *unani* or Islamic medicine, had much in common regarding basic notions of disease causation, treatment, and prevention. Each viewed the causation of disease as a complex system of 'exciting" and 'predisposing' causes, and Indian systems, like their western counterparts, only rarely made reference to divine intervention, although each system viewed moral conduct as an important factor in predisposition to disease.[24]

This renewed interest in Indian medicine first began to make itself felt in European medical texts in the early years of the nineteenth century, with the publication of several books and articles reviewing ancient Indian pharmacopoeia and treatises on traditional medicine.[25] Whitelaw Ainslie's *Materia Indica*, first published in 1826, was the first book-length example of this genre, and enjoyed a good measure of popularity among medical men in India. The tone of Ainslie's work is largely respectful, but the reader is warned that several of the remedies listed are of doubtful efficacy, or even dangerous. In Ainslie's words, 'given the state of empirical obscurity in which the science [of medicine] is still sunk in India, it will readily be believed that many substances are daily prescribed but with trifling virtues, if indeed, any to recommend them'.[26]

Nevertheless, Ainslie believed that there was still much in common between European and Asian medical systems and had 'no hesitation' in agreeing with Sir William Jones that Indian and Greco-Roman civilisations had 'proceeded from the same point'. Ainslie's reviews of Sanskritic and Persian medical works also demonstrate that he thought these systems rational, sophisticated, and useful to the European practitioners at which his book was primarily aimed.[27] Such ambivalence was typical of commentaries on Indian medicine published at this time. George Playfair's edited translation of the *Taleef Shereef*, aimed to encourage a more general use of indigenous remedies among European practitioners but, throughout, the author maintained a critical distance from the original text.[28]

Others writing in the early nineteenth century were concerned not so much with ancient medical texts, but with traditional hygienic practices still very much in evidence. James Johnson's *Influence of Tropical Climates on European Constitutions*, first published in 1812, draws heavily but selectively upon Indian medical knowledge. In this residue of ancient learning, 'this strange medley of ludicrous and ridiculous customs', the discriminating European might discern some useful knowledge. One area in which Johnson believed Indian customs had much to offer was that of dress. He noted the benefits of the turban – as a protective against sun – and the cummerbund – as a protective against chill – and advocated the wearing of analogous clothing by Europeans. Like Curtis before him, Johnson also drew attention to the inappropriate eating habits of Europeans in India, and argued that Indian dietary regimes were worthy of consideration.[29] Vigorous exercise was another European habit to be avoided in the tropics. 'The peaceful Hindoo', he observed, retires, as it were instinctively, to the innermost apartment of his humble shed, where both light and heat are excluded. There he sits quietly . . . regaling himself with cold water or sherbet, while a mild but pretty copious perspiration flows from every pore, and contributes powerfully to his refrigeration.[30]

Johnson's ambivalence towards indigenous culture is mirrored in the proceedings of learned societies during this period. In an address to the Calcutta Medical and Physical Society in 1823, the surgeon and orientalist, H. H. Wilson, argued that much could be learned from Hindu medical texts, providing that the reader was of a detached and rational frame of mind. 'Hindu notions on the subject of leprosy', he maintained,

> might form a not unserviceable introduction to the more scientific enquiries, which the better opportunities and greater experience of other members of the Society may enable them to institute. The advanced state of medical knowledge in Europe is a sufficient security, that the errors of these guides . . . will not lead us astray; whilst from their long experience . . . it is possible that some hints may be derived, which may lead us to an improved knowledge and classification, if not to a more successful treatment of the disease.[31]

One Indian notion which Wilson found eminently plausible, given the general belief in Europe and India of a connection between the stomach and the skin was that leprosy might be associated with the excessive consumption of salt or fish – a belief which was popular with medical men in India up until the end of the nineteenth century.[32]

It was their first-hand observations that gave Anglo-Indian medical men the confidence and the intellectual authority to challenge medical opinion in Europe. The Company surgeon, Charles Maclean, drew upon his experiences in India and in the Levant to challenge so-called contagionist explanations of epidemic disease, which then underpinned official policy in Europe. Maclean observed that the absence of a doctrine of contagion had spared the peoples of India and the Levant from the ravages of epidemic disease in those countries. Christian populations, on the contrary, had suffered far higher mortality as a result of their attempts to quarantine people within infected areas.[33] Maclean inveighed against prejudice in all walks of life, not just the realm of medicine. In 1798 he was expelled from India by Governor-General Wellesley for alleging corruption in the magistracy and, on returning to Britain, he secured a post on the hospital staff of the British Army only to find that his medical theories found little favour with the military authorities. Convinced that his promotion had been barred for political and professional reasons, he left the Army Medical Department in 1806, becoming a vocal critic of Wellesley and the Tory government. Maclean's medical and political views ingratiated him with Benthamite reformers like Southwood Smith, and were reported in the Whig *Westminster Review*. His so-called miasmatic theories seemed to offer would-be sanitary reformers a medical justification for the removal of noxious substances from areas of human habitation.[34]

Maclean's contemporary James Johnson, however, was no political radical, being personal surgeon to the Duke of Clarence, but he did conceive of himself as a reformer in medical terms; an independent spirit who refused to bow to the dogmas of the past. Like Maclean, he placed more value on observation than speculation, setting great store by his experiences in India as a naval surgeon. Though Johnson freely acknowledged his debt to earlier writers, such as James Lind, who had extensive experience in the tropics, and the 'immortal Cullen', he was sharply critical of the Edinburgh physician John Brown, whose ideas he considered outdated and ill-fitted to conditions in India.[35] Direct experience, for Johnson, was paramount. 'However sceptical professional men in Europe may be in regard to planetary influence in fevers', he maintained, 'it is too plainly perceptible between the tropics to admit of a doubt. I have not only observed it in others, but felt it in my own person in India, when labouring under the effects of obstructed liver.'[36]

Johnson also made use of his Indian experience in manuals written for use in Britain. In his *Economy of Health*, he made reference to India when warning against the dangers of consuming too much animal flesh, and structured his work around the 'seven phases of life' – an idea which he may have borrowed from Hindu writings.[37] Like Maclean, Johnson's ideas on disease causation also found favour with sanitary reformers keen to highlight links between filth and disease. He played an especially important role in the British cholera epidemic of 1831–2, where his 'contingent-contagionist' views on disease causation seemed to better fit the uneven spread of the disease than the strictly contagionist stance of the Emergency Board of Health. Johnson's direct experience of cholera in India conferred upon his comments an authority enjoyed by few other medical practitioners in Britain.[38]

'The tender frame of man'

By the time of Johnson's writing in the second and third decades of the nineteenth century, there had been an important shift in attitudes towards the possibility of European acclimatisation in the tropics. As already stated, eighteenth-century writers commonly expressed the conviction that European constitutions would eventually become acclimatised to life in the tropics. In the 1820s this view was no longer dominant: persistently high mortality among Europeans[39] bred a more pessimistic attitude, reflected in Johnson's view that Europeans were more indebted to the ingenuity of their minds than to the adaptability of their bodies for their survival in the tropics. 'The tender frame of man', he wrote, 'is incapable of sustaining that degree of exposure to the whole range of causes and effects incident to, or arising from, vicissitudes of climate, which so speedily operates a change in the structure, or, at least, the exterior of unprotected animals'.[40]

Accordingly, there was little prospect of Europeans colonising the tropics as they had North America, South Africa, and Australia. Europeans in India, wrote Johnson, tended to 'droop', and before long, to seek refuge in their native climate. The offspring of those who remained in India would 'gradually degenerate', morally and physically. Johnson's belief in the fundamental unsuitability of European constitutions for life in the tropics was underpinned by his theory of the origin of the human race. Unlike the orientalist William Jones, who had earlier expressed the view that humanity spread outward from a single source, Johnson believed that humankind could not be traced back to a single progenitor. For Johnson each race was distinct and the unique product of a particular environment.[41]

The dangers of the tropical environment became increasingly evident in India after 1817, in which year cholera spread outwards, for the first time, from its 'home' in Lower Bengal to decimate northern and eastern India, and ultimately much of Eurasia. The prevalence of cholera in Bengal, together with that of malarial fever, may explain why this region was so often stigmatised in colonial medical texts as being one of the most unhealthy in British India. James Kennedy's *History of the Contagious Cholera* was typical in this respect, and is worth quoting at some length:

> The stranger who visits Bengal, alive to the 'splendour of the East', discovers little to gratify his expectations . . . Weighing anchor at day-break, he leaves the treacherous 'Sand Heads' behind him, and enters the estuary of the River Hooghly . . . The sun is now gathering strength, and the malarious vapours are seen coiling themselves up from the surface of the land, which presents the unbroken aspect of an endless swamp, covered with low, black, impenetrable jungle . . . Having reached Diamond Harbour, scarcely five-and-thirty miles from Calcutta, the current of observation flows in a new channel. The pilot points to this as the place where thousands of our countrymen have been sacrificed to marsh fever. The Company's ships, in delivering their cargoes here, send many a gallant tar never to return. The malignant cholera, also, soon after its ravages were begun, travelled through the shipping at the anchorage, and carried off many victims. These remarks in passing fill the stranger with a tide of mournful emotions, and evil anticipations: his home and the expectant faces of parents, brothers, and sisters, on the one hand; his own untimely death, and their unutterable sorrow, on the other.[42]

Accepting, as most nineteenth-century writers on India did, that Europeans were incapable of becoming fully acclimatised to the subcontinent, the need to identify relatively healthy localities became more urgent. Thus, from the 1820s through to the twentieth century, medical studies of hill stations and other apparently more salubrious localities became an important feature in Indian

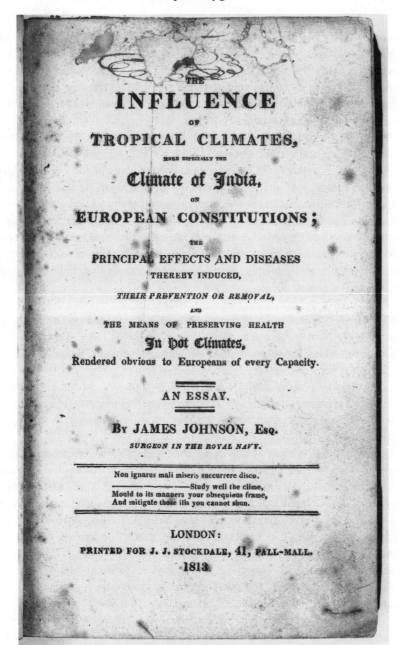

Plate 1 Title page to James Johnson's *The influence of tropical climates on European constitutions* (1813)

medical journalism and in official reports. Dr Araud writing in 1824, for instance, described Meerut in the Himalayan foothills as a desirable place for retired Anglo-Indians to end their days.[43] D. S. Young, in his 'Medical topography of the Neelgherries', a range of hills in south India, extolled the virtues of the climate there, feeling in it something of the 'serenity' described by the German scientist Alexander von Humboldt in his accounts of travels in the upland regions of South America.[44]

There can be little doubt that such sentiments were deeply felt, but this romanticising of India's hill resorts, and the many favourable official reports, served a wider purpose. As described in chapter one, in the course of the nineteenth century, service in India was an unpopular option and, for many, including medical men and women, a last resort. Many glowing accounts of hill-station life were written expressly to allay fears about the fragility and unpleasantness of life in India. However, it should be said that not all these reports were favourable: many ruled out the possibility of European colonisation of even the hills, and cautioned Anglo-Indians to educate their children abroad if they could afford to do so.

Nevertheless, belief in the salutary effects of life in the hills proved sufficiently strong that it would become official policy to station British troops new to India in hill stations or similarly healthy areas. This was a standard practice throughout the second half of the nineteenth century. When the rule of the British government replaced that of the East India Company in 1858, it also became a regular practice to shift the seat of government in the hot season from Calcutta – the capital – to Simla in the Himalayas. This tendency to seek refuge from the Indian climate tells us much about the underlying insecurities of the British in India.

However, it was not just British troops and civilians who were deemed at risk from the Indian climate. It was observed that Indian troops, or sepoys, recruited in one part of the subcontinent might fall prey to disease in another, to which they were not acclimatised. Certain regions were increasingly stigmatised as areas unhealthy not only to Europeans but to Indians. To many medical officers it appeared that unhealthy climates produced unhealthy or unwholesome races. Thus, while the Mugh tribe of the notoriously unhealthy region of Arracan were described as 'most foul feeder[s] . . . addicted to personal filthiness and to indolence',[45] the Todwars of the Neelgherries (with their more temperate climate) were 'tall, robust, and well proportioned . . . with their fine bushy beards and Roman noses' and their 'venerable, heroic appearance'. 'Many have I seen', wrote Young, 'who might have sat to Leonardo Da Vinci, when he drew his celebrated picture of the "Last Supper", without diminishing the effects of that sublime production'.[46] Since his own experience was so much in favour of the climate, Young felt that it is but reasonable to conclude that the Todwars could not have maintained their pristine vigor and present high place in the scale of animal creation, without the aid of a climate not only congenial to human existence, but such as to maintain and uphold it for ages without deterioration.[47]

In such writings indigenous peoples were idealised, made more acceptable to European tastes, and therefore subjugated in the colonial mind. Indeed, as Dane Kennedy has shown in a recent study of the ethnography of hill stations in India, the hill tribes may have existed as 'symbols of a comforting refuge from the complexities of colonial society'.[48] However, it would be a mistake to take this argument too far, for many hill tribes were regarded in a less than flattering light, and particularly those which resisted colonial economic interests, or which did not approximate to European (chiefly classical) conceptions of physical beauty.[49]

But climatological doctrines were not the only theories advanced to explain racial difference: from the 1820s physiological explanations also began to appear in medical texts. The East India Company surgeon William Twining retained much of Johnson's respect for indigenous forms of treatment and hygienic practices, and himself learnt much from Bengali medical practitioners, but felt, none the less, that certain of their remedies were suitable only for Indians. By the same token, many of the more violent forms of treatment, including bleeding and mercury, were deemed suitable only for Europeans. Although Indians were still supposed to have some degree of constitutional immunity to disease, they were often thought to be less able to endure other kinds of physical hardship.[50] Similar trends are evident in colonial medical literature outside of India. James Thomson, writing of his experiences in the West Indies, noted several physiological differences between Europeans and black slaves which manifested themselves in different susceptibilities to disease.[51]

The majority of medical men, however, continued to emphasise cultural, as opposed to physiological, differences between whites and non-whites. This was especially apparent in India in the 1830s, as some Company surgeons came to express the new creed of utilitarianism, embodied in the sweeping administrative reforms of Governor-General William Bentinck. The prevailing ethos of the 1830s is best demonstrated in the work of James Ranald Martin, presidency surgeon of Bengal and later president of the East India Company's Medical Board.[52] While Martin had some sympathy for Islamic culture, and for the 'martial races' of northern India, he expressed the commonly held opinion that Bengalis were indolent and degenerate:

> The Bengallee, unlike the Hindu of the north, is utterly devoid of pride, national or individual. His moral character is a matter of history . . . when we are looking forward with such well-founded hope to the improved results of European knowledge and example diffused among the natives.[53]

Martin had great admiration for the reforming Governor-General
Bentinck, and himself drew on James Mill's utilitarian critique of traditional
cultures:

> architecture, weaving and jewellery, says Mill, are the only arts for which the
> Hindoos have been celebrated; and even these ... remain in a low state of improve-
> ment. He might have added that all three are arts found to flourish under despotic
> Governments, and ... frequently to the exclusion of others of more general
> utility.[54]

These views could not have been more different from those expressed in Anglo-
Indian medical texts at the turn of the nineteenth century. The tolerance of
traditional structures of authority associated with Burkean conservatism and the
Company's administration in the late eighteenth century,[55] had also been
replaced by an assault on India's 'unrepresentative' and 'out-dated' institutions.
Absolute government by the Company, however, was something of an exception
to this rule, on account of its supposedly rational and enlightened principles of
government.

However, it was the Bengali's attitude towards hygiene that most concerned
Martin. 'The natives have yet to learn ... ', he wrote, 'that the sweet sensations
connected with cleanly habits, and pure air, are some of the most precious gifts
of civilization'. Nor were they impressed by the medical importance of clean
water. 'Everywhere', he claimed, 'one finds the tanks in an impure and
neglected condition'.[56] Whereas Johnson and earlier writers had found much
that was useful in indigenous hygienic practices, for Martin they had come to
symbolise all that was corrupt and degenerate in indigenous society. The Indian
people, as well as the Indian climate, were increasingly viewed as part of the
'sanitary problem'; as 'reservoirs of dirt and disease', as one government
official was to put it some years later. But, even during the height of the
reforming era in the 1830s, intervention in indigenous ways of life was rarely as
extensive or as successful as many reformers had hoped.

But what had caused Bengali culture to 'degenerate' and European
civilisation to prosper and advance? Martin did not resort to physiological
explanations, but to the more traditional position that climate determined human
character, in the same way as it exerted a profound influence upon health. 'When
we reflect on the habits and customs of the natives', he wrote, 'their long mis-
government, their religion and morals, their diet, clothing, etc., and above all
their *climate* [his emphasis] we can be at no loss to perceive why they should be
what they are'.[57] According to Martin, it was axiomatic in medical topography
that 'a slothful squalid-looking population invariably characterizes an unhealthy
country'. It was climate that enabled the Hindu 'to live heedless and slothful' and
which forced the native of Holland to be 'careful, laborious and attentive to
excess'. As justification for his climatological determinism, Martin cited the

doctrines of Montesquieu and other exponents of the view that climate impinged on human nature.[58]

Tropical hygiene in India, 1858–1914

The dim view taken by Martin of the climate and natives of Bengal exemplified the tendency, evident since the 1820s, to portray India, or at least a substantial part of it, as fundamentally pathogenic. The Indian mutiny/rebellion of 1857 served to heighten fears about the fragility of Britons in India, and to intensify this prejudice and contempt for indigenous ways of life. At the same time, the authority and influence of Anglo-Indian medicine began to wane: stagnation within the IMS, as described in the previous chapter, fostered an attitude among medical officers in which innovation in theory and practice was distrusted and discouraged.

'The embers of insurrection'

The impact of the mutiny on western medicine in India is most clearly seen in the work of the military surgeon Julius Jeffreys, whose treatise on the health of *The British Army in India* was published in 1858. Like many of his predecessors, Jeffreys took a pessimistic view of the possibility of European acclimatisation to the Indian climate. Excepting those Britons with a 'semi-tropical constitution' (i.e. of Mediterranean appearance), he believed that there were very few who could 'long endure exposure to the sun in a Tropical continent without serious damage to the Constitution'. Some degree of 'seasoning' was possible within 2 or 3 years, but, according to Jeffreys, significant adaptations in European constitutions would occur only after centuries of climatic influence. As such, 'thorough' and 'scientific' protection of the body was a necessity.[59] This vulnerability, he argued, had been noted by Indians when planning their insurrection:

> The natives of India took upon us as white bears from the cold unhealthy North, ferociously brave, but of sickly constitutions, disabling us from occupying their country without their aid. That the rebellion was long meditated, and purposely timed to commence in the hot season, I cannot entertain a doubt.[60]

He warned that 'extensive casualties amongst the soldiery from disease would . . . probably keep alive the embers of insurrection', and that urgent action was necessary to improve the health of soldiers, and to deter further disturbances.[61]

Similar fears were expressed by the Royal Commission appointed in 1859 to inquire into the health of the British Army in India and which, as described in the following chapter, exerted a profound influence on the direction of sanitary policy in the decades after the mutiny. In the civilian sphere, too, there was great anxiety about the health of Europeans owing to the negative image of India presented to the public in Britain. Recruitment problems experienced by the Indian services were compounded by the high cost of life insurance, the premiums for which increased sharply for those venturing to the tropics.[62] In addition, high profile events such as the visit to India by the Prince of Wales in 1876–7 were beset by problems caused by the onset of epidemic cholera – the cancellation of several hunting expeditions being reported in the British press.[63]

Such publications as R. S. Mair's *Medical Guide for Anglo-Indians* attempted to present a more positive image of India. 'Not many years ago', wrote Mair in 1874, 'the climate of India was looked upon as something to be dreaded. The young man proceeding to the East was expected . . . to return home, if he ever did return, a sallow, yellow-coloured invalid with his liver sadly damaged.' But the young man who had acquired temperate habits at home, and who maintained them in India, had a good prospect of enjoying a fair measure of health. Like earlier writers, however, Mair did not believe that Europeans were constitution-ally suited to tropical climates; at best, such precautions could have a mitigating influence.[64]

The health of European women and children in India was another matter which commanded special attention, since they were now thought particularly susceptible to the influence of tropical climates. Mortality figures for these two groups appear to confirm this impression: in 1889 the death rate among European women in India was just over 20 per thousand and, among children, just over 48 per thousand. By comparison, the mortality rate of European soldiers had declined to only 16 per thousand.[65] E. J. Tilt devotes a whole chapter to the effects of climate on the female constitution in his *Health in India for British Women* (1875). The vicissitudes of the tropical climate were thought to be responsible for anaemia in women, as well as causing 'frequent perturbations of menstrual activity'. Women were advised to eat very little meat, to protect themselves from the direct heat of the sun with an umbrella, and to wear a cotton or silken band around their loins.[66] Tilt's treatise had been written in response to a call from the government of India for a work on tropical hygiene and family medicine, for which a prize was awarded. Official records show that the diseases which most affected the death rate of European women in India were puerperal fever, phthisis, and enteric fever.[67]

High mortality among European children was a perennial source of anxiety among Anglo-Indians. Lady Emily Metcalfe, who had experienced life in Delhi in the 1830s and 40s, wrote of the 'terrible toll that heat and disease took yearly from the British who lived in India' and of every mother's expectation to lose 'at least three children out of every five she bore'.[68] The chief causes of death among European children appear to have been 'convulsions', diarrhoea, and 'debility'.[69] The government was especially concerned for the health of European families, since it was thought that more men would consider service in

India if they felt it was safe to bring their families with them. The government was also anxious to promote marriage among British troops in the hope that this would discourage them from resorting to prostitutes, with its attendant risk of venereal disease.[70] Some medical men believed that hill stations could play a crucial role in this respect. If troops and their families were encamped principally in hill stations, argued the army surgeon C. A. Gordon, boys and girls would be able to grow up in India relatively unharmed by the climate; with the latter providing wives for British soldiers.[71]

The majority of other medical writers, however, were less optimistic about the potential of hill stations for European settlement in India. Although the president of the India Officer Medical Board from 1873–95, Sir Joseph Fayrer, believed that the hill stations of India would 'become a permanent home to many . . . planters, landowners, and even retired . . . officers', he thought them 'too few and far between and too isolated to become the seats of real colonization'. 'The child must be sent to England', he continued, 'or it will deteriorate physically and morally', and grow up 'slight, weedy, and delicate, over-precocious . . . and with a general constitutional feebleness'.[72] Fayrer's verdict on acclimatisation seems to have been representative of medical opinion in India at this time.[73] Other writers, such as Sir William Moore, Honorary Surgeon to the Viceroy, believed that only Europeans of 'sanguine temperament' were suited to life in the tropics:

> Theoretically, it would seem possible that the European, who in type and temperament most closely resembles the condition to which climate and mode of life has converted the native of India, would be best-fitted to encounter the adverse influences of a tropical climate; and practically this appears to be the case.

But such people were apparently few and, according to Moore, notably absent among European women and children. In his experience, the latter invariably grew up 'weak and weedy', while the former were 'specially subject to tropical influences' because of the alleged effects of heat upon menstrual activity.[74] Moore recognised, like most medical men in India, that without women and children there was little chance of permanent European colonisation. Such views prevailed until well into the twentieth century, although from the late 1890s, advances in tropical medicine engendered optimism that science could render hospitable even the most hostile of environments.[75] But such views were confined largely to a small circle of medical researchers and imperial propagandists. Most Anglo-Indians, if Calcutta's *Englishman* newspaper was representative, remained profoundly sceptical of such claims.[76]

Strategies of prevention

During the 1860s and 70s, the putrefactive theory of the German chemist Justus Liebig and the waterborne theory of cholera causation of the Englishman John

Snow had begun to make some impact on the way in which 'tropical diseases' were perceived. Liebig held that diseases were caused by specific poisons, causing molecular changes to occur in the blood of an infected person. The whole process was analogous to fermentation, with the morbid poison acting in a similar way to yeast. He referred to this process as 'zymosis'. Liebig's ideas met with a generally favourable response from medical men and scientists in Britain, and William Farr, Britain's first state epidemiologist, began to categorise certain diseases (including cholera) as 'zymotic' in his annual reports.[77] Liebig's ideas could be easily incorporated within a conceptual framework which gave primacy to the action of climate and physical process in the causation of disease, and for this reason the notion of 'zymosis' rapidly gained adherents among the British medical profession in India. By 1870 it had become the standard means of classifying diseases, like cholera, which were thought to emanate from decaying organic matter.[78]

The views of Liebig's contemporary John Snow were far more controversial. The theory of 'continuous molecular action' advanced by Snow in 1853 bore many similarities to Liebig's concepts of zymosis, but, unlike Liebig, who did not posit any particular medium for the spread of cholera, Snow held that the disease was transmitted almost exclusively in drinking water. Many British medical practitioners were prepared to admit that 'bad water' might play a part in the causation of cholera, but it was quite another thing to accept Snow's claim that it was the only medium of the disease. Thus, Snow's theory was rejected as a suitable basis for sanitary action by the Board of Health's Committee for Scientific Enquiries on the grounds that it was too exclusive. Nevertheless, the 'waterborne' theory slowly gained ground among members of the British medical profession. In 1866 in an address on the 'Medical and Legal Aspects of Sanitary Reform', the respected physician Dr A. P. Stewart declared that 'the idea that Dr. Snow's views might . . . be true is now firmly fixed in the public mind . . . there are many, like myself, who could not admit their being proved they are tacitly of opinion that they are highly probable.'[79]

The theories of both Liebig and Snow underpin Edmund Parkes' *Practical Hygiene*, which became the standard text for military medical men in Britain and the colonies in the 1860s, 70s, and 80s.[80] Parkes – who had gained several years' experience in India – believed that diseases had at least two types of causes: 'predisposing' (within the body) and 'exciting' (external to the body). His most significant departure (*pace* Liebig) was the idea that these exciting causes were specific poisons, arising from putrefying matter. Different fevers were attributed to different poisons: ague to material of vegetable origin; enteric fever to material of animal origin.[81] He believed that enteric fever was transmitted in the faeces of a victim and contracted through ingestion of the infected matter. Cholera was ascribed to the action of a 'specific agent', transmitted in the stools of the victim, usually in contaminated water or food.[82]

Accordingly, Parkes believed that preventive measures should be made more specific. He paid greater attention to purification of water and to disinfection than any previous writer on tropical hygiene, and stressed the need for regular inspection of water and food for impurities and parasites.[83] Yet, Parkes felt that there should be a balance between public and personal hygiene, which took into account an individual's constitution and state of mind:

> For a perfect system of hygiene we must combine the knowledge of the physician, the schoolmaster, and the priest, and must train the body, the intellect, and the moral soul in a perfect and balanced order. Then ... we should see the human being in his perfect beauty as Providence perhaps intended him to be; in the harmonious proportion and complete balance of all parts, in which he came out of his Maker's hands.[84]

Yet, unlike the authors of earlier manuals, Parkes paid little attention to Asiatic customs, and made no mention of their utility in preserving the health of Europeans. There are no references to the dietary habits of the Hindu, but rather scientific calculations of the amount of carbohydrate, nitrogen, fats, and salts required to sustain the body in a balanced state of health.[85] Attitudes towards indigenous peoples had hardened considerably since the mutiny and the assumption of direct rule by the Crown the following year. As already suggested, it was the application of reason that allegedly distinguished British rule from oriental despotisms, and western from traditional Indian medicines. 'Besides the element of superstition', wrote the editor of the *Indian Medical Gazette* in 1868, 'there are other causes that separate the European from the Native practitioner. Both Hindoos and Mohamedans cling with blind obstinacy to the theoretical dogmas of the ancient fathers of medicine ... Their primary want', he continued, 'is that of a scientific nomenclature of disease, theirs being either fanciful ... or unintelligible to the rest of the civilised world'.[86] The increasing specificity of western etiological theory widened the gulf that had emerged between Indian and western medicine in the 1830s; a gulf that seemed unbridgeable in the atmosphere of mutual distrust which followed the rebellion of 1857.

Parkes' ideas found favour primarily with new recruits to the IMS; at the top of the medical profession in India the ideas of Johnson and Martin were still widely held, having undergone only slight modification. Senior IMS officers who had built their professional reputations upon these ideas – and who were personally convinced of their validity – were not about to abandon them overnight. Yet growing acceptance of Snow's waterborne theory in Britain, and the discovery in the early 1880s of what appeared to be the bacteria causing enteric fever and cholera, and the parasite causing malaria, made some reappraisal necessary. While many denied that the existence of such organisms had been proven or that they were causally related to disease, some attempted to assimilate new developments within existing views of the Indian disease environment. Nowhere is this approach more evident than in the writings of Sir Joseph Fayrer.[87]

Parkes' orientation was primarily physiological; Fayrer's epidemiological and universalistic. Fayrer continued to expound a 'natural-historical' approach to medicine, taking into account a wide variety of natural phenomena. In his study of cholera, published in 1888, Fayrer declared that it was his purpose to give a review of its

> history, habits, method of diffusion, geographical distribution, relation to climate, season, meteorological conditions and locality, its etiology, its effects on the human race, and . . . the methods which experience has taught us are most efficient in mitigating or preventing it.[88]

Fayrer continued to stress the uniqueness of the Indian disease environment and the distinctive behaviour of diseases in the tropics. 'The people and their habits', he wrote, 'the animal and vegetable creation, even the diseases differ from those . . . [the European new to India] has known hitherto'.[89] However, Fayrer was considerably less dogmatic than many of his contemporaries in setting forth his conclusions on the causes of epidemic disease. Assessing Snow's waterborne, atmospheric, and human contact theories of cholera causation, Fayrer admitted that he was unable to convince himself that any of these theories satisfactorily or conclusively explain all the phenomena exhibited by a cholera epidemic, or that one view can be accepted to the exclusion of the other. He was critical of those who pursued narrow and exclusive avenues of investigation:

> The cause will probably not be revealed to any one who searches with narrowed views. There is a great tendency in these days to trace all disease to a specific exterior cause, but we must not lose sight of the possibility of poisons auto-genetically developed . . . or of altered conditions of innervation.[90]

Nevertheless, Fayrer could not conceal his own bias towards the atmospheric theory, and his disinclination to accept the waterborne theory of cholera transmission to the exclusion of other factors. 'The suddenness and virulence of certain outbreaks [of cholera]', he noted, 'are remarkable, and seem to point to some factor apart from contagion or local insanitary conditions'. Rather, the evidence seemed to point to changing meteorological conditions:

> At Kurrachee, in 1846 . . . there was a sudden change in the atmosphere, the wind veered from south-west to north-east, and a thick lurid cloud darkened the air. Later in the evening cholera appeared in the thirteenth corps of the troops stationed there.[91]

'Impure water' (not necessarily water containing a specific contagion) was just one among many efficient causes of cholera, of which atmospheric changes were most important. Fayrer was supported in these views by other IMS officers

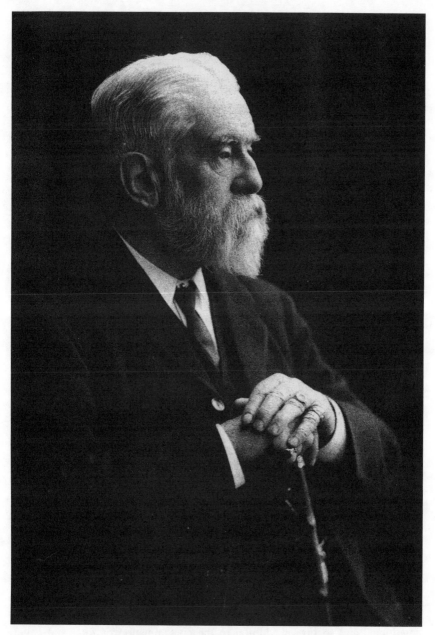

Plate 2 Sir Joseph Fayrer, 1824–1907

writing on cholera in the 1880s. Henry Bellew, sanitary commissioner of the Punjab, maintained that

> cholera does not spread from one part of the country to another along the principal lines of human traffic . . . The course and progress of cholera epidemics are wholly dependent on climatic or weather influences, aided by the . . . existing condition of the general health standard of the population.

These conditions were brought about by 'an abnormal excess of atmospheric temperature and humidity, coupled with changes in the electric condition of the air and the amount of its present ozone'.[92] Writing on the Egyptian cholera epidemic of 1883–4, Sir W. Guyer Hunter – a retired IMS officer – claimed that 'meteorological conditions had a strong influence in the generation . . . [of cholera]'. 'It is probable', he continued, 'that it is to a combination of certain conditions of a cosmotelluric character . . . that the development of an epidemic is due'.[93]

Fayrer had much the same opinion of the causation of malaria and enteric fever as he had of cholera. He was prepared to admit that specific organisms might have some role in the causation of disease, but stressed the importance of more general environmental conditions:

> The specific poisons which produce typhus, enteric fever, and some other diseases are probably as active in India and other tropical countries as they are here [in Britain], but I submit that fever with Peyerian ulceration may and does occur from causes other than faecal contamination.

In 1880 the discovery of the organisms thought to cause enteric fever and malaria gave rise to more uncertainty in Indian medical circles, but most IMS officers denied that they had any causal relation to these diseases. The sanitary commissioner with the Government of India expressed his conviction that the specific germ theory was 'inapplicable' to the history of enteric fever in India.[94] T. G. Hewlett, in his *Report on Enteric Fever* concluded that 'there seems to be no ground for believing that . . . enteric fever . . . is in all, or even in the great majority of cases, due to a specific poison derived from the intestines of a previously infected person'. This was also the view of Drs T. R. Lewis and D. D. Cunningham, special scientific assistants to the Indian government.[95]

Fayrer, Hewlett, and others, were concerned that undue emphasis on a specific organism, whether or not it had any role in the causation of enteric fever, would prejudice existing sanitary measures which took into account weather, insanitary conditions, and so on, in addition to the contamination of food and water. According to Hewlett 'the question of whether this poison is of specific or non-specific origin is not of such supreme importance as the recognition of the fact that . . . it is connected with insanitary conditions, and that . . . the surest way to prevent its development is to correct in every station all sanitary defects'.[96]

Specificity in disease causation, then, was associated with the dangers of an exclusive sanitary policy.

Prior to Alphonse Laveran's discovery of Plasmodium in 1880, European medical men were virtually unanimous in their opinion on the causation of malaria. Though some had speculated that the disease was caused by microscopic 'animalcules', the vast majority attributed malaria to 'miasma' arising from rotting vegetable matter because of malaria's connection with particular localities.[97] At first, Laveran's claims were greeted with widespread scepticism, and in some cases great hostility.[98] But following confirmation by Italian and American scientists in the mid-1880s, the concept of a 'specific factor' began to be accepted. But in India there was more dogged resistance: as late as 1894, according to Ronald Ross, 'the great bacteriological discoveries of Koch and Pasteur were scarcely recognised, or were ridiculed, and Laveran's was almost unheard of'.[99] This may have been something of an exaggeration, design to cast Ross' own work in a more favourable light, but it was not, probably, too far from the truth. Ross' statement is confirmed by the editor of the *BMJ*, who, in 1894, complained that Laveran's work had been virtually ignored by medical officers in India.[100]

Laveran's work was neglected in India not simply because he was a foreigner – although hostility to 'interference' from outside undoubtedly played a part. His emphasis on a specific causal agent was incompatible with the more holistic notions of disease causation associated with the 'natural historical' model, which continued to dominate medical thinking in India, long after it had become unpopular in Britain. Malaria had long been regarded as being at the 'non-contagious' end of the disease spectrum because of its apparent dependence on locality. Holistic concepts of disease causation were also difficult to dislodge because of their wider social and political significance. They underpinned traditional anti-malarial measures like the removal of vegetation from the immediate vicinity of European settlements. These measures probably did little to prevent disease, but at least served to comfort those who lived there – they were an art of the possible.[101] Laveran's claim threatened to undermine the theoretical basis of existing preventive measures, and was also potentially damaging to medical men who had built their reputations as experts on malaria.

Though hostility to Laveran's discovery continued for many years, there was growing acceptance in the 1890s of the specificity of Eberth's bacillus, and of its causal relation to enteric fever (by then sometimes referred to as 'typhoid'). Confirmation of Eberth's work in Europe, especially by Widal, Sanorelli and A. Chantemesse at the Institut Pasteur was crucial in this respect.[102] But a decade after the discovery of *B. typhosus*, the sanitary commissioner with the Indian government – W. R. Rice – reported that, although 'practically all bacteriologists agree[d] that Eberth's bacillus . . . [was] a necessary factor in the causation of the disease', the question of how it was conveyed was 'still unresolved'. In Rice's estimation, the dominant view was that the bacillus passed into the alimentary canal in drinking water or in 'other ingesta contaminated by the dejecta of a previous case'.[103]

Only a small minority continued to attribute the causation of enteric fever to general environmental factors,[104] though some influential authorities still held that there was a strong racial predisposition to enteric fever. Darker-complexioned Britons were thought to be less susceptible to the disease because of their physical resemblance to indigenous peoples.[105] It was an established fact that Indian troops were less prone to enteric fever than their British counter-parts,[106] but in the first half of the nineteenth century such differences had been explained in terms of different cultural practices. A similar transition from cultural to biological explanations of racial differences is met with in dietary surveys conducted in nineteenth-century India.[107]

There was even less agreement on how best to prevent the disease. Most IMS officers, including Rice, were adamant that no option should be closed as long as key epidemiological problems remained unresolved. In 1896 Robert Harvey – sanitary commissioner with the Government of India – warned against over-reliance on bacteriologically based prevention, on the grounds that it was too exclusive. Harvey continued to recommend a 'natural-historical' approach in assessing the behaviour of enteric fever: 'besides utilizing the aid of the chemist and bacteriologist, we must learn the geological source and history of . . . water, and must go in search of the conditions surrounding and affecting the source and the storage'.[108] However, as is shown in the following chapter, a growing number of IMS officers were urging greater attention to water supplies,[109] while a minority came to advocate preventive measures based on the new science of bacteriology, such as the typhoid inoculation developed by Almroth Wright at the Royal Army Medical School.

Conclusion

The opposition of Sir Joseph Fayrer and the majority of IMS officers to specific methods of disease prevention illustrates the continuing vitality of a distinctive Anglo-Indian medical tradition which emphasised the distinctiveness of the Indian disease environment, and which had its roots in eighteenth-century notions of climatic determinism. The reluctance of most IMS officers to incorporate new scientific ideas may also be attributed to the internal problems of the service (considered in chapter one) and, in particular, its ethos of anti-intellectualism, its failure to reward or encourage innovation, and its increasing unpopularity with medical graduates in Britain.

However, the historical importance of Anglo-Indian medical theory lies not so much in where it stood in relation to European ideas and practices, but in its significance for relationships between Indians and Europeans. Tropical hygiene simultaneously shaped and reflected British attitudes towards India and its indigenous inhabitants. By the early nineteenth century, guarded optimism about the prospect of European acclimatisation in the tropics had given way, in the face of persistently high mortality among Europeans, to a widespread pessimism about European colonisation of the subcontinent. At the same time, medical texts came to reflect the prevailing ethos of utilitarianism, and the increasing gulf between European and Indian culture. No longer was there a sense that anything of value could be gleaned from indigenous medical texts or hygienic practices. The Indian people, their 'filthy' habits, and 'degenerate' life styles, were now identified as part of the sanitary problem – anxiety about which intensified in the wake of the mutiny of 1857. Yet, as is shown in the following chapter, the desire to control and to contain indigenous sources of infection was only partially realised in colonial sanitary policy.

3

The foundations of public health in India: crisis and constraint

On account of the peculiar habits of the people, which, in most respects, are dirty in the extreme, ammendment in the conservancy of a great portion of native towns is almost hopeless, and, under the most favourable circumstances, must necessarily be a very gradual process; but, with regard to the towns and villages in the vicinity of and adjoining European stations, immediate improvement should be strictly enforced. (Stewart Clark, *Practical Observations on the Hygiene of the Army in India*, London, 1864)

Public health policy following the assumption of rule by the British Crown was dominated by the lingering shadow of the mutiny. The events of 1857–8 exposed the vulnerability of British troops in India to disease as well as to Indian hostility, but at the same time underscored their importance as the guarantors of British rule. The mutiny also demonstrated that the new administration ignored indigenous sensibilities at its peril, and fostered an understandable reluctance to interfere with Indian cultural practices in the name of public health. Herein lay the dilemma facing colonial administrators in the decades after 1858: how to sanitise those elements of the indigenous population which threatened the health of European troops without provoking a backlash which might threaten the stability of British rule. This chapter looks at the ways in which the colonial administration attempted to resolve this problem in several key areas of sanitary policy, and at the consequences of these attempts for relations with the indigenous population, and for competing concepts of government within the European community.

The military

Army hygiene in India was the beneficiary of the growing concern with the health of troops evident in Britain since the Crimean War and the findings of the Royal Commission in 1857, which reported that mortality rates in the British

60

Army at home were greater than among the civilian population.[1] Two years later, in the wake of the mutiny, a similar commission was set up to inquire into the health of the army in India. The effectiveness of British troops during the mutiny had been severely hampered by the ravages of epidemic disease, particularly cholera, which had also claimed many lives among European civilians besieged at Lucknow and in other north Indian towns.[2] Medical officers noted that, after years of neglect, the East India Company's board of directors were at last taking a proper interest in the health of their troops.[3] However, it fell to the British government, rather than the Company, to rectify the defects of military hygiene in India. The Royal Commission on the Sanitary State of the Army in India, appointed in 1859,[4] recorded a death-rate of 69 per 1,000 among British troops in the years running up to the mutiny (over three times as high as the worse death-rate of any regiment in Britain) and identified the underlying causes as inadequate sewerage and water supply, poor drainage, and ill-ventilated and overcrowded barracks. In its report of 1863, the commission recommended the creation of distinct areas of European habitation (military cantonments and 'civil lines') regulated by sanitary legislation similar to that in Britain, and situated in accordance with the topographic principles laid down by J. R. Martin, president of the India Office Medical Board and member of the commission. Martin, who we encountered in the previous chapter, advocated that troops should be sent in rotation to hill stations above 5,000 feet.[5]

Discipline and disease

The location of British troops in India was a matter of some urgency for, as a consequence of the mutiny, it had been decided to increase the number of British in relation to Indian troops in the proportion of 3 to 1. The obvious flaw in the plan, as envisaged by Martin, was that, if British troops were stationed in the hills, it would be difficult for them to respond effectively to an uprising in the plains.[6] Accordingly, the Indian government concluded that only a small proportion of the numbers contemplated by the commission should be garrisoned in the hills – no more than one third of the total force at any one time.[7] There were also doubts about the salubrity of many hill stations: medical officers warned that there were 'numerous examples of elevated positions being unfavourable to health', especially those which rose abruptly from alluvial or jungle-covered tracts. In such places, malaria was 'conducted upwards as if by a series of inverted funnels'.[8] Darjeeling, Naini Tal, and Lantour, were all thought to be unhealthy in this respect, and with a similarly high incidence of diarrhoea and dysentery.[9]

Relocation aside, it was believed that much could be done to prevent the worst ravages of the Indian climate. As discussed in chapter 2, Anglo-Indians attached great importance to diet and clothing in adapting to the Indian climate, and there was no shortage of opinions ventured about such matters in manuals of military hygiene. One innovation was the heat reflective, ventilated cavalry helmet proposed by the army surgeon Julius Jefferys in 1858.[10] The other principal concern when selecting garments was the avoidance of 'chill': a sudden change in temperature associated with the onset of gastric disorders, and most notoriously cholera. Every soldier in India was issued with a flannel waistband – or 'cholera belt' – to protect his abdominal region from the vagaries of the climate; a practice which continued into the twentieth century.[11] Uniform also varied according to season, and in the decades after the mutiny it became increasingly common for the British soldier to wear white clothes or khaki during hot weather, and a serge or cloth uniform during the cold season.[12]

After 1858 there was also far more attention to the subject of military nutrition. Florence Nightingale described as 'extraordinary' the practice of giving soldiers in India the same diet (regardless of season) as in Britain. Every day, the British soldier in India received 1 lb of meat, 1 lb of bread, 1 lb of vegetables, 4 ozs of rice, tea or coffee, as well as his entitlement to beer and spirits.[13] During the 1860s, however, this began to change, as the diet of British soldiers came to be regulated by the guidelines established by Edmund Parkes in his capacity as professor of military hygiene at Netley. Parkes advocated a diet balanced between nitrogenous substances, fats, carbohydrates, and salts. He also stressed the importance of inspecting cattle for the presence of diseases like anthrax, and of meat for the presence of parasites.[14] The diet in India was generally more nitrogenous and less rich in starches than that of soldiers in Britain, but fresh vegetables were sometimes in short supply and scurvy was not unknown in some garrisons in India. There was some concern over this in the 1860s when, following the report of the American Army Sanitary Commission on the health of troops during the civil war, fresh vegetables were shown to be invaluable in protecting against wound infection and disease.[15]

However, beyond these basic principles, there was little agreement as to what, exactly, should constitute the soldiers' diet. Much depended on personal preferences and experiences. The army surgeon Charles Gordon, for instance, believed that soldiers in tropical countries should drink a cup of coffee before going on early morning duty to protect against chill.[16] Robert Caldwell expressed the commonly held view that too much rich food or over indulgence in fruits could lead to intestinal disturbance and even dysentery,[17] but E. C. Freeman thought that curry, 'on account of the aromatic and antiseptic substances it contains' was 'a most wholesome article of diet', the use of which should be encouraged as much as possible. He alluded to the widespread belief that there was 'some connection between the comparative disuse of curry by Europeans in India and the increase in enteric fever'.[18]

The most controversial component of the soldier's diet was, by far, his allowance of beers and spirits. Soldiers were permitted up to a gallon of spirits every 20 days, a quart of strong beer every day, and one or two drams of rum or arrack (an Indian spirit). In addition, they were able to purchase arrack and other Indian liquors for a modest price in the local bazaar. The free availability of liquor, together with the boredom of barrack life, and the sense of isolation in an alien and often dangerous environment, were contributory factors in the extremely high incidence of alcoholism among British troops in India.[19] 'There is a good deal of intemperance among soldiers everywhere', wrote Florence Nightingale, 'but I very much doubt whether the same amount of tippling ever goes on in the British Army in this country as appears to be encouraged by the canteen system in India'.[20] Drunkenness was still, according to Charles Gordon, the 'most prevalent vice in India' in 1866, and a major factor in the incidence of hepatitis, heat apoplexy, phthisis, and especially venereal disease, among British soldiers. Such concerns eventually led to restrictions on the issue of spirits in canteens, and the establishment of more alternative recreational facilities.[21]

These reforms were accompanied by a decrease in the number of convictions for drunkenness in the early 1870s, but the reduction was short lived. The introduction of short service[22] in 1875 put an end to the gradual decline in the proportion of young, unmarried men in the British Army in India, which had followed the mutiny. The percentage of under 25s in the army in India increased from 33 in 1877 to 55 in 1898. It had long been recognised that such men were more likely to acquire the vice of intemperance in India than their older fellows, and after 1875 the incidence of alcoholism in the British Army in India began once more to increase.[23]

Rising alcoholism gave rise to grave concern among civilians, particularly in religious circles. In his *Notes on Hygiene with Hints on Self-Discipline for Young Soldiers* (1882), the Rev. J. G. Cole combined moral and medical sanctions in a crusade against alcoholism and promiscuity. 'It is chiefly through our careless-ness and neglect of personal management', he warned, 'that our whole system from the brain downwards gets out of condition. How soon is the body punished and the mind deranged by an intemperate habit!'[24] But such warnings had little effect: alcohol was still freely available in the bazaars and convictions for drunkenness in the army continued to increase until the turn of the century. From that time the incidence of alcoholism appears to have declined slightly, but largely as a result of the smaller number of new arrivals in India during and following the South African War of 1899–1902.[25]

An equally important factor in the health of troops in India was the sanitary condition of barracks. Here, the sanitary commission had revived an issue which had lain dormant since the early 1850s, when it had been raised by the inspector-general of hospitals Sir John Hall. Hall had complained that rules regulating the space allotted to each soldier in barracks were rarely followed and were, in any case, inadequate. He recommended a surface space of 50 square feet and that

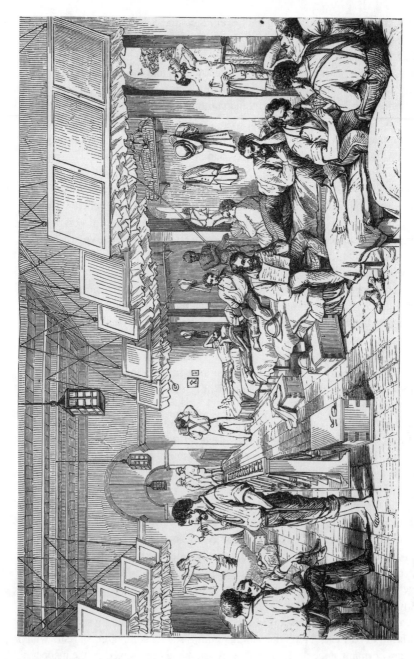

Plate 3 Troops at rest in an Indian barracks, from Florence Nightingale's *Sanitary state of the army in India* (1863)

beds be arranged singly to give each soldier more private space.[26] Yet the plans of medical officers were quashed by the indifference and parsimony of the military authorities.

Too often, historians have accepted uncritically Florence Nightingale's condemnation of army medical officers in the Crimea and in India. In some cases her criticisms were justified, but more often the efforts of medical officers were eclipsed by the testimonies of Nightingale and members of official commissions, who attributed sanitary progress to their own intervention.[27] Nightingale was able to succeed where army medical officers had failed only because of the public clamour for sanitary reform which followed the Crimean War and the mutiny. As Charles Gordon, deputy inspector-general of hospitals for the British Army in Bengal put it in 1866, medical men had long 'raised their voice in condemnation' of sanitary conditions in military cantonments in India, but 'their warnings, so often uttered, continued to be disregarded until a few years back, when the public demanded inquiry into the various causes of the sickness and mortality that prevailed in our army'.[28]

Following the commission's report, the new cantonment authorities established under the Military Cantonments Act of 1864 began to rebuild barracks to allow for 1,000 cubic feet of space for each soldier – 400 more than in Britain. Barracks were to be supplemented by separate ablution rooms and latrines, whereas formerly both functions had been performed within a single building.[29] But the issue of barrack construction was not without problems, there being some dispute between the Indian and British governments over the amount of floor space to be allocated to each soldier. The former, presumably for reasons of economy, felt that 90 square feet per man was sufficient for barracks in the plains, whereas the latter insisted on 100, though agreeing to a proposal by the Indian government to reduce this to 77 square feet in hill stations.[30] Married quarters were also to be improved: instead of existing provisions for married soldiers and their families in shared barracks, each family was now to be allocated two rooms of its own wherever possible.[31]

A central concern in the construction of new barracks was ventilation: the lack of windows and air vents in existing barracks and the inefficiency of the punkah were thought to be contributory factors in the high incidence of cholera and malaria among British troops. Better ventilation was a key feature of the new barrack architecture, and bullock- or steam-operated fans were introduced in a few cantonments to replace the traditional punkah.[32] Another innovation in barrack architecture was the regulation that each new construction should have two stories (the upper one being reserved for sleeping) in the belief that air at low level was damper, and more liable to be malarious.[33]

The construction of new barracks made considerable headway in the decade after the commission's report.[34] According to J. L. Ranking, sanitary commissioner of Madras, 'vast advances' had been made in this direction by 1868, the new barracks being 'palatial in their accommodation when compared with the old class of buildings'.[35] However, the continuing vulnerability of British troops is demonstrated by the fact that they still suffered mortality rates far higher than their Indian counterparts. During the cholera epidemic which swept northern India in 1867, European troops experienced a cholera mortality rate of almost 14 per 1,000, whereas Indian troops died at the far lower rate of 3 per 1,000. In fact, the death-rate from all diseases except fever was lower among Indian troops than among Europeans.[36]

These stark differences almost certainly reflect the different living conditions of British and Indian troops. While the former inhabited overcrowded and insanitary barracks, the latter generally lived in separate accommodation with their families. Indian troops were given a hutting allowance with which to construct their own dwellings; and which, as Florence Nightingale put it, was 'no doubt a most excellent thing for their health'.[37] But it is important not to idealise conditions in 'native lines'; these huts were often ill-ventilated and badly built (owing to the pittance allowed for their construction), and often with little or no provision for sanitation.[38]

Improvements to barracks continued – absorbing a high proportion of military sanitary expenditure – throughout the 1870s and 80s, although aggregate expenditure fell over these years.[39] From the mid-1870s, however, concern over military accommodation was eclipsed by concern over water supplies and sewage disposal within cantonments. The Army Sanitary Commission and other observers such as Florence Nightingale expressed grave reservations about the purity of water supplies in cantonments. Arrangements for raising and distributing water from wells were little different from 1,000 years before: water was raised in leather sacks by bullocks, emptied into troughs, and then conveyed by Indian water carriers – or 'bheesties' – to the barracks. This procedure exposed the water to contamination at several points, and, without filtration, the water was often cloudy and unappetising, and regarded in some cantonments as undrinkable.[40]

In 1870, with the construction of new barracks well under way, the Indian government ordered the supply of new pumps and filters for wells in military cantonments. Initially, these measures were confined to selected wells in European lines, but were eventually extended to stations housing Indian troops. The filters were developed by the IMS officer Francis MacNamara, and constructed from alternate layers of sand and charcoal.[41] Their effectiveness, however, was questionable, and they were found to corrode very quickly, leading to their replacement by similar filters made of stone in the mid-1870s.[42] By this time, the military authorities acknowledged that there was a strong link between the spread of cholera and water supplies.[43] In 1877 the commander-in-chief of the British Army in India, Major-General F. Roberts, issued orders for the prevention of cholera which stressed that 'the utmost attention must be paid

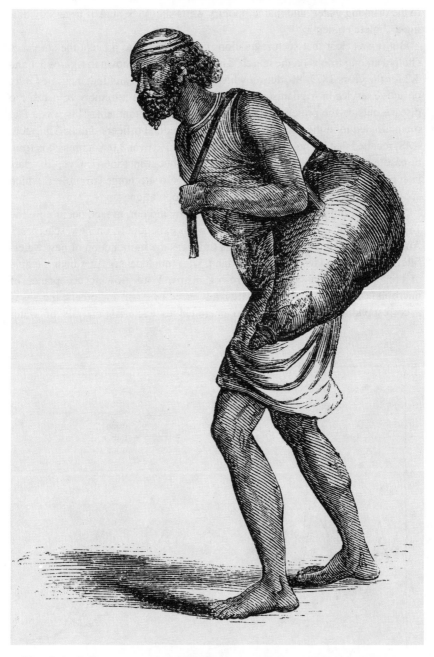

Plate 4 An Indian water carrier of 'Bheestie', from Florence Nightingale's *Sanitary state of the army in India*

to the drinking water' and that temporary wells should be sunk if necessary during a cholera epidemic.[44]

But it was clear that such regulations could do little to prevent the spread of cholera among troops on the march. The high mortality shown in figures 3.1 and 3.2 for the years 1877–80, during which time the British and Indian armies were on active service in Afghanistan, reveal that troops were extremely vulnerable to disease outside the protective environment of the cantonment. This was a fact often alluded to in the personnel accounts of medical officers. James Thornton, IMS, recalled that his regiment of 750 men recorded over 3,000 admissions from disease and 100 deaths during operations in Bhutan in 1866–7. Over 20 years later on the North-West Frontier his regiment again succumbed to cholera, which appeared to have spread from the indigenous population.[45]

Substantial improvements in the water supply did not, in fact, occur until the 1890s, when there was a marked increase in expenditure on new schemes.[46] Another important development at this time was the introduction of new water-filters, such as the Pasteur–Chamberland, with much denser filter beds capable of preventing the passage of micro-organisms. With growing acceptance of microbial theories of disease causation advanced by Koch and others, there was a corresponding move away from chemical to bacterial analysis of water

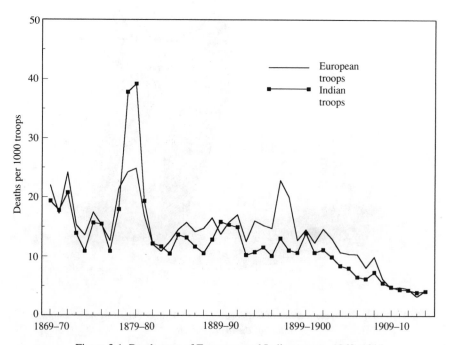

Figure 3.1 Death rates of European and Indian troops, 1869–1914

supplies, although there was still a feeling that bacterial analysis could not entirely replace a sound geological knowledge of a water course.[47] The practice of boiling water during cholera epidemics also became standard.[48] Yet, as figures 3.1 and 3.2 demonstrate, these measures appear to have made little impact on the health of British troops until the turn of the century.

The problem of drainage in military cantonments was equally pressing and perhaps more intractable, given that drainage depended greatly on conditions outside of military stations. In 1863, when Nightingale made her observations on the evidence given to the royal commission, she noted that, in many cantonments, there was 'no drainage whatever, in any sense in which we understand drainage'. At Fort St George in Madras the main drain of the town was 80 yards distant, and the fort itself 'swamped in offensive effluvia'.[49] In 1868 the fort's drainage was still 'indifferently provided for', being left largely to natural means, except in the immediate vicinity of barracks.[50] By the turn of the century, however, drainage schemes had been completed in several cantonments with favourable results,[51] but in some stations effective drainage was apparently 'out of the question'. In Delhi, the river Jumna annually washed the walls of the fort during the rainy season and, as the flood receded, many miles of the surrounding country were left covered with stagnant pools in which mosquito larvae 'bred by the millions'.[52]

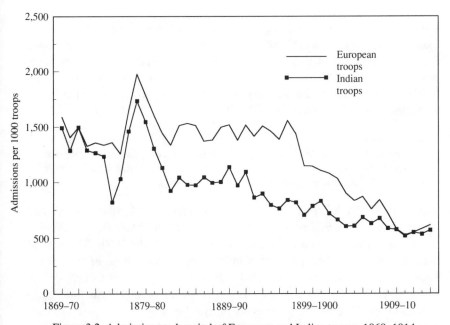

Figure 3.2 Admissions to hospital of European and Indian troops, 1869–1914

Drainage did begin to improve in some cantonments in the 1880s, but the more favourable mortality and morbidity trends evident among British troops around the turn of the century are probably due as much to specific measures designed to control the spread of enteric fever. In the 1900s, in the light of research conducted by Robert Koch, it was generally acknowledged that 'in all probability water plays only a minor role in the dissemination of enteric fever', and that the priority should be to 'deal effectively with the earliest patients'. This meant isolation of patients in separate wards, thorough disinfection or destruction of contaminated linen, and the burning of faeces from infected persons. The early identification of cases was the key to this new system of military hygiene, with bacteriologial diagnosis playing an important part. In the early 1900s, each cantonment acquired a small 'laboratory' in which blood samples could be tested for the presence of typhoid or the newly discovered paratyphoid bacilli.[53]

There was also greater attention to the preparation of food, since it was now thought that poor food hygiene was one of the principal reasons for the high incidence of enteric fever (or typhoid as it was increasingly known) in army camps. Many British regiments soon dispensed with their Indian cooks and domestic assistants in the belief that their 'disregard' for hygiene was at the root of the problem.[54] 'Nothing seems more right and suitable to the native mind', wrote Captain E. C. Freeman, RAMC, in 1899, 'than that the same man and the same broom should attend to the cookhouse and the latrine'.[55] Europeans were generally sceptical that they would see 'any appreciable change' in the habits and customs of Indians, especially their apparent 'disregard for ordinary acts of cleanliness', and their 'indifference to the most suitable locality for compliance with certain natural wants'.[56] Robert Caldwell's experience as a military medical officer in the North West Provinces had convinced him that lower-class Indians were 'walking disseminators of the most repulsive forms of filth'. 'The European in India', he wrote in 1905,

> is constantly exposed to the risk of either swallowing or inhaling excremental refuse conveyed by dust, flies, water, or food, or which clings to the clothing and person of his immediate attendants, and which is transferred from fetid fingers to all kinds of articles of intimate use.[57]

Bacteriological theories of disease causation, then, served to particularise, and perhaps to heighten, European anxieties about the medical dangers of the Indian people. An increasing fatalism was also evident during the 1900s. The general belief that there was little prospect of Indians being educated out of their 'filthy habits', and that they were 'saturated with infection', even cast doubt on the effectiveness of measures to control disease within the vicinity of cantonments.[58] Surgeon-Captain A. E. Grant, professor of hygiene at Madras Medical College, noted with regret that years of daily contact with a people, the mass of whom, rich and poor, regard such matters [as sanitation] with perfect composure or indifference have inoculated these officers with the fatalistic virus to such a degree that they have been known to imply . . . that the attempt to sanitate Indian towns is a mistake, an interference with the laws of nature.[59]

The development of inoculation against typhoid, however, seemed to offer the possibility of protection against the disease regardless of sanitary conditions in military stations. The vaccine had been developed and tested by Almroth Wright, professor of pathology at the Royal Army Medical School, Netley. Having unsuccessfully attempted to persuade the British Army to introduce inoculation on a trial basis in 1896, Wright induced soldiers in India to come forward for inoculation while serving as a member of the Indian Plague Commission. The experiment, if Wright's data is to be believed, was a success, with only 44 cases of typhoid appearing among the 4,502 who volunteered for inoculation. But Wright had failed to secure first the permission of the military and colonial authorities, who were outraged at his action.

There appears to have been deeply ingrained resistance to the new measure in government circles and in the IMS. Despite promising, if not conclusive, trials in British mental hospitals and, later, during the South African War, the Medical Advisory Board of the War Office continued to be suspicious of inoculation and refused to introduce it, even on a voluntary trial basis, until 1904. In the wake of high mortality from typhoid in the South African campaign, the board's reluctance to introduce inoculation precipitated a national outcry. *The Times* denounced the decision as 'a serious example of the ignorance of . . . scientific methods . . . against which the public services of this country are condemned to strive'. Wright resigned from his chair at Netley in 1902, and continued his campaign from his new post at St Mary's Hospital in London.[60]

Antipathy towards Wright had several roots. Among British army officers, and even at Netley itself, Wright was regarded with suspicion since he was not, himself, a military man. Wright had been a civil servant before joining the Army Medical School in 1892, and continued in that capacity throughout his period at Netley. Moreover, while he gained the affection and loyalty of his students, Wright was intolerant of the school's restrictive rules, and soon alienated himself from its military administration. Also, in the days before a standardised dosage had been agreed upon, inoculation could often be a painful experience, and for this reason was generally unpopular among troops. An ex-pupil of Wright's – Colonel L. W. Harrison – wrote to him of his 'great difficulty' is persuading soldiers of a cavalry regiment in India to undergo inoculation.[61] The attitude of troops towards inoculation was an important consideration given the recruitment problems experienced by the services at this time.[62]

Another reason for opposition to inoculation was the fear of pursuing too exclusive a sanitary policy, compounded by the additional cost of supplying and administering the vaccine. E. Roberts, RAMC, writing in 1906, stressed the need to present a complete picture of the disease and a comprehensive programme for its elimination.[63] R. H. Firth, RAMC, also continued to advocate a system of prevention which took into account factors predisposing an individual to disease, and the effects of local climate and water supplies.[64] Others withheld judgement on the value of inoculation pending an inquiry by the War Office, which did not report its favourable conclusions until 1912.[65]

The contagious diseases acts

One of the most persistent problems facing the military authorities was the high incidence of venereal disease among British troops. Vying with malarial fever, venereal disease was one of the two most important causes of admissions to hospital among British troops in India throughout the nineteenth century. In 1870, for example, there was an admission rate from venereal disease of 52.5 per 1,000 troops, with each soldier spending on average 22 days in hospital in the course of the year.[66] Venereal disease was an important drain on manpower in Britain too, but in India the situation was even worse since the vast majority of men and around two-thirds of officers were unmarried, with prostitutes providing a vitally important form of relaxation. The military authorities recognised the inevitability of this behaviour and felt that to forbid access to prostitutes would, to borrow Ronald Hyam's phrase, turn cantonments into 'replicas of Sodom and Gomorrah'.[67] Yet the problem posed by venereal disease had clearly to be addressed.

In the late eighteenth and early nineteenth century, concern over venereal disease led the East India Company to give its guarded approval to the establishment of 'lock hospitals' for the compulsory treatment of 'diseased women'. However, the civil authorities charged with administering these hospitals found their duties distasteful, recognising that the system of inspection was degrading and that the standard treatment which used mercury was extremely hazardous. By 1835 the system had been discontinued throughout India.[68] However, abolition of the hospitals was accompanied by an increase in venereal disease among troops and, in 1852, after much protest from the military authorities, a scheme of inspection and compulsory treatment of hospitals was introduced in Madras city. But other areas resisted pressure from the military and, even in Madras, the local magistrates were often unwilling to allow medical officers to examine women.[69]

The military authorities were more successful after 1858 in the light of fears generated by the mutiny. The Royal Commission recommended that the lock hospital system be introduced with a greater degree of compulsion than hitherto, and the secretary of state endorsed this opinion. The Cantonments Act made provision for the medical inspection and regulation of brothels and, in 1868, the system was formalised and extended under the Contagious Diseases Act (CD Act), modelled on similar legislation passed in Britain 2 years earlier. The act could be introduced in any locality specified by a local government, providing it had the sanction of the governor-general.[70] Outside of cantonments executive responsibility for the enforcement of these measures lay with civil surgeons, municipal health officers, or specially appointed superintendents of lock hospitals. Overall responsibility for lock hospitals lay with the provincial sanitary commissioner.[71]

The enforcement of the CD Act varied greatly from one area to another and opinions differed as to its severity. In his report of 1870, the superintendent of lock hospitals in Calcutta concluded that the 'Indian Act was more stringent than the British one' since it applied to the 'whole civil population of Calcutta where the military element is very small' whereas, in England, the act was confined to garrison towns such as Aldershot. Moreover, in England, the police were

> entirely interdicted from interference, and the Act is worked only by a limited special establishment sent down from the metropolitan police for the purpose . . . In Calcutta, on the other hand, the administration of the Act is entrusted to ordinary local police and every police officer is authorized to arrest, without warrant, any common prostitute who has failed to register or to attend for examination.[72]

Six years later, however, the lieutenant-governor of Bengal expressed his approval of the fact that the commissioner of police for the presidency did not, as a rule, enforce the penal provisions of the Act, but found it sufficient, in most cases, to warn and to discharge. Of 2,359 women arrested for failure to register in 1870 only 301 were brought before magistrates.[73]

Yet there is little doubt that the superintendent's fears were justified, since the Indian subordinate police were notorious for extortion and other abuses of power.[74] Indeed, the City of Bombay went so far as to employ women to mingle among the prostitutes and act as 'spies' in order to detect attempts at extortion by the police.[75] The health officer himself was firmly of opinion that 'no native subordinate to [his] Department ought to have anything whatever to do with the working of the provisions of the Act',[76] while the superintendent of lock hospitals in Calcutta felt that its administration should be entrusted to a special force rather than the ordinary police.[77] Thus, the Indian CD Act may have been far more punitive in its operation than Ronald Hyam has suggested in his controversial *Sexuality and Empire*.[78]

Opinion on the efficiency of the CD acts was equally mixed. The lieutenant-governor of Bengal believed that the act had been largely successful,[79] and the Indian government insisted that

> the working of the lock hospitals has, on the whole, been productive of good, both in diminishing the prevalence and mitigating the severity of venereal diseases among registered prostitutes and European soldiery, and the amount of good thus

affected is sufficient to warrant the maintenance of the system with such improvements as may be found practicable.[80]

But this optimism was not shared by the sanitary commissioner with the Indian government who pointed out that 'in spite of a very general introduction of the rules for the prevention of venereal disease among European troops, the results have hitherto been a failure'. In many instances, he explained, it was 'almost impossible' to say when or where the disease had been contracted, and added that many cantonments had, in fact, made little effort in this direction.[81] In his view, the only hope for improvement lay in the concentration of the regulations in areas of a smaller and more practicable size, and to establish better co-operation between civil and military authorities.[82]

Following especially high levels of venereal disease among European troops in 1877 and 1878, a special committee was appointed to look into the effectiveness of the act.[83] It was found that it provided no definition of the term 'common prostitute', that it made no provision for the compulsory registration of prostitutes on conviction, and that it gave the police insufficient powers of arrest. In the light of the report, and the governor-general's refusal to sanction more stringent regulations, the Bengal government decided to restrict the area to which the CD Act applied.[84]

In Bombay financial considerations proved more important in determining the future of the CD legislation. Owing to severe financial difficulties in 1871, the Bombay Corporation – with the concurrence of the Indian government – allowed the CD act to lapse, and regulations were not reintroduced until 1880.[85] In that year, in the face of increasing pressure from the lieutenant-governor and the rear admiral commanding the fleet at Bombay, the municipality defied government policy and agreed to sanction a grant of Rs 15,000 towards the provision of a lock hospital. It was not, however, in a position to realise this sum, owing to a shortage of revenue, and the act remained a dead letter in Bombay. The Bombay government also took punitive action, withholding Rs 15,000 of its annual grant towards the city's police expenditure.[86]

At the same time, there was increasing criticism of the CD Acts in Britain and India from religious groups such as the Salvation Army, which were concerned that the acts implicitly condoned immoral behaviour. Some exponents of an authoritarian, interventionist, approach towards public health such as the Calcutta Health Society vigorously defended the legislation,[87] but it was denounced 'in the name of God and humanity' by evangelical organisations in India, and meetings were held specially to condemn the measures. A meeting at Calcutta's Exeter Hall learned 'with astonishment and grief that the system of licensed impurity has been established by British authority in over seventy places in India', including the principal centres of population.[88]

The CD Acts were also unpopular with many Indians,[89] although not universally so. In 1875, the *Hindoo Patriot* declared its support for the act in Calcutta and expressed its pleasure that its provisions appeared to have led to some improvement in the health of European troops.[90] More typically, though, the Indian press was vocal and persistent in its opposition to the CD Acts. The *Bengalee* condemned the act as 'a useless piece of legislation' which had been attended by 'a degree of oppression . . . which far outweighed any benefits which might be supposed to have accrued from it'.[91] It pointed out that the act had been 'a powerful engine of tyranny in mofussil towns in the hands of an unscrupulous police and unscrupulous neighbours':

> If the neighbours have any grudge against a woman of the town – if the paramour has quarrelled with his mistress, or if the Police underling is anxious to extort some money from one of these unhappy creatures – straight away a complaint is lodged that the woman is carrying on the business of prostitution, the summons is issued, conviction follows, the woman is fined and ordered to be sent to the lock-hospital for examination, which in the case of a Hindoo means loss of caste and a depth of degradation which it is impossible to describe.[92]

As a result of the combination of these pressures, the acts were suspended in 1881 on the orders of the Liberal viceroy Lord Ripon. During the Liberal administration of 1886 the British act was repealed, and the Indian act 2 years later.[93]

But the repeal of the CD act did not mark the end of the medical inspection of prostitutes in India. The new Military Cantonments Act of 1889 incorporated a deliberately catch-all clause which provided for

> the prevention of the spread of infectious or contagious diseases within a cantonment, and the appointment and regulation of hospitals . . . for the reception and treatment of persons suffering from any disease.[94]

The provisions of the act could be, and frequently were, interpreted to permit the inspection and compulsory treatment of prostitutes. The Liberal government in Britain was determined to end this flagrant violation of its orders and, in 1894, directed the Indian government to limit the scope of the Cantonments Act. Accordingly, in 1895, the government passed legislation stating that no rule under the Cantonment Act of 1889 should contain any regulation permitting the medical examination or compulsory treatment of prostitutes suspected of having venereal disease.[95]

However, in 1897 the Conservative secretary of state Lord Hamilton, concerned about the continuation of high levels of venereal disease among British troops in India, decided to overturn the policy of the previous administration. He instructed the viceroy, Lord Elgin, to repeal the 1895 Act and to draft new rules permitting medical inspection to be reintroduced in cantonments – a move which was extremely unpopular with the Indian community. The *Bengalee* had 'a vivid recollection of the nameless horrors practiced by an unscrupulous

Police in the name of the Contagious Diseases Act', in which many Hindus had lost caste.[96] But the official mood in 1897 was one in which indigenous opinion on the matter of the CD Acts counted for very little, being eclipsed by the more pressing problem of the plague epidemic which had swept across the Bombay Presidency, and which threatened Bengal and Madras. In the same month as the *Bengalee* made its protest, the Epidemic Diseases Act was passed by the Indian government, placing a wide range of custodial powers at the disposal of provincial governments.[97] In such circumstances the cantonment legislation was passed with relatively little publicity and, as Kenneth Ballhatchet has put it, 'the military authorities won the last battle in a long campaign'.[98] Yet it was a campaign in which the military's control over the indigenous population had been confined within the walls of the cantonment by the combined forces of economy, moral indignation, and Indian opinion.

'Reservoirs of dirt and disease'

Sanitary policing

Improvements in water supplies, barracks, and the introduction of more specific preventive measures, all contributed a great deal to the mortality decline among British and Indian troops, but the health of soldiers was not considered in isolation. Physical segregation was never total, and military cantonments and their environs were host to a variety of tradesmen, vendors, servants; all of whom were viewed as potential threats to the health of troops. The tendency to view Indians as part of the 'sanitary problem' confronting Europeans had been evident since at least the 1830s, but the mutiny heightened anxieties on this score, producing demands for the sanitary surveillance and regulation of the Indian population; at first within, and then without, the military cantonment.

Bazaars on the edge of cantonments were singled out for special criticism in the evidence given to the royal commission. The bazaars, according to Florence Nightingale, were 'simply the first savage stage of social savage life'. They had 'no regular system of drainage, no public latrines . . . and no sufficient establishment to keep them clean'. They suffered from 'overcrowding, bad ventilation, bad water supply, filth, foul ditches . . . jungle and nuisances'. In short, the bazaars were 'one immense privy'; a danger to their inhabitants and European troops alike.[99]

The Military Cantonments Act of 1864 was the Indian government's response to these concerns. The act provided for a system of sanitary policing under the overall charge of military medical officers: regulations were laid down governing land use, nuisances, drainage, and unlicensed trades, but the extent to which these measures were enforced is questionable.[100] In 1868, following a severe cholera epidemic the previous year, the Army Sanitary Commission recommended that there should be a further inquiry into the sanitary state of military stations in India, and that a 'more rigid system of sanitary police' be introduced. Wary of provoking civil unrest, the Indian government resisted the move, but final authority lay with the British government, and the scheme was introduced on a trial basis in a few cantonments in the Bengal Presidency.[101] However, the matter was not pursued further and the Indian government allowed the scheme to lapse.[102] There was even opposition on financial grounds to the extension of the water analysis scheme established by Francis MacNamara in Calcutta.[103] The lieutenant-governor of Bengal thought it 'undesirable to institute any such experiment, the results of which would probably be indeterminate, while the expense attending it would be uncertain.'[104]

Problems also attended the sanitation of bazaars. As late as the 1880s, there were doubts as to the legality of interfering with bazaars on the edge of cantonments, and most local authorities had not drawn up bye-laws for their regulation.[105] Indeed, conditions in the vicinity of cantonments were causing great anxiety among medical officers, particularly the pollution of water supplies by Indian villagers living upstream. They protested that they were powerless to intervene outside the confines of their station, and called for the formation of special committees to inspect neighbouring villages and to compel the residents to follow sanitary regulations similar to those in force outside the cantonment.[106]

In 1877 permission was granted by the Indian government and the committees were empowered to inspect all villages within a 5 mile radius of the eight cantonments initially involved in the scheme. The committees could insist that wells be repaired, refuse be collected, latrines be provided, and that a scavenging staff be engaged. It was recognised that these measures would involve 'large expenditure' and that they would necessitate 'much interference on the part of the police' in the daily affairs of villagers. But the Indian government thought the risk posed to the health of troops by conditions outside cantonments sufficiently great to warrant such measures, although it decided to cushion the blow in the short term by drawing the necessary funds from the military budget.

In the long term, however, it was envisaged that the money would be drawn from revenue raised by the imposition of a conservancy tax on the villagers concerned.[107] Military imperatives were, then, vitally important in the process by which sanitary policing was extended into rural areas: Indian villages were seen as the foci of epidemics which, sooner or later, would take their toll among British soldiers. In the words of the sanitary commissioner with the Indian government it was a 'good thing to secure the cleanliness of the immediate environment of troops, but they will never be safe as long as the native population and its towns and villages are left uncleaned to act as reservoirs of dirt and disease'.[108] But, if the indigenous population was to shoulder the burden of sanitary expenditure, greater concessions had to be made to local élites in terms of representation on local bodies. This was the essence of the reforms introduced by the viceroy Lord Ripon in the mid-1880s, and which form the subject of chapter 7.

Vital statistics

The 'keystone in the arch of sanitation', as one health officer described it, was the registration of births and deaths.[109] The registration of deaths in cantonments was sanctioned under the act of 1864, while in the civil sphere it was made the responsibility, first of the sanitary commissions, and after 1868 of the provincial sanitary commissioners. The latter had the difficult task of co-ordinating an array of registration officers from civil surgeons to the Indian subordinate police.[110] This scheme was to provide the basis for an annual aggregate of the vital statistics of the civilian Indian population, or 'general population', as they were referred to in official reports, after 1869. However, it was recognised from the very beginning that these statistics would provide no more than a rough indication of age-specific mortality, since many Indians were apparently ignorant of their own age. Given the enormity of the task facing the registration agencies with regard to deaths alone, plans to extend the system of birth and marriage registration which already existed in the Central Provinces and Burma were held in abeyance for the time being.[111]

In the countryside the administrative area of death registration was the police circle, with the chief police officer, or *mohurrir* as he was known in the North West Provinces, the circle registration officer. Village headmen were responsible for reporting deaths to the registration officer, classified according to race and religion, causes of death, age (approximate to between 5 and 10 years), and name of village. In the towns, where in some cases death registration had begun in the 1850s, officers were specially appointed by the municipality or the cantonment committee. Jails and lunatic asylums submitted separate returns.[112]

The urgency with which death registration was introduced owed much to military imperatives, and military factors continued to shape its development. In 1870, owing to high rates of cholera among European troops, the Army Sanitary Commission urged all large cities in India to produce weekly returns of deaths in the hope that this might afford warning of an impending epidemic. Some provincial governments such as the Punjab, the Central Provinces, and Berar complied, but others protested that to publish death-rates more often than on a monthly basis was practically impossible, unless financial support was forthcoming from central government to employ additional staff.[113]

Anxiety about the health of troops also lay at the heart of the Indian government's attempts to centralise information in the hands of its sanitary commissioner – J. M. Cuningham. Cuningham wanted mortality statistics to be passed directly to cantonment authorities, via the quartermaster-general, and ultimately to his office, by-passing civil surgeons and provincial sanitary commissioners. But while most medical officers shared the government's concern with the health of troops, many were vehemently opposed to any diminution of their own authority.[114] William Walker, a civil surgeon in the North West Provinces, felt that

> Dr. Cuningham's proposal to introduce a system of centralizing information in the Sanitary Commissioner with the Government of India, seems to me to ignore not only the Sanitary Commissioners with the Local Government, but to shadow forth an interference with the power of the Local Government to deal with an epidemic as circumstances may seem to call for action.[115]

This was precisely the point: the Indian government was concerned for reasons of public order to prevent the imposition of custodial measures such as cordons sanitaires, and Cuningham's proposals effectively deprived provincial governments and medical officers of the initiative in dealing with epidemic disease. Yet, opposition from local administrations, and, no doubt, the impracticality of operating death registration without the participation of local medical officers, meant that death returns continued to be processed first at provincial level.

But death registration was already experiencing enormous difficulties. Part of the problem stemmed from the system's reliance on the subordinate police and others who lacked even the most rudimentary medical knowledge.[116] As the sanitary commissioner of Bombay put it, 'death registration is effected by the agency of uneducated men, and is generally admitted to be far from accurate'.[117] Even within cantonments, death registration was, in 1874, still 'far from satisfactory', prompting the sanitary commissioner with the Indian government to comment that the time had come for 'the compulsory registration of all births and deaths within cantonments to be strictly enforced'. In 1869 a clause had been added to cantonment regulations obliging the head of every family to report a death in his household within 24 hours but, according to the sanitary commissioner it had been little acted upon. Similarly, compulsory provisions had been made by only a small number of municipalities; again, with mixed results.[118] Cuningham wrote that 'in many parts of the country the registration of deaths is as yet so imperfectly conducted, that any detailed analysis of the results would be merely a waste of time and labour'. 'The want of educated medical practitioners', he continued, 'and the ignorance and apathy, not only of the people themselves, but also of the village officials by whom reports are made, all offer obstacles to correct registration'.[119]

The registration of births progressed even more slowly, varying greatly from province to province. In the Bengal Presidency it was confined to a few areas in 'Bengal proper', the North West Provinces, and the Punjab; in Oudh it was not attempted at all. It was, then, extremely difficult for medical men to ascertain demographic trends among the Indian population, although some rough estimates were attempted. The sanitary commissioner for the Punjab reported that in 'normal years' the birth rate exceeded the death rate by one third, but that in 1875, due to an 'unhealthy season', they had been roughly equal.[120]

In the coming years the inadequacies of the registration agencies became even more apparent. In Bombay the health officer complained that the Indian police who had been charged with registration of deaths had consistently failed to report deaths and to fill out properly the forms provided. 'I have had to report ten of the sepoys to the Commissioner of Police', he lamented, 'whose patience I have very severely taxed'.[121] In Berar there was some attempt to reform the system by removing responsibility for registration from the district super-intendents of police and placing it under civil surgeons, in the hope that they would demand a higher standard of medical accuracy from their subordinates.[122] But for many medical men the burden of extra administrative work was far from welcome, although, in 1877, sanitary commissioners were relieved of some statistical work in order that they might devote more time to registration.[123]

Though dissatisfied with the progress of registration, the Government of India was reluctant to press it as a compulsory measure, and directed that where cantonments and municipalities chose to introduce such measures, they should not be enforced to the detriment of relations with the indigenous population. The registration of births and, especially, deaths impinged on some of the most sensitive areas of family life and had, for obvious political reasons, to be handled with tact. Accordingly, all provincial governments except Bombay resisted appeals by the Indian Famine Commission to make compulsory the registration of deaths in rural areas as well as in all towns. The Indian government believed that 'the time has not yet arrived when the registration of births and deaths should be made generally obligatory by law', and advised that the best course of action was to leave the matter to the discretion of local officials.[124]

The Bombay government, however, felt that the time had come for a change of policy, and agreed with its sanitary commissioner that 'petty fines in Municipalities, if levied judiciously will no doubt have a good effect; and any gentle pressure of this kind put on the *people* will tend to better registration'.[125] Bombay continued to be the only provincial government to permit the introduction of compulsory registration in rural areas, even though it was acknowledged in the 1890s that progress was generally very slow. In 1893 the Bengal government compared its sanitary commissioner to 'a skilled workman labouring with indifferent tools'.[126] The following year, the sanitary com-missioner with the Indian government reported that the 'returns are still far from accurate', the 'machinery for recording events imperfect', and the subordinate staff 'neither by intelligence nor education well qualified for their duties'.[127] Nevertheless, there had been some improvement on previous years, since whereas births had been registered in only 45 towns in Bengal in 1886, a decade later they were registered in almost every town in the province.[128]

Any improvement apparent in 1896 was, in most areas of India, short lived. The devastation caused by the plague epidemics of 1896 onwards, and by severe famines in western and central India, meant that medical and other agencies were stretched to the limit, and to the detriment of registration.[129] However, plague did result in a number of reforms in the system of registration. The Epidemic Diseases Act passed in 1897, as a measure to control the spread of the plague, empowered provincial governments to make provisions for the inspection of corpses and the compulsory notification of all cases of, and deaths from plague.[130] Opposition to corpse inspection and other measures led to their being discontinued in most areas, but the usefulness of compulsory notification of infectious disease had been confirmed, strengthening the hand of those in the medical profession who had been calling for such measures to be introduced.[131] The Indian Plague Commission also recommended that more municipal health officers be employed, and that one of their principal duties should be to supervise the registration of births and deaths. However, it was recognised that any dramatic improvement in the accuracy of death registration was unlikely, since it was estimated that no more than one third of the population of Calcutta and other large cities had access to a qualified (western) medical practitioner.[132]

In Bombay, which had suffered more than any other city from plague, a number of individual registration initiatives followed closely upon the report of the Plague Commission in 1901. The city's new health officer John Turner pointed out that of 24,068 deaths registered in the previous year, only 569 certificates had been provided by qualified medical practitioners, and 2,599 by infectious diseases hospitals, leaving the vast majority to be supplied by medically unqualified persons.[133] In a proposal to the Bombay Corporation, supported by the professorate of Grant Medical College, Turner argued that more medically qualified men should be appointed by the municipality for the work of registration, and that a system of compulsory notification of all diseases be introduced. After some deliberation, the corporation accepted a watered-down version of Turner's proposal, by which all cases of tuberculosis, malaria, and certain infectious diseases notified to the city's health department would be published in the press and as hand bills, but without any compulsory provision to this effect.[134] The corporation had apparently received protests from the city's medical profession that 'compulsory notification of malaria and tuberculosis would entail a hardship on medical men'.[135]

Turner was unable to effect any further concession from the municipality, or to engage substantially more medically qualified staff in the process of registration, and the accuracy of returns continued to leave much to be desired.[136] In rural areas of India the progress of registration was even more disappointing. Delegates to the All-India Sanitary Conference in 1911 regretted the reluctance of people in rural areas to register births and deaths, the inaccuracy of reporting by village headmen, and the problems faced by local boards in maintaining registration establishments on insufficient funds.[137] With the 'keystone' in the arch of sanitation far from secure, the superstructure itself afforded scant protection to the millions of Indians outside of military cantonments.

Vaccination against smallpox

Vaccination was one of the earliest but one of the most controversial forms of colonial medical intervention in India. Jennerian vaccination was introduced into India in 1802 and promoted with considerable enthusiasm by European officials like the governor of Bombay, Lord Elphinstone. It has been suggested that, at a time when the British were seeking to consolidate their hold on newly conquered territory in India, the East India Company promoted vaccination of Indians in an attempt to create an impression of colonial benevolence.[138] Vaccination also, perhaps, symbolised the progress of western civilisation, and it is noteworthy that Elphinstone's ambitious plan of 1827 to vaccinate the inhabitants of rural Bombay was conceived amid the stirrings of utilitarian reform in India.[139] Equally, vaccination provided a means of surveying and understanding the indigenous population, and was especially important in the absence of an efficient or universal system of birth and death registration.[140]

During the early years of the campaign it was hoped that vaccination would gain the acceptance of the Indian people, and that they would eventually take it up for themselves, thus reducing the charge on the colonial exchequer.[141] However, such a view seems surprisingly optimistic in view of the considerable opposition which vaccination had met with in Britain.[142] Aside from technical limitations, such as the shortage of lymph and cowpox crusts which had to be imported from Britain,[143] there were enormous cultural and political barriers in the path of vaccination in India. Probably the most significant of these was the fact that arm-to-arm vaccination – the dominant form of vaccination in India until well into the 1890s – was considered ritually polluting by Hindus since it entailed the transfer of bodily fluids from low caste or 'untouchable' vaccinifers.[144] Neither was the widespread belief in the smallpox deity *Sitala* – which was propitiated annually in ceremonies throughout India – easily displaced by the secular process of vaccination.[145]

Vaccination had also to compete with a deeply entrenched and near-ubiquitous form of inoculation against smallpox which, unlike vaccination, was sanctioned by Hindu and Moslem religions. In eastern India, inoculation had its own special practitioners known as *tikadars*, or 'mark-makers', who received payment for their services. Although British medical men had displayed some sympathy for the practice prior to the introduction of vaccination,[146] inoculation was afterwards regarded with hostility and almost universally derided as inefficient and dangerous.[147] In 1844 the superintendent of vaccination in Calcutta went so far as to report that 'smallpox is annually introduced into Calcutta by a set of inoculators', while the IMS officer S. P. James, in 1909, still maintained that many smallpox epidemics could be traced to the activities of such men.[148]

Most importantly, the extension of vaccination suffered from the contradictions of colonial medical policy itself. On the one hand, vaccination of the indigenous population was militarily and economically desirable; on the other, it involved great cost and the strong possibility of creating civil unrest through interference in indigenous cultural practices.[149] According to the inspector of hospitals for Bengal, prejudice against vaccination existed not only among 'the lower and ignorant classes, but also among some supposed to be better informed, and considered to have good social positions'.[150] Thus, while much was done to encourage the indigenous population to come forward for vaccination, the government shied away from demands that it should be made compulsory, even within the more strictly regulated confines of military cantonments.[151]

Where vaccination was introduced gradually and with due regard to indigenous sensibilities, it was thought that the measure might gain acceptance, and provide an excellent means of 'impressing other sanitary matters on the attention of the people'.[152] But a minority of reform-minded medical officers favoured the introduction of compulsory general vaccination against smallpox. John Lumsdaine, health officer of Bombay, justified the proposal on the grounds that 'as far as the masses are concerned it would be a distinction without a difference, for it is now the general belief that it is compulsory'.[153]

By 1872 Lumsdaine had mustered enough support among the European community to effect the introduction of a bill in the Bombay legislative council providing for compulsory vaccination in the City of Bombay for all children under 14 years of age. The Indian government viewed this development with alarm and warned the Bombay government that 'in all sanitary legislation in this country it is essential that the people should first be alive to the benefits of the proposed law. It would be much better to postpone compulsory vaccination . . . until the benefits of vaccination are more fully appreciated.'[154] The official position was clear, and the attempt to pass the vaccination bill was shelved for the time being. 'All that the Government can hope to do', wrote J. M. Cuningham, 'is to confer the benefits of vaccination on a certain very limited number of persons' and 'to show the people by experience what vaccination professes to do'.[155] This was a clear departure from the view, embodied in the paternalistic administrations of Elphinstone and others, that public health was a responsibility of the state.[156]

Another obstacle to a more extensive and effective vaccination programme was the vaccination establishment itself. The subordinate staff involved in vaccination could not be trusted to produce accurate statements of their work and neither, it seems, could some of their superiors.[157] In 1884 a deputy sanitary commissioner in the NWP was removed from his post to military duties for falsifying vaccination returns in Jalaan District.[158] Nor was there much reason to suppose that the accuracy of vaccination statistics improved in the coming decades. In 1892 the inspector-general of vaccination for Madras noted in his annual report that in six circles the deputy inspectors had failed to verify even 50% of vaccinations, while one deputy was fined and another dismissed for irregular behaviour.[159] Indeed, in most hill districts of the province there was 'no proper supervision exercised over Deputy Inspectors', while great difficulty was experienced in obtaining suitable (subordinate) staff on existing rates of pay.[160]

The administration of vaccination was further complicated by the fact that it was carried out by two independent organisations: the special vaccination establishment and the provincial dispensaries. The organisation of vaccination also differed from province to province. In the North West Provinces and the Punjab there was a superintendent responsible to government for vaccination only. In Bengal there was also a superintendent of vaccination, but he was subordinate to the Medical Department and with more limited functions. In the Central Provinces, Berar, and Burma, the post of superintendent was combined with sanitary commissioner. The latter arrangement being the one preferred by the Indian government, since it was more useful for gathering information about the health of the people, and for publicising sanitary measures among them.[161] The Central Provinces eventually became the model for the amalgamation of the vaccination and sanitary departments throughout British India in 1880.[162]

Frustration with the slow progress of vaccination led to renewed demands that it be made compulsory within certain areas. In 1877, after much deliberation, the Bombay government decided to act contrary to advice from Calcutta and passed a Vaccination Act embodying the provisions of the Bill of 1872. A similar act was passed in Karachi in 1879.[163] In the face of increasing demands from the European community, and with no serious unrest evident in either Bombay or Karachi, the Indian government reluctantly took steps to enable other administrations to do the same. Its Compulsory Vaccination Act of 1880 empowered provincial governments to introduce into certain towns and cantonments compulsory vaccination for children over 6 months old, with the sanction of a fine of Rs 1,000 or six months imprisonment for a parent or guardian who did not bring their child to be vaccinated.[164]

But the act did not mark a clear break with the policy of gradualism and cautious intervention espoused by the Indian government in the 1870s. The viceroy Lord Ripon felt that the act was of such a permissive nature that it gave the inhabitants of each locality the opportunity to state their objections, and he seems to have first sought the agreement of eminent Indians such as the Hon. Sayyad Ahmed, a member of the legislative council.[165] The introduction of compulsory vaccination was also favoured by the Bengali newspaper the *Hindoo Patriot*, which claimed in an editorial of 1878 that it was only 'the ignorant and bigoted who still oppose it'.[166] However, compulsory vaccination was still a controversial measure, with some prominent Indians like the Parsi philanthropist Sir Jamsetji Jijibhai refusing to bring forth their children for vaccination.[167] The Madras government was also wary of making vaccination compulsory in Madras City, and did so only after much protest from its European inhabitants, and in the wake of a severe outbreak of smallpox in 1884.[168] In fact the majority of provincial administrations were reticent about implementing the act, and it was introduced into only 441 towns and cantonments by 1906, representing 7% of British India's total population.[169]

The limited extent to which compulsion was introduced was probably a reflection of continuing indigenous hostility towards vaccination, outside of a small, western-educated, urban élite. In 1888 the sanitary commissioner of Bombay wrote of the refusal of many parents to allow vaccinators to take lymph from their children, and noted that thousands of villages in the Bombay Presidency had not yet even been visited by a vaccinator.[170] In 1880, the surgeon-general of Bengal also noted the persistence of 'extravagant beliefs and prejudices' against vaccination in his province, and the continuing popularity of inoculators, especially in the hill districts.[171]

Another problem surrounded the use of vaccine made from calf lymph, introduced on an experimental basis in Bombay in the late 1850s. There was, initially, considerable opposition to the practice from orthodox Hindus who objected to what they saw as a violation of their sacred animal, and an attempt to introduce vaccination with calf lymph into Karachi had to be abandoned in 1880 because of civil unrest.[172] Nevertheless, many medical officers, such as the sanitary commissioner for Hyderabad, continued to advocate the measure on the grounds that it was 'popular with the native public, who, as a rule, dislike to give lymph from their children's arms, and especially . . . those fastidious caste men who object to lymph taken from the arms of low caste children'. The stock of calf lymph, he argued, could be increased indefinitely at comparatively little expense, although he recognised that the method did have certain drawbacks; principally, the shorter lifespan of calf lymph and the fact that it caused greater inflammation.[173]

W. J. Simpson, health officer of Calcutta, was another enthusiastic advocate of calf lymph, claiming high-caste Hindus had been gradually reconciled to the practice, and that only certain tribes in up-country areas consistently opposed it.[174] However, the Nepalese and the Lepchas, who inhabited the hill districts of Bengal were equally opposed to arm-to-arm vaccination, and were generally unwilling to permit their children be used as vaccinifers.[175] The Indian government and provincial governments also had reservations. As the secretary to the Indian government pointed out, 'the cost of producing all the animal vaccine that would be wanted would be prohibitive'. In the early 1890s the issue was further complicated by the growth of Hindu opposition to the killing of cows by Muslims.[176]

A measure of official reticence over the use of calf lymph was the decision by the Madras government to remove a deputy sanitary commissioner from his position with the Sanitary Department for distributing calf lymph without having first obtained permission from government. The offending officer, W. G. King, claimed that there had been nothing in the Madras *Manual of Vaccination* to prohibit such a course of action, and his supporters ensured that the matter was taken up at the highest level in Britain. Having persuaded the British government of the injustice of King's removal from office, the secretary of state Lord Kimberley intervened on his behalf, forcing the Madras government to reinstate him, this time as the new sanitary commissioner, with a salary increase of Rs 400 per month.[177]

It was, perhaps, the King decision that led other provincial governments to extend their production of vaccine from calf lymph. It was also true that, in many instances, vaccination with animal lymph *was* more acceptable to Indians than the old system of arm-to-arm vaccination. From November 1893 the use of calf lymph became the stated policy of the Bengal government,[178] while in the Central Provinces it was found that many objections to the use of animal lymph could be overcome if the matter was obtained from buffaloes instead of cows.[179] The same method was adopted in Assam, but some problems were initially experienced in the production of the vaccine.[180] By 1911 the manufacture of vaccine from animal lymph had allowed British India to become self-sufficient in vaccine, with the Vaccine Institute at Belgaum producing over 600,000 doses annually.[181] Laboratories such as the King Institute in Madras had also done much to improve the quality of animal lymph and its preservation.[182]

This expansion of production permitted a substantial increase in the number of vaccinations performed yearly from the late 1890s. From less than 5 million per year in 1887, the number of vaccinations rose to over 9 million in 1905.[183] However, it is necessary to regard these figures with some scepticism, for, as the secretary to the Indian government warned,

> the percentage of success claimed for primary operations [in Bengal] is . . . incredibly high, and is due, it is feared, to deception practised on civil surgeons. In other provinces Vaccinators and Inspectors have been detected in bringing forward for inspection the same children for a number of years in succession.[184]

These reservations seem to be consistent with the fact that, although the number of vaccinations had increased considerably in the 1890s and early 1900s, there was no corresponding decrease in mortality from the disease. In British India as a whole, the number of smallpox vaccinations performed annually increased from 6.2 million in 1891–2 to 8 million a decade later. Yet deaths from smallpox actually increased over this period, from 101,721 in 1891–2 to 115,445 in 1901–2, falling significantly only after 1909.[185]

The plague epidemics of 1896 onwards also did much to hinder the progress of vaccination. Plague created an additional burden on vaccination establishments which were already insufficient to reach many people in rural areas; and, in the atmosphere of mutual distrust and panic which followed the outbreak of the disease in India, rumours circulated to the effect the vaccination was responsible for transmitting the plague.[186] Indeed, there is evidence that opponents of vaccination actually became more vocal in India in the wake of plague. In a series of letters to the orthodox Hindu newspaper the *Amrita Bazar Patrika*, in 1912, a correspondent warned that strict enforcement of vaccination in Japan had led to an increase in smallpox, and urged that general sanitary reforms were a better preventive against smallpox than vaccination.[187] The *Indian Public Health and Municipal Journal* also noted an increase in opposition to compulsory vaccination at this time.[188] In addition to suspicion of colonial motives in promoting vaccination, there was also resentment among Indian Moslems of the fact that many vaccination establishments were comprised almost entirely of Hindus.[189]

Vaccination, then, by 1914, was still clearly culturally unacceptable to many of the Indian people, although this was not, probably, the most significant factor in the slow progress of vaccination. Where vaccination was introduced with the co-operation of community leaders there is some evidence that resistance to the measure could be overcome in time.[190] A more significant factor was the basic inadequacy of the vaccination programme. Vaccination establishments simply had not sufficient resources to reach many of the infants who required vaccination on a regular basis. Thus, although the numbers of those vaccinated increased, the disease was never denied a fresh supply of victims among the new-born in areas which relied on the occasional visits of travelling vaccinators.[191] Equally important was the fact that smallpox was never made a notifiable disease in India. As with the issue of compulsory vaccination, the lack of action in this regard was a measure of the government's fear of provoking a backlash from its subjects, and of the practical difficulties of enforcing such measures even in the best-protected urban areas.

The civilising mission

The political uncertainties of the post-mutiny era fostered a mood of caution among British administrators in India: legislative intervention in public health, or in any other sphere which impinged upon deep-rooted religious or cultural practices, was kept to a minimum. In addition to public order considerations, sanitary legislation of the kind enacted in Britain was never a realistic option in India, given the immense area to be policed and insufficient medically trained personnel to ensure its enforcement. It was as an alternative, or as a precursor to legislative intervention that popular education in hygiene came to attract the attention of sanitary reformers late nineteenth-century India.

Sanitary education formed part of the strategy of cautious intervention advocated by the Indian government, though initiatives in this direction came not chiefly from the government, but from voluntary bodies funded on a charitable basis.[192] For the most part the government was sympathetic to these voluntary initiatives, but was reluctant to involve itself directly in their administration. Nevertheless, voluntary bodies promoting vernacular education in western hygiene drew enthusiastic support from the Anglo-Indian community and from sections of the Indian élite. Though government patronage of these schemes rarely extended to financial support, certain spheres of their activity were slowly brought within the remit of local or provincial government. By the 1910s the climate of opinion created by the activity of voluntary bodies also began to have some influence upon the public health policy of the Indian government.

The dispensary movement and sanitary education

The establishment of charitable dispensaries from the 1830s was one of the earliest attempts to provide western medical care for the Indian people. It was soon realised that these institutions could perform useful public health functions, in addition to their curative work. Dispensaries became local centres for vaccination against smallpox and for conveying western ideas about sanitation and hygiene; and 'local sanitary amendments, such as the digging of tanks and wells, fencing them off, and filling up holes' apparently followed the opening of dispensaries in different parts of Bengal.[193] Many of these dispensaries owed their existence to Indian philanthropists, who provided the money for the building of dispensary houses and a monthly sum for their maintenance.[194] By the 1860s, the fortunes of the landed notables who had sponsored these schemes were waning, and increasingly the sources of philanthropy became more diverse. In some cases 'native doctors' and medicines, and even the dispensary itself, were provided by government;[195] sometimes by commercial organisations, like the Bengal Coal Company,[196] and sometimes by subscriptions from Europeans.[197] However, from 1870, as part of a move to reduce public expenditure, the colonial administration sought to distance itself from the running of dispensaries, which it felt should rely increasingly on local funds. The Government of Bengal resolved that:

> The utility of dispensaries has now become so fully acknowledged that there is no necessity for the state to offer assistance to such an extent as when the movement was recent . . . The accumulation of balances further shows that there is no difficulty in obtaining locally even more money that suffices to meet the wants of these institutions as at present conducted.[198]

Financial devolution left dispensaries dependent on local revenues which were subject to substantial fluctuation and regional variation, and dispensary provision varied accordingly. However, the total number of such institutions increased considerably in the decades after 1870: in 1867 there were only 61 dispensaries in the province of Bengal, with 17,000 in-patients and 318,895 out-patients,[199] but by 1900 over 500 had been established in Bengal, attracting in excess of 50,000 in-patients and 2,296,617 out-patients.[200]

The increasing number of persons treated at dispensaries was one of the more impressive achievements of colonial health policy in India, but the extent to which contact with dispensary staff provided an education in public health is harder to gauge. The presence of dispensaries in some cases apparently encouraged a desire for vaccination among the Indian people,[201] while in towns like Puri, the presence of the dispensary was thought an important factor in the adoption by Indians of western sanitary practices.[202]

In the majority of cases, dispensary staff set a good example to their patients,[203] but doubt was cast on the competence of some. On inspecting Bograh dispensary, the deputy inspector-general of hospitals for Bengal found that the medical officer in charge was an opium eater and totally unfit for his post.[204] According to the superintendent of Marrickgunge dispensary, 'the insubordination and carelessness shown by native doctors when away from control is so uniform that it is only by periodical inspections and really knowing the actual state of the branch dispensaries that these institutions are made useful to the community'.[205] It is, of course, necessary to take account of racial prejudice when evaluating the testimony of European medical officers. Nevertheless, it is likely that conditions were far from perfect in many dispensaries; particularly as local dispensary committees usually met infrequently, making effective management of such institutions difficult.

One notable area in which dispensaries failed was in the treatment and vaccination of women. In 1869, the superintendent of dispensaries for Bareilly District spoke of the 'great difficulty' he and his staff had in persuading women to attend dispensaries;[206] and, in 1871, only 18% of those attending dispensaries in Bengal as in-patients or out-patients were women.[207] From the 1880s, however, there were attempts to make dispensaries more acceptable to Indian women otherwise prevented from attending by the seclusion of purdah. Writing in 1900, the inspector-general of hospitals for Bengal claimed that most dispensaries in the province had now

been improved . . . in connection with the privacy of women. In all places the object has been to have a separate delivery window for females, which shall open, if possible, into a separate waiting-room for that sex. Privacy for women has been held by me to be a most important condition of success.[208]

But the results of these initiatives were disappointing. Although many more women were attending dispensaries in Bengal (some 587,092 in 1901) than in the 1870s, this was simply a function of the growing number of such institutions in the province. In fact, in 1901, the percentage of women attending dispensaries had increased by only 0.3% on that of 30 years before.[209]

Outside of dispensaries, the government's role in sanitary education was confined largely to the distribution of literature on basic hygiene. J. M. Cuningham's *Sanitary Primer* was translated into many Indian languages and became a set text in Indian schools. Tens of thousands of copies were distributed in the 1870s and 80s. In 1887, 3 years after Cuningham's retirement from the post of sanitary commissioner, his primer was replaced with an alternative source of wisdom on sanitary matters, the former being considered 'too elementary' even for junior classes. The Indian government's attention had been directed to a publication by the Madras Christian Vernacular Education Society, entitled *The Way to Health*. Like Cuningham's *Primer*, it stressed the evils of fatalism and the simple precautions which might be taken against ill-health. But *The Way to Health* paid more attention to the causation of specific diseases than Cuningham's text, and, unlike its predecessor, presented cholera as an essentially waterborne infection.[210] However, its tendency towards over-simplification, and its anachronistic notions of disease causation, may not have been the only reasons for the withdrawal of Cuningham's *Primer*. In 1882, with Cuningham still *in situ* at the Sanitary Department, the Government of Assam requested that it be replaced by a booklet written by an Indian – Babu Jadu Nath – on account of its simpler phraseology and 'native standpoint'. Yet, the Indian government refused to sanction its withdrawal, presumably not wanting to undermine confidence in its sanitary commissioner.[211]

It is significant that the text which eventually replaced Cuningham's was published by a missionary organisation. Non-official, and especially religious, organisations invariably made the running in matters of sanitary education. Hygiene was an important element of their 'civilising mission', in which moral and medical teaching went hand in hand.[212] Public and personal hygiene was a matter of Christian duty, and sanitary manuals like *The Way to Health* inveighed against the moral as well as the medical dangers of alcohol and other forms of intoxication.[213] Missionaries were perhaps better placed than government officials to observe on a regular basis the cultural practices of Asiatic peoples and to devise methods by which western principles could be introduced. However, the moralising tone and the air of cultural superiority conveyed in missionary texts may have limited their appeal to an Indian audience.

The veil of the 'zenana'

The most striking aspect of non-official activity in the sphere of public health education was its preoccupation with the health and sanitary education of Indian women. Prior to 1870 there had been few initiatives in this direction, but it had often been noted that women were seldom admitted to hospital or sought western medical attention. In the 1860s there were a number of attempts to remedy this situation, concerned chiefly with the training of Indian midwives (*dais*).[214] The question of how best to gain access to one-half of India's population, so far largely untouched by western civilisation, became increasingly important to missionaries in the 1870s and 80s. The provision of medical relief was seen as one of the few ways by which western ideas could penetrate the veil of the *zenana*.

At the same time there was a growing supply of female medical practitioners from Europe and North America who, unlike their male counterparts, would not be barred from attending purdah women. Missionary work provided one of the few openings to newly qualified women in Britain and the United States.[215] Female practitioners from America began to set up missions in India in the 1870s, while the first British medical woman to practise in India – Miss Fanny Butler – was despatched by the Church of England Zenana Missionary Society in 1880. Prior to 1880 some medical work was undertaken by female missionaries without medical qualifications; for example, the work of the Society for Female Medical Education in the East.[216] The establishment of these organisations suggests that the health of women in the British Empire had become an issue of some importance in Britain as well as in India.

Another indication of growing public concern over the health of women was the support declared by Queen Victoria for a proposal by Mr Kittridge of Bombay to raise funds for British medical women willing to give their services in India. The scheme, which was supported by several prominent Indian gentlemen, also hoped to raise enough money to establish a medical course in India; the total required being estimated at Rs 30–35,000. These proposals were greeted with enthusiasm by the *Bombay Gazette*, which was pleased to report that over Rs 33,000 had been received in subscriptions in the 3 weeks since the scheme was announced.[217]

However, Kittridge's proposal raised the question of what kind of medical education should be made available to women, and hence of their professional status in relation to male practitioners. Initially the government of Bombay approved a proposal by Dr Van Dyke Carter – principal of Grant Medical College – to institute a 3-year course specifically for women. In many respects the course was similar to that leading to the Licentiateship of the London Society of Apothecaries, and did not provide special instruction in diseases peculiar to women or in obstetrics. This move was heavily criticised by the *Bombay Gazette*, which argued that women should be admitted to existing courses of instruction, including the 5-year MB degree. Otherwise, it claimed, Indians would lack confidence in the ability of women medical graduates.

Ultimately a compromise was reached, in which women were restricted, initially, to taking the diploma suggested by Dr Van Dyke Carter, but after 3 years would be admitted into the full university course to study for the final 2 years of the degree.[218] This did not augur well for future relations between male and female medical staff. The *Indian Medical Gazette* wished the movement 'every success', but was of the opinion that 'women are better fitted for nursing rather than doctoring, and that educated nurses would fulfil the requirements of this country better than full-fledged lady doctors'.[219] It is significant that the years 1883–4 marked an intensification of the campaign for medical registration in India. Male practitioners were concerned that the inclusion of Indian women in the medical profession would lower its status in the eyes of Europeans.

Despite the reservations of IMS officers, the movement for the training of British and Indian female practitioners began to gain ground, capturing the imagination of the British public,[220] the Anglo-Indian community, and a section of the western-educated Indian élite. Two years after the Bombay scheme was established, Queen Victoria enquired of the new viceroy – the Marquis of Dufferin – whether or not it could be extended to include the whole of British India. The Indian government, while reluctant to involve itself directly in such a scheme, was willing to provide the services of one clerk and to permit IMS officers to supervise its operation.

The new organisation was entitled the National Association for Supplying Female Medical Aid to the Women of India; known more commonly as the Dufferin Fund, after its first president the Countess of Dufferin. Queen Victoria became the fund's patron, affording it a good deal of publicity. It aimed to provide the salaries of British medical women willing to work in India, and scholarships for Indian women wishing to train in western medicine. By 1888 eleven medical women were employed by the fund, six of whom were of Indian origin.[221] The launch of the Dufferin Fund was greeted with enthusiasm by the Anglo-Indian community in general, but there was still some reservation on the part of the IMS. 'We wish it every success', wrote the editor of the *Indian Medical Gazette*, 'as it promises to provide skilled nurses and midwives for Indian women [but] as concerns the education of native girls as doctors, we are not quite so clear or sanguine'.[222]

The impetus behind the fund was not simply the humanitarian desire to extend medical relief and knowledge of hygiene to Indian women, but to proselytise western values more generally. Europeans regarded the *zenana* as a bastion of ignorance and superstition; as the *Bombay Gazette* put it:

> western ideas will continue to spread in India, partly because of our eagerness in disseminating them, partly because of the eagerness of the more advanced native races in spontaneously embracing them. But here is a field in which native custom is stronger than any effort that might be made to shake it, even if we are

sufficiently confident in the superiority of western customs to make the effort . . . If native women are to have medical attendance worthy of the name it must be the attendance of women versed in the art of medicine and skilled in its act.[223]

Female doctors, then, were considered essential to the success of the civilising mission, but, even where medical missions or voluntary hospitals were able to call on the services of female practitioners, it proved difficult to penetrate the *zenana*. Writing of her experiences at a dispensary for women in Hyderabad, a British doctor acknowledged that the city's inhabitants were 'liberal-minded' and 'receptive of new ideas', but that it was still difficult to dispel their fears about hospitalisation. The mythology of the 'magic bullet' surrounding western medicine could also be counterproductive. 'Frequently', she complained, women using the dispensary 'cease attending after a few days, believing that if English medicine does any good, it ought to do so in a very short period'. More importantly, the institution of purdah itself continued to hamper the work of medical missions. 'Some of the men', she wrote, 'are still extremely reluctant to allow their wives and daughters to make periodical visits to the hospital, fearing perhaps that they will create a love of going out, which would be extremely inconvenient to such domestic tyrants'.[224] The treatment of purdah women was also frustrated by a rule in the Dufferin Fund's constitution which required its hospitals to undergo regular inspection by male doctors from the IMS.[225]

Nevertheless, the fund received sufficient subscriptions from Indians as well as Europeans to enable it to open branches in London and in most Indian provinces. In 1886 the *Bombay Gazette* expressed pleasure at the 'impressive list of contributions from the chiefs and princes of western India, and from other wealthy representatives of the native races'.[226] According to the *Hindoo Patriot*, the women of India were under a 'deep debt of gratitude' to Lady Dufferin for founding such a 'noble institution' which had so far proved 'remarkably successful'.[227] Though some of the initial momentum began to fade in the coming years, the fund's finances were still in a 'satisfactory' state in 1891. So far, reported the *Indian Medical Gazette*, 11 lakhs of rupees had been invested in the fund, yielding an annual income of Rs 50,000. Income from private donations and subscriptions for the year 1891 totalled almost 1 lakh of rupees. Thirteen female practitioners (holding qualifications higher than the LMS) were now employed by the association, and 27 women of the 'assistant-surgeon' class who held a variety of 'certificates' and 'diplomas'. Twenty-one of the latter were Indians, and another 204 medical students sponsored by the fund had yet to qualify. Over 400,000 women were said to have received medical aid at its hospitals and dispensaries.[228] By 1892 there were 10 provincial branches of the fund in India and 120 local and district associations administering 48 hospitals. These were supervised by a central committee in London.[229]

However, the effectiveness of the fund remained limited inasmuch as it courted well-to-do Indians and drew its patients almost exclusively from the Indian middle class.[230] The *Moslem Chronicle* thought the association 'one of the noblest institutions for behoof of womanhood in India', but regretted that the fees charged at its hospitals and dispensaries were

> not only exorbitantly high, but quite out of any reasonable proportion to the demand that the public has on their services. This, it need hardly be urged, makes their services open to the 'privileged few', while the great majority of people . . . are simply banned from taking benefits of the trained knowledge of lady doctors.[231]

According to Surgeon-General C. R. Francis, speaking at the Indian Medical Congress in 1891, 'the stronghold of custom and prejudice was in the home', and the training of medical women had so far done little to overcome it.[232] In general it was acknowledged that western notions of hygiene had made little impact on the vast majority of Indian people. In 1894 the Army Sanitary Commission observed that

> it is only needful to read the reports of the Deputy Sanitary Commissioners, who have spent the best part of the year amidst the people in their towns and villages, to be convinced that, as taught by us, sanitation is still almost everywhere unknown or, if heard at all, is disliked as a new-fangled, troublesome and expensive innovation. The people prefer to live and die as their forefathers lived and died – to be left alone.[233]

Similarly, in his account of his experiences as a civil surgeon on the North West Frontier in the early twentieth century, Henry Holland lamented that 'it is slow work to educate the people in ways of health; to overcome prejudice, ignorance and apathy; to gain a community response to the value of preventive measures'. In Holland's view, these remarks applied not only to the illiterate rural masses, but equally to 'the intelligentsia of cities in the East'.[234]

The inability of the Dufferin Fund to effectively penetrate the *zenana* may have owed much to the increasing suspicion with which it was regarded during the 1890s. The influential *Bengalee* newspaper, which represented Hindu professionals in the province, felt that the fund had not done enough to secure the employment of Indian women in supervisory positions. Of the 11 fully qualified doctors employed by the association in 1890 not one was an Indian, despite the fact that several Indian Christian women had obtained medical degrees. The *Bengalee*'s editor hoped that this 'slur to native worth' had not been intentional,[235] but in its annual report issued early the following year, the central committee of the fund defended the exclusion of Indian women on the grounds of age and experience, and saw 'very strong reasons' for continuing to employ women from Europe. It was now clear, according to the *Bengalee*, that the fund meant 'deliberately to exclude our countrywomen from occupying posts of high responsibility' and to perpetuate 'those unjust race-distinctions which act as a great hindrance to the advancement of the Indian people'.[236]

Relations between the fund's employees and their male counterparts in the IMS were equally fraught. In 1904 the *Indian Medical Gazette* wrote of the fund's 'inefficiency', which it ascribed largely to the 'defective education' of its staff. It also noted that its financial position had worsened considerably, and that many of its hospitals were experiencing problems with the lack of privacy afforded to patients.[237] The numbers of Indian women coming forward to train as hospital assistants and apothecaries was equally disappointing, low pay and lack of proficiency in English being blamed for this state of affairs.[238] There was also considerable dissatisfaction among the fund's European employees. In 1907 an Association of Medical Women was established in India along the lines of the one already existing in Britain. Two years later, in an attempt to end male dominance of the association, it made a representation to the effect that at least one female practitioner should be given a seat on its central committee and that its secretary should in future be a woman. A sub-committee of the fund alleged that medical aid and advice for women in India was totally inadequate.[239]

However, some progress had been made in training Indian women as midwives. The Victoria Memorial Scholarship Fund established by Lady Curzon in 1903 had, by 1912, set up centres in 14 different provinces and trained 1,395 midwives. Provincial governments now also made small contributions to the education of women. The Government of the United Provinces granted 6 scholarships annually to enable women to complete a 2-year course of instruction at Agra Medical School.[240]

By 1913, after much criticism in the British press, the Indian government decided to assume a more direct role in the finance and administration of the Dufferin Fund. The lack of special provision for the health of Indian women had formed the subject of editorials in *The Times* and the *Daily Chronicle*, and medical women themselves had memorialised Secretary of State Lord Morley and his successor, in 1910, Lord Crewe.[241] The need to train more Indian women in medicine had now been largely accepted by medical practitioners in India. Speaking at the second All-India Sanitary Conference in 1912, Dr Souza, health officer of Lucknow, saw women as vital to the success of sanitary education:

> we all know the influence exercised by women in India in domestic sanitation, and if any good is to accrue from our efforts, we have not only to detect diseases in children, but approach their mothers and instruct them in prevention and treatment of diseases.

A proposal from Miss Benson, an employee of the Dufferin Fund for 'the formation of a women's domestic sanitary service' in India was also well received.[242]

Though it decided against the creation of a state service similar to the IMS, the government approved a grant of Rs 1,500,000 (£10,000) per annum for a reconstituted service administered by the central committee of the Dufferin Fund, to be called The Women's Medical Service for India. Recruitment in India would be conducted by a sub-committee which included the DGIMS and the viceroy's personal surgeon; and in Britain by a sub-committee which included 1 medical man and 2 medical women. The central committee itself now included a female medical member, and the salaries of women holding qualifications higher than the LMS were placed on a par with those of male civil surgeons.[243] Thus, the professional concerns of female medical personnel had been taken into account, but their political demands had not.

One consequence of the women's health movement was a growing interest in maternal and infant welfare. The first initiatives in this direction were made in Bombay, Delhi, and Karachi, where small maternity homes were founded, and free or cheap milk distributed by voluntary organisations.[244] But no systematic attempts were made to address this subject until 1914, with the establishment of the Lady Wellington Scheme. Initially funded by subscription, the scheme employed 12 female health visitors to attend poor women in the city of Bombay. They offered advice on matters of personal hygiene and, if necessary, persuaded women to attend a municipal maternity home, or one of the homes established under the scheme. Two such institutions had been established by 1916, one of which was taken over by the municipality in 1918.[245]

The medical education of British and Indian women was only one part of the attempt to spread the sanitary gospel. Another aspect of this campaign was the formation of sanitary associations in a number of the larger Indian cities: a direct consequence of the plague epidemics of 1896 onwards. The Bombay Sanitary Association (BSA), founded in 1904, had by 1912 attracted Rs 800,000 in grants from the provincial government and the Bombay Corporation, and in donations from the public. The BSA funded a course in elementary hygiene, enabling graduates to qualify as sanitary inspectors, and 201 students completed it between 1904 and 1912. Health visitors were also employed by the association to advise the city's population on sanitary matters. They made weekly reports to the BSA's secretary, who informed the city's health officer of any insanitary conditions.[246]

Another important feature of the campaign for sanitary education concerned the teaching of hygiene in government-maintained schools. In 1908 the editor of the *Indian Public Health and Municipal Journal* warned that 'unless the rudiments of Hygiene . . . [were] drilled into . . . [children] at school it . . . [would] be difficult for them to grasp sanitary problems when they . . . [grew] up'. Not a single government-maintained school in India provided systematic instruction in hygiene, he complained, and in such circumstances it was not surprising that 'false views as regards inoculation against plague and other beneficial sanitary measures' had been formed.[247] A *Catechism on Hygiene* for elementary schools was published later the same year,[248] but it was not until

1914 that the curriculum in Indian schools was revised to provide for the teaching of sanitary science at all levels.

More attention was also paid to the subject of physical education. 'The surest and best way of preventing the physical deterioration so manifest in our juvenile population . . . ' wrote Bombay's health officer John Turner, was to make physical education compulsory in secondary schools, and to instruct both teachers and pupils in the 'laws and essentials of healthy living'. 'Owing to the ignorance of the parents', he continued, 'the care of the home needs to be supplemented . . . The State being the ultimate guardian of the child, should participate in the guardianship of health.'[249] However, medical examination of schoolchildren (introduced in Britain in 1907), despite repeated demands by the sanitary profession, was not established in India until 1914, and then only on an experimental basis. It was placed on a permanent footing in Bombay in 1917, though with a manifestly inadequate establishment of only two inspectors.[250]

Conclusion

Public health provisions in British India grew out of, and continued to be shaped by, anxieties aroused by the Indian mutiny of 1857; particularly the unhealthy state of British troops. An infrastructure of public health evolved in response to these concerns, at first within the confines of military cantonments and then, increasingly, without the camp. But the desire to sanitate the Indian population, most evident among the military and certain officers of the IMS, was held in check by financial considerations, logistical difficulties, and by opposition from British humanitarians and Indian élites. The 'civilizing impulse' was forced to express itself in more subtle forms – in sanitary education and in the activities of the Dufferin Fund – but such organisations had little success in penetrating the veil of the *zenana*, and in inculcating western principles of hygiene.

Yet, if the 'civilizing mission' was largely a failure, public health measures such as smallpox vaccination and the registration of deaths provided means – however imperfect – of knowing the population. The expansion of smallpox vaccination in the late nineteenth and early twentieth centuries was also beginning to effect a decrease in mortality from the disease in some areas of India, although the inadequacies of the vaccination establishment and continuing suspicion of the measure ensured a constant stream of infection, particularly in rural areas. The main focus of colonial medicine remained the military cantonment, where much was done to improve the health of British and Indian troops. Mortality rates among both British and Indian soldiers began to fall significantly, if unevenly, from the early 1880s. But disease continued to constitute a greater obstacle to military efficiency than Curtin, Headrick, and others have suggested. Sickness among British soldiers remained alarmingly high until the turn of the century, and military hygiene still left much to be desired outside of the cantonment. Both the British and Indian armies suffered high losses from disease when conducting campaigns in the northern frontier provinces, where the army fell prey to epidemics among the indigenous population; a problem which will be considered at greater length in the following chapter.

4

Cholera theory and sanitary policy

Statistics are the Sibylline Books of modern times; and when they are the outcome of true registration . . . they are an unerring guide for the future. (James Lumsdaine Bryden, *Reports Bringing Up the Statistical History of the European Army in India*, Calcutta, 1876)

The evil results of the contagion theory, as interpreted in other countries, have been shown, not only in the rigours and hardships of quarantine . . . but in the panic and demoralization which have degraded and deranged society generally. (Sir Joseph Fayrer, *The Natural History and Epidemiology of Cholera*, London, 1888)

Before 1817, cholera had been confined to Lower Bengal, with sporadic outbreaks among the rural population, but not among European enclaves in towns, or in military stations. In that year, however, the disease spread outside of its 'home' in Bengal to claim the lives of many thousands of Indians and Europeans in northern and eastern India, and, in the following years, in the presidencies of Bombay and Madras. As described in chapter 2, the outbreak of what appeared to be a new disease – *epidemic* cholera – made a profound impression on Europeans, arousing more fear and interest than any other disease.[1] In the wake of further outbreaks of the disease, debate raged over the causation of cholera and how best to prevent it.

No disease was more important, and no disease so little understood, as the 'epidemic cholera'. Hindu literature referred only to cholera in its sporadic, endemic form, while European practitioners conjectured variously that the disease was caused by the electrical state of the atmosphere;[2] by the operation of climate on the soil, providing the right conditions for the germination of the cholera 'seed';[3] by contagion;[4] or by transmission of the cholera germ in water (Snow's theory). Such questions acquired a fresh relevance after the mutiny, during which British troops had been seriously depleted by the disease. The dominant view in the 1860s was that cholera was essentially a 'disease of locality', its causes being similar to those of malaria; although an increasing

99

number subscribed to Snow's waterborne theory, which was then gaining in popularity in Britain.

But the causation and spread of cholera was not debated in an atmosphere of academic detachment. As in Britain, cholera theories had profound implications for sanitary policy, and political and professional interests impinged directly on medical theory.[5] In India the debate over cholera was intertwined with the issues of internal and maritime quarantine, and with questions of government finance. The government came to adopt an official position on cholera which vindicated its policy of limited intervention in public health and its opposition to the quarantines imposed against India following the Constantinople Sanitary Conference of 1866. The increasingly dogmatic stance of the Indian government drew it into conflict with foreign governments, and with members of the medical profession in Britain and India. In many respects the cholera debate was part of a wider debate about how best to govern India; about the role and responsibilities of the colonial state.

Official doctrine and its critics

'The special geography of Hindoostan'

To enter the realm of medical theory in India in the 1860s and 1870s is to enter the abstract world of Dr James Lumsdaine Bryden: India's premier epidemiologist and the government's chief adviser on epidemic cholera. Bryden (1833–80) left his native Scotland in 1856 after taking the LRCS and a gold medal in the MD degree at Edinburgh University. After a short spell in the military wing of the IMS, and only 4 years as a civil surgeon in the Bengal Presidency, Bryden became the first person to occupy the post of statistical officer to the newly formed Sanitary Department.[6] During his time as a civil surgeon, Bryden became fascinated by cholera: East India Company administrators estimated that over one-and-a-quarter million people died annually of the disease between 1817 and 1831; some 18 million in total.[7] Having gained first-hand experience of cholera in Bengal, where the disease was endemic, Bryden was well placed to observe its seasonal fluctuations and its seemingly law-like behaviour under Indian conditions.

Soon after being appointed statistical officer, Bryden was commissioned by the government to investigate the phenomenon of epidemic cholera. His main tasks were to establish the limits of the geographical distribution of the disease, the duration of epidemics, the influence of meteorological conditions and, most importantly, its mode of propagation and spread. Bryden's enterprise was such that he and commentators in the medical press came to refer to it as a 'natural history' of cholera.[8] Cholera, like other natural phenomena, had to be viewed in relation to other factors, and over a considerable period of time. This idea had its roots in eighteenth-century natural philosophy, with its emphasis on adaptation to the environment, and understanding natural phenomena from an historical perspective.[9]

Newtonian physics underpinned the Enlightenment notion that nature was a coherent and interconnected whole and that most, perhaps all, physical phenomena were governed by natural laws.[10] Bryden believed that the essential nature of these laws was beyond human understanding, but that they were capable of being measured and manipulated for the benefit of humanity.[11] The task of the 'natural historian' was to gather as much data as possible relating to the object of the study and its physical surroundings. From these data he would attempt to deduce the law governing the phenomena under observation. It was an attempt to impose order on the natural world; in Bryden's case, on an alien and seemingly hostile environment. In this respect, Bryden's statistical reports formed part of a much wider endeavour. Together with the geological, botanical, zoological, and meteorological surveys of India, medical men aimed to understand the Indian environment and render it habitable and bountiful for Europeans.[12]

The Enlightenment tradition filtered down to Bryden through three sources: his medical training at Edinburgh, from existing work on tropical hygiene and medical topography in India, and the legacy of William Farr, compiler of abstracts at the Registrar General's office in London. Farr, who was appointed in 1839, had made a number of successful deductions about the course of epidemics from epidemiological data.[13] His work almost certainly provided the model for Bryden in India. He adopted Farr's Liebigian nosology and his statistical methods, and shared his conviction that all physical phenomena were essentially law-abiding and capable of being predicted.[14] For Bryden and Farr the statistical method was central to practical sanitation– 'an unerring guide to the future'.[15]

But Bryden differed from Farr in one crucial respect. By 1866 Farr's observations had led him to believe that cholera was spread in contaminated drinking water, but, until his death, Bryden remained convinced that cholera was an air- and not a waterborne disease.[16] Bryden believed that there were two processes at work in the generation of epidemic cholera. The first was that the pathogenic organism – which he likened to a seed – underwent a cycle of reproduction and decay which was quickened or retarded by certain environmental conditions. The second was the phenomenon of epidemic spread itself, in which cholera seeds were transported beyond the endemic area by monsoonal air currents. With this in mind, Bryden produced a topography of cholera, representing graphically the limits of epidemic influence.

Meteorological conditions were the key determinants of these epidemic zones, affecting both the vitality and the mobility of the cholera seed. He maintained that the 'vehicle is in all cases, and whenever epidemic advance is in progress, a humid atmosphere'. The prevailing wind was the agency which directed the course of an epidemic, and determined its limitation in geographical distribution.[17] The perennial coincidence of certain meteorological phenomena combined with the fact that India was the only country in which the disease was endemic gave rise to the belief that India was epidemiologically unique. 'It is the special geography of Hindoostan', insisted Bryden, 'the regularity with which the seasons come forward year after year, and the normality of the limit of the meteorological agencies in every year that causes its surface to become mapped into normal areas'.[18] But these agencies might not operate outside the sub-continent. In Europe, according to Bryden, cholera might be spread by contagion instead of monsoonal air currents.

Bryden's views on cholera causation were shared by other senior IMS officers. The sanitary commissioner with the Indian government from 1866 to 1884, James McNabb Cuningham (1829–1905), was another Edinburgh graduate, and was personally well disposed to Bryden's airborne theory and his attempt to adduce a general law of cholera dissemination. In the opinion of his obituarist, Cuningham 'relied more on statistics than on research' and was 'apt to throw cold water on strivings towards the truth by local inquiry and clinical and pathological investigation'.[19] In Cuningham's hands, Bryden's localist/ atmospheric theory of cholera epidemics became a powerful tool against advocates of quarantine and those who pressed government to intervene more directly in public health.

Dissent

The government's most persistent critic was Annesley Charles DeRenzy (1828–1914), sanitary commissioner of the Punjab. A partisan of Snow's water-borne theory, DeRenzy mounted a concerted attack on Bryden's hypothesis and on the government for its inaction in the sphere of public health.[20] DeRenzy drew his inspiration and his model of sanitary reform from Britain, and cited metropolitan authorities in his attacks upon the colonial medical establishment. 'I had two special reasons for examining Dr. Bryden's theory', he explained in a letter defending one of his annual reports,

> first it is calculated to severely retard sanitary progress . . . second, it has been the basis of the action of the Government of India against cholera . . . To substantiate the first reason, I have only to refer to almost every review of Dr. Bryden's book. It will suffice to quote here the opinion of one whose authority is universally admitted, Dr. Parkes. He says – 'Dr. Bryden's views strike at the heart of the usual preventive measures.'[21]

Parkes, like most medical men in Britain, had come to believe in the efficacy of more specific measures against cholera. He recommended chemical examination of drinking water, and its purification by the addition of substances like alum and filtration through sand and charcoal.[22] Bryden saw no need for special attention regarding the water supply. He thought it detracted from the main object of sanitation: the removal of filth, in which the cholera seed was thought to propagate. The only additional measure deemed useful against cholera by Bryden was the improvement of barracks and European dwellings to guard against aerial incursions by the disease. His recommendations appear to have been translated into government policy and are, perhaps, reflected in high levels of sanitary expenditure on improvements to military accommodation at this time.

DeRenzy recognised the need for adequate accommodation for troops in India, but protested strongly against other items of sanitary expenditure, especially the large sums of money expended on the administration of the Contagious Diseases Act. He believed that the money would be better spent on improvements to the water supply in cantonments, and in grants to municipal commissions.[23] Prior to DeRenzy's crusade, very few IMS officers singled out the water supply as the 'favoured' medium of cholera, and DeRenzy readily acknowledged that Bryden's theory held sway among medical men in India.[24] In the 1860s Francis MacNamara (1831–1899), professor of Chemistry at Calcutta Medical School and chemical examiner to the Indian Government, stood virtually alone in his support for Snow's waterborne theory and in his attempts to persuade government to give it a fair hearing. In the late 1850s, MacNamara had also initiated, and later improved, a large water supply scheme in Calcutta. As with DeRenzy, who in many respects took up his mantle, MacNamara's efforts did not ingratiate him with the colonial authorities. In the words of his obituarist, MacNamara died 'without any mark of approbation from the Government he had served so long and so well'.[25]

DeRenzy and the Indian government first crossed swords in 1870, over the former's unfavourable review of Bryden's treatise on cholera. 'Dr. DeRenzy', protested the government's sanitary commissioner,

> does but scant justice to Dr. Bryden's remarkable work; and it appears to me that if such a proceeding be generally followed, it will lead to very inconvenient results. I would therefore strongly recommend that the Sanitary Commissioners refrain from criticizing the views held by other officers of the same Department.[26]

But DeRenzy did not refrain from criticising Bryden and, in 1872, the Indian government made a formal protest to DeRenzy's superiors. DeRenzy was 'instructed to adhere strictly to the orders of the Government of India in the presentation of future reports'.[27] His failure to do this led ultimately to his being transferred from civil to military duties at a remote station in Assam.

Indeed, Dr. DeRenzy appears to have courted unpopularity on a grand scale. As well as the government of India, he had incurred the wrath of his local newspaper, the *Indian Public Opinion and Punjab Times*, which accused him of neglecting his duty during a cholera epidemic in the province, during which he had been in the hills collecting statistics for his cholera research. The *Times* referred to 'his fallacious statistics and wild schemes', and his 'love of the hills when his duty was in the plains'. A correspondent to the newspaper, Dr Taylor, also imputed that DeRenzy had lacked courage in departing from Amritsar during an outbreak of the disease. Outraged by these allegations, DeRenzy took the *Times* to court, suing the newspaper for Rs 1,000, but obtaining damages of only Rs 500; a verdict which suggested that the newspaper's claims had not been entirely without substance.[28] More significant are the nature of the claims themselves: DeRenzy seems to have been portrayed as a zealot, or at least as some kind of crank, whose views on cholera were unrepresentative of Anglo-Indian opinion.

But DeRenzy was not alone in his criticism of government, or in his support for Snow's waterborne theory. 'At no time', wrote the secretary to the Bengal government, 'has controversy on the causation of the disease [cholera] run higher than at the present'.[29] Unfortunately for Cuningham, who was at that time defending his new department from critics within the general IMS, much of this dissent came from within its own ranks. 'For the production of cholera', wrote the sanitary commissioner for the Central Provinces, 'two conditions are necessary – the presence of a special contagion, and a susceptibility to its influence'. He believed that cordons sanitaires combined with more general sanitary measures were the best means of preventing the spread of cholera.[30] The sanitary commissioner of the North West Provinces also took a contingent–contagionist stance on cholera causation. 'The chief prevalence of the disease in a cluster of villages', he concluded, 'seems to point to contagion as one cause of the spread, whilst prevalence in isolated centres of population may point to local insanitary conditions as the cause of the outbreak'.[31] Dr Coates, sanitary commissioner for Bengal, was similarly of the opinion that 'to limit the cause of cholera to any one factor and its entrance into the system would be unwise. Notwithstanding this . . . my conviction has become stronger and stronger that there is a connection between impure water and the disease.'[32]

There were dissentient voices, too, among officers of the general IMS. 'Dr. Bryden', wrote the editor of the *Indian Medical Gazette* in 1872,

> with a bold combination of the philosophy of Aristotle and Pythagoras has, in recent years, furnished us with a striking illustration of a reversion to a metaphysical stage of scientific thought . . . He rejects the tedious system of elaborating principles and well observed instances. Principles thus obtained are secondary truths.[33]

He felt that Bryden's mode of inquiry, though nominally empirical, tended towards unnecessary and somewhat inflexible theorising about the 'laws' which seemed to govern cholera. The *Gazette*'s editor concurred in DeRenzy's view that the existence of local factors in cholera causation was not inconsistent with the communicability of the disease, but expressed regret that he had detected some acerbity in his tone. 'When will doctors', he lamented, 'learn to differ amiably'.[34]

In Britain, too, since the Army Sanitary Commission's unfavourable report of 1863, there was concern that the Indian government was not doing enough to protect British troops from disease.[35] Some, like Florence Nightingale, extended their critical gaze to conditions outside military cantonments. Nightingale advocated a more interventionist sanitary programme financed by local taxation. To those with more experience of conditions in India, her notions must have appeared hopelessly optimistic:

> Caste prejudices have been alleged as insuperable stumbling blocks in the way to sanitary improvement, but a curious and cheerful instance of caste prejudice being overcome is this: when the water supply was first introduced into Calcutta, the high caste Hindoos still desired their water carriers to bring them the sacred water from the river; but these functionaries, finding it easier to take the water from the new taps, just rubbed in a little . . . and presented it as Ganges water . . . The natives are always ready to be taxed, as far as obtaining, at least, a purer and more plentiful water supply goes.[36]

However, Nightingale would have found considerable support in India for her view that 'forced removals of sick, especially of women, for quarantine purposes, and other restrictions set the people against everything that is done under the plea of public health'.[37]

A *'disease of locality'*

These criticisms came at a time when the Indian government was attempting to distance itself from matters of public health. From 1870, under the administration of Lord Mayo (governor-general from 1869 to 1872), the political climate was in no sense conducive to sanitary reform. Mayo had inherited a large budgetary deficit from the expansionist regime of Lord Lawrence (1863–9) which he sought to remedy by increasing taxation and reducing public expenditure.[38] A key part of Mayo's strategy, and one which received the full backing of the first Gladstone government, was his Resolution on Provincial Finance of 1870. Its aim was to give provincial governments an incentive to cut public spending by devolving upon them certain heads of income and expenditure previously controlled by the Indian government.[39] Provincial governments, in turn, were keen to see the burden of sanitary expenditure shouldered by the municipalities and, with this in mind, the elective principle was reintroduced in municipal commissions in some of the major towns.

The other issue which focused attention on cholera at this time was the controversy surrounding the epidemic of 1867: the first major outbreak of the disease since the report of the Royal Commission in 1863. Originating in Hurdwar in the North West Provinces, where thousands of pilgrims had gathered for the *Kumbh Mela* (an annual religious fair), the epidemic appeared to spread outwards along the routes of returning pilgrims, affecting towns and military cantonments. The direct threat posed to the health of European troops, and the demand by delegates to the Constantinople Sanitary Conference that the Indian government make sanitary provisions at places of pilgrimage within India, led the government to launch an inquiry into the causes of the 1867 epidemic.[40]

The two persons chosen to conduct the enquiry were Bryden and Dr John Murray (1809–98), inspector-general of hospitals for the North West Provinces. Bryden's nomination was not surprising, given his position as statistical officer to the Sanitary Department, but Murray was something of an unknown quantity, having hitherto displayed no special interest in cholera.[41] Much to the government's annoyance, the two investigators came to very different conclusions about how the disease was spread. Some sections of their joint report reveal the meteorological bias of Bryden, while others reflect the contingent–contagionist perspective of Dr. Murray. 'It cannot be regarded as mere coincidence', wrote one of its authors (presumably Murray),

> that in thirty-five districts of Upper-India . . . the epidemic should have gradually appeared in one place after another, immediately after the return of a body of pilgrims stricken by the disease . . . Without a doubt, the germ of epidemic cholera appears to reside in the evacuations of a person suffering from the disease.[42]

Murray went on to recommend strict regulation of the water supply and restrictions on population movement as preventives against cholera. He envisaged a system whereby special camps supplied with pure water and hospital accommodation would be set up at regular intervals to and from religious gatherings, averting the need for pilgrims to enter cantonments or towns in search of accommodation or sustenance. Murray also believed that there was a role for conventional cordons sanitaires whenever 'unusual danger' threatened.[43]

Murray's recommendations, which were reiterated by the MacKenzie Committee commissioned by the Madras government, appear to have been rejected by the Indian government on grounds of cost.[44] However, public order considerations were almost certainly as important, since there is some evidence to show that even the basic sanitary measures introduced at the *Kumbh Mela* were not popular among pilgrims. According to Drs Bryden and Murray:

> the mass of the people attributed the outbreak to the fact that the authorities buried filth in trenches close to their tents . . . It is not to be wondered at that an ignorant and terror stricken multitude should have seized on the chief feature of the arrangements as the cause of all their troubles.

It was claimed that pilgrims viewed the epidemic as divine retribution by the goddess Kali, in whose hands they had hitherto placed their fate.[45] Radhika Ramasubban, however, offers a different interpretation. She argues that pilgrims attending the *Kumbh Mela* were impressed with the sanitary measures implemented at Hurdwar, and cites the MacKenzie report as evidence.[46] But the MacKenzie committee, which called for stricter sanitary regulation of pilgrimages, had an interest in highlighting only the more favourable indigenous responses to sanitary measures at the *Kumbh Mela*. The report of Bryden and Murray may be the more reliable testimony, in that it constitutes an agreement between two observers with quite different views on how best to prevent the spread of cholera. Bearing in mind Murray's recommendation that the sanitary regulation of pilgrimages should continue, it was not in his interest to draw attention to indigenous hostility towards measures at Hurdwar. That said, the two testimonies need not necessarily conflict. On analogy with other aspects of western medical intervention, it is probable that indigenous opinion was divided: a small minority of western-educated Indians being in favour of the measures, but with the majority unable to comprehend their utility.[47] The lack of Indian enthusiasm for sanitary regulation of pilgrimages is also suggested by continuing opposition in the Indian press. The high-caste *Hindoo Patriot*, for example, declared that 'any interference in them would be felt as a great hardship by the people' and supported J. M. Cuningham in his opposition to those who implicated pilgrimages in the spread of cholera.[48]

Fear of provoking civil unrest through heavy-handed intervention in the lives of Indians also lay behind the Indian government's increasing opposition to the use of quarantine and cordons sanitaires. On this issue, for a variety of medical and practical reasons, the majority of medical officers were at one with the government. Advocates of the atmospheric theory of cholera dissemination associated with Bryden, and of Snow's waterborne theory, agreed that there was no medical logic in quarantine, and thought it unnecessarily damaging to trade. Some also had humanitarian objections to the use of custodial sanitary measures. The sanitary commissioner of the Punjab, for instance, was unable to find words 'sufficiently strong' to express his disapproval of the forcible removal of the sick from their homes to hospital during a cholera epidemic in the province in 1872.[49]

Such measures appear to have been common practice in India in the years following the severe cholera outbreak of 1861; cantonment authorities being especially concerned to prevent the disease spreading among troops in the light of the mutiny.[50] But, by 1870, the government was in a position to reflect on the factors which had led to the mutiny and considered it politic, for reasons of public order, to discontinue cordons sanitaires. Colonial administrators were also concerned not to provide a precedent for custodial action at a time when they were being pressed on the issue of maritime quarantine. Yet, in 1873, 3 years after the resolution on cordons sanitaires, there were still several cantonment authorities which had not abandoned the practice, and, as late as 1877, there were reports of quarantines being established against cholera at several military stations in Madras.[51] Indians wishing to enter cordoned towns were sometimes detained for up to 10 days. Military men were among the foremost advocates of custodial legislation in India, and, as previously described, it was largely due to their anxieties and persistence in the matter that Contagious Diseases legislation was not allowed to lapse as quickly as many civilian administrators would have liked.

In opposition to cordons sanitaires, the Indian government's sanitary commissioner J. M. Cuningham drew attention to the fact that no evidence had been produced to show that such measures were effective. 'The whole history of the epidemic', he argued, 'point[ed] to the danger of locality', and the only sensible response was the evacuation of troops to places thought to be free from cholera.[52] The government's favoured strategy against cholera was preventive action in the form of 'general sanitation', or 'practical sanitary action' as it was sometimes known. 'Cholera', wrote Cuningham, 'is to be dealt with on the same general principle as all other diseases . . . Every sanitary defect must be sought out and, as far as possible, remedied. [Cholera] is favoured by filth, overcrowding and every other condition adverse to health.'[53] The responsibility for public health, in Cuningham's view, lay with individual municipalities and cantonment authorities. 'There can be no question', he advised government in 1873,

> that the municipalities must form the centres from which education in sanitary matters should spread among the people, and there is no more important duty for the Sanitary Commissioners to discharge than that of encouraging . . . and creating the desire for sanitary improvements.[54]

This was an important departure, for it was now clearly recognised that the success of sanitary measures lay in co-operation with the indigenous population. The emphasis on education, of course, was also a means of transferring responsibility for sanitation onto the municipalities and the people themselves.

Cuningham knew that the epidemiological evidence regarding cholera was still very much open to interpretation. Investigations in Britain and India seemed to implicate the water supply in outbreaks of cholera, but there were counter instances and, until such time as a causal organism was identified, evidence for the waterborne theory remained purely circumstantial.[55] While uncertainty remained, it was possible to counter Snow's waterborne theory by an appeal to some other scientific authority. With Bryden coming under increasing criticism, the Indian government cast its eyes abroad, as if to gain an impartial vindication of its stance on cholera causation. It found a champion in the German hygienist Max von Pettenköfer, whose 'sub-soil water' theory of cholera causation had already achieved widespread international recognition. Pettenköfer's theory did allow for the communicability of a hypothetical cholera 'germ', but placed most emphasis on the local factors thought to be necessary for its propagation. The most important of these factors was the presence of a porous soil and abnormally high levels of ground water.[56] Pettenköfer's preoccupation with locality and with environmental factors was well suited to the Indian context. Cuningham also saw that, if it were shown to be correct, Pettenköfer's theory would place Indian sanitary practice on firmer foundations. The government's use of scientific expertise, then, was highly selective: etiological theories did not so much determine, as provide, a justification for existing sanitary policies.[57]

Thus, in 1870 a scheme for the registration of sub-soil water levels was instituted in Madras, being extended to other provinces the following year.[58] However, the results of sub-soil water registration fell short of vindicating Pettenköfer. The first year of registration had been one which was 'unfortunately immune' from disease, so no significant correlation could be established.[59] Nevertheless, the government persisted with its programme, insisting that while Pettenköfer's theory had not been proved it had not yet been disproved either.[60] Provincial sanitary commissioners, many of whom had already been converted to the waterborne theory, were reluctant to continue the scheme. 'It is not clear', commented A. C. Lyall in 1874,

> on what grounds the Sanitary Commissioner for Bengal considers it unnecessary to continue . . . the sub-soil water registration. It is now generally admitted that local conditions are intimately concerned with the presence or absence of cholera . . . Variations in sub-soil water level should continue to be registered on an improved basis.[61]

By 1875 the registration scheme was becoming an embarrassment to the government. Its arch critic DeRenzy had the 'honour to report' that 'the observations on sub-soil water level made to test Professor Pettenköfer's theory . . . have not led to any clear or decisive results'.[62] There was also opposition to Pettenköfer from medical men outside the Sanitary Department, though limited sources make it impossible to gauge accurately its extent. The *Indian Medical Gazette*, which claimed to represent medical opinion in India, begged Pettenköfer 'before he again attempt[ed] to lay down the law regarding the diffusion of cholera in India . . . to consult authorities who can give him reliable information on the subject'.[63] It was understandable that medical men in India would have felt devalued as a result of their government's decision to consult a foreign 'expert'. Moreover, the IMS had long valued experience of conditions in India over and above theoretical speculation. The *coup de grâce* was delivered to sub-soil water registration by the Army Sanitary Commission in 1879. It noted that registration had failed to produce any significant results and that 'no general theory' could account for the incidence of cholera in different parts of India.[64]

Statistical epidemiology formed by far the greatest part of the government's 'enquiry' into cholera. Yet related questions, such as the existence or identity of a causal organism could not be entirely ignored. Most of the research undertaken by IMS officers in this regard was reactive and generally negative in character, its chief purpose being to disprove the existence of a specific pathogen. The only systematic investigations carried out to test the 'germ' hypothesis were those undertaken by D. D. Cunningham of the IMS and T. R. Lewis of the Army Medical Department. They were appointed special scientific assistants to Cuningham in 1874, though both had been working on cholera for some years.[65] Of particular importance was the question of whether certain micro-organisms found in human blood in conjunction with certain diseases were causal agents or merely 'epiphenomena': bodies which appeared to increase as a *consequence* of disease. Lewis concluded that such organisms had no causal relationship to cholera and were 'not uncommonly . . . associated with no physical disturbance of the normal condition'. That Lewis understood the wider significance of his work is clear from his comment that

> should the views now commonly advanced [on the existence of pathogenic micro-organisms] prove to be correct, the theory and practice of medicine would be radically affected, and possibly the future action of the state with regard to disease be materially modified.[66]

In order to place the Indian cholera debates in context, it is useful to consider how the views of the various parties were reported in the British medical press. As early as 1870, the *Lancet* expressed an unfavourable opinion of Dr Bryden's theory, arguing that human intercourse was of 'primary importance' in the diffusion of cholera.[67] The following year it threw its weight solidly behind DeRenzy, recommending his *Report on the Sanitary Administration of the Punjab*. 'It is so clearly written', wrote the journal's editor, 'that we have occasion to do little other than strictly follow it . . . We regard it as an uncommonly good one.'[68] Cuningham's *Report on the Cholera Epidemic of 1872* was not so well received. 'Its conclusions', claimed the *Lancet*, 'are at variance with all the prevalent doctrines, and the author does not hesitate to combat every hypothesis that had been advanced regarding the nature, origin and development of epidemic cholera'.[69]

Neither did Cuningham's address to the Royal Medical and Chirurgical Society in London in 1874 ingratiate him with the metropolitan profession. His manner, protested a correspondent to the *BMJ*, had been 'arrogant' and 'dismissive of all cholera research in Britain over the last 100 years'.[70] 'Dr. Cuningham', wrote the editor of the *Lancet*,

> spoke of contagion as if it were a self-operative Frankenstein giving laws to itself . . . Hardly less extraordinary was the fallacy that because India was the home of cholera . . . observations made there had a pre-eminent advantage over observations conducted elsewhere.[71]

The respected physician Dr Netten Radcliffe had a similar view of Cuningham's work. 'The contagion of which Dr. Cuningham spoke', he maintained, 'was not the contagion understood in this country; the water-theory had not the faintest resemblance to what is meant here . . . Dr. Cuningham judged of the contagion of cholera as if it were operative in the same way as smallpox.'[72] By narrowing down all notions of 'contagion' in this way, Cuningham hoped to place official theory beyond falsification.[73] So long as Cuningham continued to contrast cholera with smallpox he was able to hold up its 'preference' for certain localities and the absence of cases among those who tended the sick, as evidence against its communicability.

Return to the mainstream

The cholera commissions

Thus, through the 1870s official medical doctrine in India diverged increasingly from medical opinion in Britain. This was still the case for much of the 1880s, although, from the middle of the decade, following Robert Koch's claim to have discovered an organism causing cholera, there began a major shift in the official Indian position on cholera and in the means by which the disease was investigated. Robert Koch (1843–1910) and the German Cholera Commission arrived in Calcutta in December 1883. The commission had already spent several months making clinical examinations of cholera patients in Egypt. There it had identified vast quantities of a particular bacterium in the intestines of persons suffering from cholera, but it was by no means clear whether these organisms bore any causal relation to the disease.[74]

In Calcutta the commission was the guest of J. M. Cuningham, in his last year as sanitary commissioner. The commission was provided with a small laboratory and such equipment as the Calcutta Medical College could afford.[75] In February, after isolating the 'Egyptian' bacillus from a water-tank in Calcutta, the commission announced that they had discovered the causal organism of cholera. Several cases of the disease had very recently occurred among people who regularly drew their drinking water from the tank.[76] Koch's assertion contradicted everything Cuningham and his superiors held to be true of cholera; moreover, his claims were made on the basis of evidence gathered in India itself. The isolation of the cholera bacillus called into question Cuningham's professional competence, and threatened to undermine the theoretical basis of the government's sanitary policy. This memorandum by Surgeon-General Fayrer, president of the India Office Medical Board, is one of the clearest statements of the official reaction to Koch's claims:

the doctrine of contagion . . . is still maintained by many influential authorities on the Continent and here; the former loudly insisting on quarantine and charging us with conniving at the introduction of cholera to Europe, rather than interfere with our own mercantile interests . . . That a bacillus in association with cholera has been detected there need be no question . . . but that the cause of cholera has been discovered any more than it was before . . . I believe to be a dangerous and unverifiable statement, inasmuch as it will tend to emphasize the views of contagion and the importance of quarantine already so much insisted on.[77]

Fayrer's memorandum draws attention to one of the chief weaknesses of Koch's argument. Koch had successfully demonstrated the existence of the 'comma bacillus' and its association with cholera, but he had not proven conclusively that it was the cause and not merely a consequence of the disease. Koch's theory rested solely on his ability to show that large numbers of the bacillus were present in the intestines of an infected person, and absent from persons free from infection. Another weak link in Koch's theory was his inability to reproduce the disease in animals; though, on this score, he was able to draw analogies with other diseases widely supposed to be 'contagious', like leprosy and typhoid.[78]

Nevertheless, Koch's assertions were taken sufficiently seriously by the British government to warrant the formation of a team of researchers to investigate his findings. The English Cholera Commission, which comprised the distinguished London-based bacteriologists Edward Klein and Heneage Gibbes, was to work in conjunction with the Sanitary Department, but remain free from official interference. The two doctors received Rs 400 per month in payment for their services, up to Rs 50 for expenditure on scientific equipment, and free passage on board a P & O steamer to Bombay.[79] Much to the satisfaction of both the British and Indian governments, the commission concluded that 'the comma bacillus in acute typical cases of cholera [was] by no means present in such numbers and with such frequency as to justify Koch's statement that the ileum contains almost a pure cultivation of cholera bacilli'.[80] These conclusions cast doubt on the strongest part of Koch's thesis – his presence/ absence argument. According to E. R. Lankester in a letter to *The Times* in November 1884, Koch stood 'self-condemned'. He had not reproduced the disease in man or animal, and yet he had 'staked his reputation on the dogmatic assertion that the comma bacillus is the cause of cholera'.[81]

From 'locality' to laboratory

But, for the most part, Koch's auditors accepted his claim that the comma bacillus was the causal organism of cholera. As Coleman puts it, 'the evidence [by analogy with other diseases] was persuasive if not conclusive'.[82] At the same time, it appeared to the Indian government that the controversy would be resolved in the laboratory rather than on the basis of purely epidemiological evidence. It was this realisation that prompted it to improve facilities for medical research in India. The inadequacy of existing provisions had been highlighted by the visit of the English Cholera Commission, which had conducted its enquiry in a makeshift laboratory in the Calcutta Medical College.[83]

In December 1884, in accordance with a directive from the India Office, the Indian government sanctioned at a cost of Rs 15,000 the construction in Calcutta of India's first medical laboratory. It realised that the enquiry into cholera might 'extend over a considerable period of time'.[84] In his capacity as special scientific assistant to the sanitary commissioner, D. D. Cunningham was appointed director of the laboratory, a post he would hold in conjunction with his professorship of physiology at Calcutta Medical College. With his track record of opposition to cholera 'contagion', Cunningham, another Edinburgh graduate, was the obvious choice.[85] These developments were a clear departure from the statistical epidemiology of the 1860s and 70s. Increasingly, the attempts of senior IMS officers to 'save the phenomena' of local causation led them into the unfamiliar world of bacteriology. Few IMS officers had experience of microscopical research, and even fewer had been trained in bacteriological techniques.

It was no mere coincidence that the year of Koch's discovery saw the foundation of India's first journal of medical research. The first editor of *Scientific Memoirs by Medical Officers of the Army of India* was Surgeon-General B. Simpson (1831–1923), Cuningham's successor as sanitary commissioner. The journal's first edition carried an article by D. D. Cunningham, 'On the relation of cholera to schizomycete organisms', which purported to demonstrate that bacilli in the intestine of cholera patients might assume several forms, varying according to temperature, acidity and so on. Cunningham claimed that this discovery undermined Koch's claim to have identified a fixed species of bacillus in association with cholera. Cunningham was well aware that he had arrived at a conclusion 'in direct conflict with the majority of pathological bacteriologists'.[86]

Three years later, Cunningham continued his assault upon Koch, arguing that the comma bacillus was a comparatively 'feeble' organism unable to survive for long outside the human body. If this did not disprove Koch's theory, it seemed to place a great deal of emphasis on the environment necessary for the generation of cholera. 'If the choleraic commas really be the essential cause of the disease', he argued, 'then the facts would lead us to regard their agency in the production of epidemics as entirely subordinate to . . . local conditions'.[87] In 1889 Cunningham reiterated his belief that 'no contagionist theory will account for the phenomena of epidemic diffusion', and that Pettenköfer was correct in insisting on 'the primacy of local conditions'.[88]

By 1894, Cunningham had conceded that the comma bacillus was, in fact, a distinct organism associated with the 'choleraic condition', but refused to acknowledge that it was the sole, 'efficient' cause of the disease. Cunningham now advocated a modified version of Pettenköfer's theory which allowed for the action of 'two distinct poisons'; one manufactured in the intestinal tract, the other in the outside environment. Certain 'environmental' factors – particularly humidity – gave rise to a 'cholera poison' which was capable of producing the disease in an individual only if comma bacilli were present. If none were present, exposure to the 'cholera poison' would result in nothing more than mild ptomaine poisoning.[89] In this way Cunningham was able to square growing international acceptance of the role of the comma bacilli with the Government of India's insistence on the importance of local factors in the production of cholera. It was a theory which was also capable of explaining the limited success of the cholera inoculation developed by Waldemar Haffkine, while preserving a central role for 'general sanitation'.[90]

The fact that most discussion of the cholera controversy was limited to official journals and reports makes it difficult to generalise about the extent to which Koch's findings were accepted by the IMS as a whole. Editorial statements in the *Indian Medical Gazette*, at the time when Koch's discovery was first made public, display a certain sympathy with Koch's endeavours, but acknowledge that the matter was still far from resolved.[91] But the conclusions of the English Cholera Commission tilted the balance decisively against Koch. 'That Dr. Koch has certainly not proved that the comma bacillus . . . is the [cause of cholera] must now be regarded as clear', insisted the *Gazette*, 'indeed his supporters have now withdrawn so far from their position as to admit this; and they now simply allege its diagnostic importance'.[92]

In order to assess to what extent these pronouncements were representative of the views of the British profession as a whole it is perhaps wise to consider the personal viewpoint of the journal's editor, Kenneth MacLeod. MacLeod, editor of the *Indian Medical Gazette* from 1871 to 1892, was a public advocate of the waterborne theory and critical of Pettenköfer, Bryden, and the Indian government. In his assessment of Pettenköfer's work, MacLeod had shown himself hostile to interference from 'outsiders' who presumed to understand cholera better than the IMS itself. This may partly explain his lukewarm reception of Koch's thesis. Nevertheless, as editor of the *IMG*, and as a distinguished medical man in his own right, MacLeod's views would have been influential in shaping medical opinion in India.[93]

But it was only after 1893, following Georg Gaffky's analysis of the Hamburg cholera epidemic the previous year, that Koch's theory came to command almost universal assent among medical men in Europe. Gaffky had established the critical role of drinking water in the spread of the epidemic, providing firm epidemiological evidence to support Koch's hypothesis.[94] But official acceptance of Koch's theory in Germany, as Richard Evans has shown, owed as much to political factors as to the force of scientific logic.[95] At the same time, Koch actually opposed maritime quarantine, since he believed that cholera invariably spread to Europe overland from India. For this reason, Koch's theory was attractive to the British government and, increasingly, to the other European powers whose traffic in the Mediterranean, and through the Suez Canal, had increased markedly in the 1880s and 90s. This situation made liberalisation of international quarantine regulations possible in the 1890s and, in order to secure broad agreement, the British government began to pressurise the Indian government to make certain concessions regarding sanitary improvements on board Indian ships. Thus, the economic threat, which had been one of the most important imperatives behind official doctrine on cholera, was removed. There was now also laboratory evidence in support of Koch's hypothesis. In 1894 the Russian bacteriologist E. Metchnikoff, working at the Institut Pasteur in Paris, induced cholera in himself after drinking water containing comma bacilli. He also claimed to have reproduced cholera in rabbits, providing the 'proof' which Koch had hitherto been unable to attain.[96]

These developments convinced most European medical men of the validity of Koch's theory,[97] which also received confirmation from epidemiological evidence obtained in India.[98] But Cunningham clung to his position that the comma bacillus had a 'definite causal relation' to cholera only under certain conditions within the intestinal tract. These intestinal conditions were themselves, in certain circumstances, influenced by the 'external environment'.[99] The breadth and complexity of Pettenköfer's theory provided the basis for compromise: in its modified form, it seemed to allow for both the existence of a specific causal organism and for the influence of certain environmental factors.

Increasingly, the question became one of emphasis. As Ira Klein puts it, in the mid-1890s 'it was no longer fashionable to deny completely the germ theory of disease'.[100] But within this new framework there was still disagreement over the media in which the cholera bacillus was spread, and particularly over the measures required to prevent it. These disagreements are best illustrated by the dispute between W. A. Roe – sanitary commissioner for the Punjab – and W. R. Rice – sanitary commissioner with the Indian government – over measures to arrest the disease. Roe, a microbiologist, maintained that preventive measures should be focused specifically on the bacillus' chief mode of transmission; the water supply. Rice, however, believed that there were many sources of infection and continued to favour a broad, non-exclusive approach to sanitation.[101] By the early twentieth century these conflicts had been largely resolved, with wide agreement among medical men in India on the utility of specific measures against cholera, but as merely one part of a more general sanitary programme.[102] No longer was there thought to be any fundamental contradiction between the aims of research scientists and those who struggled on a day-to-day basis with practical sanitation.

Conclusion

The response of the Indian government to epidemic cholera embodied many of the contradictions and tensions of British rule in India. The protection of Europeans, and especially European troops, necessitated some degree of intervention in the lives of indigenous peoples, but any such action carried with it the risk of civil unrest. The government, therefore, proceeded with caution, resisting demands from foreign governments and the military for the introduction of more drastic and custodial measures. The government's fiscal policy was another important factor in its reluctance to meet these demands. After 1870, the government effectively washed its hands of public health, devolving its responsibilities in that department to provincial and municipal administrations, which were often financially ill-equipped to deal with the demands placed upon them.

In order to maintain its policy of detachment from public health, the government was prepared to go to extraordinary lengths, manipulating the flow of information and theoretical discussion in official circles, and dealing harshly with medical officers who stepped out of line. Medical experts were carefully selected and employed to defend the government's position: they effectively defined the limits of medical intervention under British rule, or, at the very least, provided a rationale for the government's inactivity. But the rigidity of official doctrine between 1870 and 1890 brought Anglo-Indian medicine into disrepute, and served only to diminish the government's credibility abroad.

The medical establishment's return to the mainstream in the 1890s owed much to the fact that it had chosen to fight Koch on his own ground – the laboratory. After the existence of the bacillus had been accepted in India, the disease was defined largely in terms of its presence and, thus, received its identity from the laboratory. However, the gradual modification of cholera theory, which occurred in the 1890s, shows that the comma bacillus was integrated into a *pre-existing* etiological framework, in which a 'pre-laboratory' hierarchy of causes was maintained.

5

Quarantine, pilgrimage, and colonial trade: India
1866–1900

The better classes of Muslims are a source of strength and not of weakness to us.
They constitute a comparatively small but energetic minority of the population,
whose political interests are identical with ours. (John Strachey, *India: Its
Administration and Progress*, London, 1903)

From 1866 through till the end of the century, no aspect of British medical
policy in India was more important than the issue of maritime quarantine, with
its implications for colonial trade and for the annual pilgrimage of Indian
Muslims to Mecca and Medina. The quarantine controversy provides an index
of the changing and often conflicting priorities of the British government and
colonial administrators in India, and sheds fresh light on the nature of the
colonial regime's relationship with indigenous élites.

The British and Indian governments had a common interest in maintaining the
free passage of troops, mails, and merchandise between the two countries, but
their experience of epidemic disease, and of the effects of maritime sanitary
legislation, varied considerably. India, regarded as the source of the cholera
epidemics that had afflicted Europe since 1830, suffered more than Britain from
the effects of maritime quarantine imposed after the Constantinople Sanitary
Conference of 1866. Unlike their counterparts in London, colonial administrators were directly concerned with the annual pilgrimage of Indian Muslims to
Mecca, singled out at sanitary conferences as the chief vehicle for the transportation of cholera to the West.[1] The Indian government had to weigh the
demands of the European powers for the medical inspection and quarantine of
pilgrims against the likely reaction from India's 60 million-strong Muslim
community. The government was particularly sensitive to Muslim opinion at this
time, for since 1870 it had pursued a policy of 'co-operation' with Muslim
leaders, by asserting the 'common interests' of both parties.[2] The vast majority
of Indian Muslims were hostile to the idea of quarantine, which they considered
a grave indignity as well as an inconvenience, but Muslim leaders backed

European demands for stricter sanitary measures on board pilgrim ships and in Indian ports. Lower-class Muslims were generally opposed to any such restrictions on grounds of cost, and as unnecessary infringements of their liberty. Although these concerns were viewed sympathetically by politicians in London, they were regarded as subordinate to Britain's wider economic and strategic interests. Within a few years of the Constantinople conference, the British and Indian governments were at loggerheads over the question of maritime sanitary policy.

Cholera

In the wake of a severe cholera epidemic in southern France, the French delegation to the Constantinople Sanitary Conference proposed that a sanitary service be established to administer quarantine against pilgrims arriving from India and other countries infected with the disease. They envisaged that the service would be administered by a board of health based in Suez, comprised of representatives from all the countries concerned. The stations, which would all be located in the Ottoman possessions, would be run by the Turkish authorities under the guidance of European doctors nominated by the board. The proposal was opposed by the nations with responsibility for sizeable populations of Muslims – namely Britain, Russia, Persia, and Turkey – but was accepted on a majority vote.[3] The Indian government, not permitted a separate delegation at the conference, nevertheless found a champion in one of the British delegates, Dr Goodeve, who had held a senior post at Calcutta Medical College. He opposed the new arrangements on three grounds: their potentially adverse effects upon trade; the likelihood of an unfavourable reaction from pilgrims; and continuing uncertainty over how cholera was spread. Goodeve, like most British doctors in India at this time, held the view that cholera was a disease of locality: one which arose from an unhealthy combination of general environmental conditions. This notion of cholera causation, which saw the disease as confined within certain geographical limits, provided a convenient rationale for the Indian government's opposition to quarantine long after such notions had been rejected by the medical profession in Britain, and even by the majority of well-informed medical men in India.[4]

The Indian government also faced international criticism of its failure to provide adequate safeguards for the health of passengers on board pilgrim ships. European delegates pointed to the lack of sanitary provisions on these vessels, and to the chronic overcrowding to which all but the wealthiest of pilgrims were subjected.[5] The first positive response to these criticisms came from provincial administrators in India, who began to urge central government to amend the existing Native Passenger Ships Act. Provincial officials were generally more sensitive to public opinion than their colleagues in central government, and were

painfully aware that quarantine measures had already aroused the hostility of
the mercantile lobby in Bombay and other Indian ports.[6] Initially, the Indian
government resisted calls for legislative intervention, because the introduction
of sanitary legislation might incur the hostility of lower-class Muslims. Such
measures, it was felt, might be construed as unnecessary interference in the
religious duties of its subjects. Four years elapsed before the government
thought it expedient to pass new legislation. The Native Passenger Ships Act
of 1870 required that ships hold a clean bill of health and a certificate to
show that they were not overcrowded before they were permitted to leave
India.[7]

It is not fully clear why government chose to intervene in 1870, though one
important consideration was undoubtedly the desire to appease Muslim élites.
Muslim leaders, and in particular those of the Khoja community in Bombay,
were much opposed to quarantine, and had made it clear that they held the Indian
government, through its inaction in sanitary matters, as partly responsible for its
imposition. Insanitary conditions on board pilgrim ships provided a justification
for quarantine in middle-eastern ports. The appalling sanitary state of pilgrim
vessels had been highlighted by the *Batchman Sirusker* scandal of 1869, when a
vessel of that name returned to Madras full of dead and half-starved pilgrims.[8]
From 1870 the demands of Muslim leaders began to receive a more sympathetic
hearing. The Indian government had embarked on a policy of 'collaboration'
with Muslim leaders, viewed as potential allies in its attempt to counter the
increasingly vocal Hindu middle class. The government's strategy combined
dialogue and appeasement with educational and political reforms, culminating in
the granting of separate electorates for Muslims after 1909. A second factor may
have been the opening of the Suez Canal in 1869. Though an undoubted boon to
commerce, the opening of a passage between the Mediterranean and the Red Sea
brought with it the less attractive prospect of infected persons being conveyed
direct into European ports. The Act of 1870 may have been an attempt to
anticipate demands for a reconstituted sanitary service, or for more stringent
measures at Mediterranean ports.

Surprisingly, however, the epidemiological implications of the canal were
not discussed at the next sanitary conference, held in Vienna in 1874. It was
presumed that the existing sanitary board at Suez would make adequate
provisions should a major epidemic occur in India.[9] Nevertheless, the Vienna
conference had its fair share of controversy, and marked the first real clash of
interests between the British and Indian administrations over the quarantine
issue. Lord Salisbury, then secretary of state for India, viewed the free passage
of troops and mails in the Red Sea as a *sine qua non* for any international
agreement on the Red Sea's sanitary policing. To this end, he was prepared to
agree to terms to which Goodeve, sensitive to colonial interests, had already
expressed the 'gravest objection'.[10] Salisbury had conceded that regulations

concerning sanitary provisions and overcrowding on pilgrim ships should be tightened. Aware that such measures might be misconstrued by lower-class Muslims, Goodeve argued that the limits on overcrowding demanded by the majority of delegates were unrealistic, and that they would make the voyage prohibitively expensive for many pilgrims. He pointed to the Government of India's 'exemplary' record in maritime legislation, and to the inadvisability of binding itself to any rigid system, when the nature of cholera transmission was still far from certain.

Another term accepted by Salisbury, and which particularly angered the Indian government, was a clause making quarantine in the Red Sea dependent on the incidence of cholera in the port from which a vessel had set sail.[11] Bombay, the principal outlet for India's western trade, was afflicted with cholera to varying degrees between May and August, and the somewhat arbitrary criterion of an 'infected port' gave cause for concern lest trade be disrupted for anything up to 4 months each year. The Indian government also objected to the establishment of new and more permanent quarantine stations in the Red Sea (first suggested in 1866), for which it was expected to contribute the largest portion of the initial outlay.[12]

Without support from Britain, the Indian government was in no position to oppose these terms. Its only realistic course of action was to demonstrate its willingness to tackle the problem of disease in India and on Indian ships, thus abrogating the need for stringent quarantine in the Red Sea. But the 1876 Native Passenger Ships Act, which introduced medical inspection of pilgrims prior to embarkation, failed to reassure the European Powers, and served only to provoke the Bombay Chamber of Commerce, which objected to the delays and extra running costs incurred by the new arrangements.[13]

In the same year an outbreak of bubonic plague in the Gulf states added another dimension to the vexed question of quarantine: the Egyptian Board of Health quickly imposed a quarantine of 15 days against all ships arriving from the region. Viewing the situation with alarm, the Indian government imposed a similar quarantine, hoping to allay international fears that the disease might spread to Bombay or Karachi, which traded regularly with the Gulf.[14] But a blanket quarantine against Gulf shipping was economically undesirable, and the government began to consider other ways of tackling the problem of sanitary regulations in Indian ports. One such initiative was the port health officer scheme instituted in Calcutta in 1876, and extended to other ports in 1878.[15] Based on the British scheme established on the recommendation of John Simon, the port health officer was charged with responsibility for the sanitary condition of the port and its environs, and with the medical inspection of ships. Instead of quarantining all persons arriving from infected ports, he was to isolate and detain only those suspected of carrying infectious diseases. This procedure was applicable only to diseases supposedly alien to India, such a bubonic plague and yellow fever. The economic rationale behind the new system was clearly spelled out by Calcutta's first port health officer:

> the mercantile community fully appreciate the necessity for the appointment of a Health Officer . . . and understand that, in view of the increasing number of ships visiting Calcutta, and the more rapid communication with Europe by the Suez Canal, the only alternative would be the introduction of a regular quarantine.

Later, in 1882, medical boards were added to the government's sanitary armoury; their purpose was to monitor the level of infectious disease in Indian ports. They were an attempt by the Indian authorities to establish some kind of control over the definition of an 'infected port'.[16]

It is illuminating to compare these measures with those in force in the 'white settler colonies'. In a recent article on smallpox in colonial Australia, Alan Mayne has shown how medical and political priorities in Sydney and Melbourne had, by the 1880s, begun to diverge from those of Britain. Like India, the colonies of Victoria and New South Wales discontinued a system of quarantine in the mid-1870s in favour of medical inspection and selective isolation. But, in contrast to both Britain and India, the Australian colonies continued the old practice of regularly proclaiming overseas ports 'infected places', and subjecting arrivals from them to lengthy quarantine. In 1881, for example, the government of Victoria ordered a quarantine against all vessels from China and, in the same year, the Government of New South Wales introduced selective measures against ships thought to be carrying Chinese. In the Australian settler colonies, according to Mayne, quarantine practice was influenced by racial prejudice, and became an important instrument of immigration control.[17] In India, however, there was no immigration issue, and the government had nothing to gain from imposing quarantine against any nation. The volume of trade was much greater in Bombay and Calcutta than it was in Melbourne or Sydney, making restrictions of the kind regularly enforced in Australia both impracticable and economically undesirable. But, in responding to conditions peculiar to their colonial context, both India and the Australian colonies implemented medical policies which diverged from the metropolitan model, and which, in the case of India, sometimes conflicted with metropolitan interests.

The upheavals of the mid-1870s were followed by a period of quiescence in the quarantine debate, but in 1881–2 the issue acquired fresh significance following the Turkish government's declaration that pilgrims wishing to take part in the forthcoming Hadj would have to secure a 'passport' from their country of origin, proving that they were in possession of sufficient funds to make the return voyage. Pilgrims without a passport would be expelled from the Ottoman possessions. The declaration was a response to the growing problem of destitute pilgrims who had failed to make provision for their return voyage, and who had become a burden on the Turkish authorities.[18] Passports were to be issued only to those pilgrims who could prove – on arrival in Jeddah – that they were in possession of the Rs 40 necessary to pay for the return voyage. The sum was to be deposited at the British consulate.[19] Wary of confrontation with its Muslim subjects, the Indian government shied away from implementing the scheme, and was supported in its stance by the Anglo-Indian press. The *Bombay Gazette* denounced the scheme as unworkable and as likely to reflect badly upon government:

> Our Mohamedan subjects are very suspicious of anything which affects their religious practices, and it is important, therefore, that while Government should take every possible precaution for their protection, it should not lend any aid to schemes proposed by the Turkish Government.[20]

But, with the pilgrim season only a few weeks away, and faced with a total ban if it did not comply, the government had no real option other than to implement the scheme. Before doing so, the government sought and secured the compliance of the Mohamedan Association, which had long been concerned about the welfare of destitute pilgrims at the Hadj.[21] However, the measure proved deeply unpopular with the majority of pilgrims, who did not comprehend the reasoning behind the new regulations. The 'weight of opinion', concluded the government, was opposed to the scheme, and it decided, in the interests of public order, to withdraw it the following year. Difficulties in enforcing the new regulations led the Turkish authorities to abandon the scheme in 1882, but relations between the Turkish and Indian governments remained strained for several decades. Equally, the passport issue reminded the Indian government of the limits to its interventionist capacity.[22]

The post-mutiny preoccupation with public order and financial stringency lay at the heart of the Government of India's non-interventionist approach to sanitation in the 1870s and 80s. Only when compelled to do so by international opinion, or by unusual economic and political conditions at home, did the government risk interference in the cultural and religious practices of its subjects. It was especially anxious to avoid confrontation with Muslims in 1882, since this was the first year in which pilgrims were to be detained in the new quarantine station on the island of Kamaran, at the southern entrance to the Red Sea. Until then, Indian pilgrims had undergone periodic quarantine in makeshift camps at Jeddah. Although the camp had been envisaged in 1866, the Turkish authorities had delayed building it because of the great expense involved.[23] Provisions at the camp reflected the reluctance with which it had been constructed, and an exorbitant head tax was levied on each pilgrim in order to recoup the cost. Immediately after the arrival of the first pilgrims, complaints began to reach the British consulate in Jeddah. The water was scarce and brackish, the food expensive, fuel and cooking facilities in short supply, the accommodation insufficient, and the camp guards violent and abusive. The

Mohamedan Association, the voice of India's Muslim élite, expressed its outrage in a petition to the Bombay government, demanding that it take steps to ensure that quarantine at the station would no longer be considered necessary.[24] The new arrangements were equally unpopular with shipping companies trading in the Red Sea. One captain protested that he had been forced to pay over 13,000 piastres to secure a bill of health, and a further 23,000 for the disinfection of his cargo of rice, some of which was stolen in the process.[25]

The Turkish sultan, however, had provided the anti-quarantine lobby in India with just the evidence it needed to make a powerful case against such restrictions. Seizing its chance, the Indian government launched an immediate inquiry into conditions at Kamaran. It reported to the secretary of state that 'pilgrims were subjected to oppression and extortion amounting to positive cruelty' and that 'the whole arrangement seemed to be designed solely for the pecuniary benefit of the Turkish authorities'.[26] As for cholera, the Indian government could now argue with some force that conditions at Kamaran were just as, if not more, conducive to the dissemination of cholera than those in Indian ports. The editor of the *Bombay Gazette* claimed that 'more sickness occurs on the island of Kamaran than during the voyage. On board ship pilgrims are tolerably well cared for. At Kamaran they [the pilgrims] are turned onto a desert island without an adequate supply of water or shelter from the sun.'[27]

Of greater concern to the British government were the quarantines imposed against India following a severe outbreak of cholera in India in 1882. These quarantines disrupted the flow of troops and merchandise between Britain and India, adversely affecting the economies of both countries. India, however, was hardest hit by the restrictions: over half of her imports were supplied by Britain, which was the principal importer of Indian raw cotton, the country's chief export at that time. The quarantines were received with howls of indignation in the Anglo-Indian press. The *Bombay Gazette*, champion of the city's European commercial class, was anxious to play down the incidence of cholera, and lamented the effects of quarantine at Suez:

> A steamer in quarantine is not only forbidden to allow a passenger to set foot on shore but cannot even take the canal pilot on board ... These vexatious restrictions are so oppressive that companies running steamers regularly have had to send out steam pilot-boats to Suez ... and in many cases trading steamers were held back to the detriment of commerce and to the positive loss of owners and shippers.[28]

A less damaging, though irksome, quarantine had been imposed by the Portuguese authorities at Goa, to the south of the Bombay Presidency. 'The fright in Goa is so great', observed a correspondent to the *Gazette*,

> that the Governor-General ... does not shake hands with any gentleman arriving from British India ... I trust the Bombay Government will send a letter of protest

against this ridiculous quarantine, which is a nuisance to our merchants and ship-owners . . . There is no epidemic cholera or choleraic fever in Bombay.[29]

The economic problems experienced as a result of quarantine in 1882 were particularly acute as the year had been a poor one for trade. Depressed markets in Britain had seriously damaged Bombay's export economy, which, according to shipping experts, was 'devoid of animation'.[30] The *Gazette* and the Indian government denounced the quarantine as an example of European jealousy of Britain's colonial trade, and as having no basis in medical fact. 'There are many, indeed most, well-informed persons who believe cholera is not contagious', protested the editor of the *Gazette*.[31] In claiming this he had, perhaps deliberately, misrepresented medical opinion on cholera. Since the late 1860s most British-trained medical men had come to believe, though in the absence of concrete proof, that cholera was transmitted by man, albeit indirectly in drinking water contaminated with the faeces of an infected person. It was true, however, that the majority of British doctors agreed that quarantine was impracticable and a useless hindrance to trade.

Deeply concerned at the situation in Bombay, the viceroy, Lord Ripon, urged the secretary of state Lord Hartington to demand the lifting of restrictions at Suez and elsewhere.[32] Similar demands were made at Westminster. Sir Charles Dilke, then under secretary for foreign affairs condemned the quarantine and called upon his fellow ministers to exert pressure on the Egyptian government.[33] In marked contrast to its response to the pilgrim issue, the British government reacted almost immediately to the commercial and strategic threat posed by quarantine at Suez. In March 1882, less than one month after the quarantine at Suez had been imposed, Granville, the foreign secretary, informed his representative in Egypt that:

> Her Majesty's Government are not prepared to acquiesce in the recurrence of such arbitrary and capricious acts of the International Board as have of late caused enormous losses to shipping; and they can no longer assent that an irresponsible body should have the power of making unreasonable laws which disturb the whole Eastern trade of Great Britain and unduly impede her communications with India.[34]

But the effects of quarantine were more deeply felt in India than they were in the metropolis. Although the value of India's foreign trade rose rapidly between 1876 and 1890, merchants and manufacturers in India were having problems adjusting to the abolition of the favourable import tariff in 1882, forced upon them by the British government under pressure from Lancashire mill-owners.[35] Bombay's mercantile and manufacturing community had experienced considerable uncertainty as a consequence of wildly fluctuating exchange rates.[36]

In India, the government did its best to cover up the severity of the cholera epidemic afflicting Bombay and its hinterland. Yet, in view of the unsuccessful

record of the Indian authorities in preventing the spread of cholera to the Middle
East, it was thought necessary to introduce some new measure to allay the fears
of the Egyptian board. With this in mind, the Bombay government announced in
1882 the formation of a medical board, comprising the principal of Grant
Medical College, the surgeon of the European general hospital, and the health
officer of the city. It was the board's duty to 'report . . . whether the trifling
cholera usually to be found [in Bombay] had assumed an epidemic form'. In
such an event, the board would enforce the medical inspection of all passengers
and crew leaving for Aden or Suez.[37] Through the board, the Bombay government hoped to retain some control over the definition of an 'infected port' and
reduce delays in shipping to a minimum. But the government's attempts to play
down the cholera menace were frustrated in August 1882 by an outbreak of
the disease on the SS Hesperia, which was carrying over 500 pilgrims from
Bombay to the Holy Land. The vessel docked at Aden where it was immediately
placed in quarantine. After 10 days and no further cases the vessel was allowed
to proceed, but the Constantinople Board of Health, which had responsibility
for surveillance at Red Sea ports, was far from satisfied and quarantine was
immediately imposed against ships from Bombay and Aden. Outraged, Ripon
denounced the measure as 'groundless', and protested the 'great hardship' it
would bring to pilgrims and the mercantile community of Bombay.[38]

The British government's response was to set up a special committee of the
Foreign Office, which advised that a 'quarantine committee' be set up within the
Egyptian Board of Health, where the number of Egyptian nominees would be
equal to the number of delegates sent by the European Powers. The logic behind
this suggestion lay in the Egyptian government's vulnerability on the question of
its national debt, which had led to the establishment of 'dual control' by Britain
and France in 1879. Britain hoped to gain more favourable terms from a
reconstituted Board by exercising its influence over the Khedive. It was thought
that 'a restoration of the responsibility of the Egyptian Government [over that
of European delegates] would do much towards relieving British trade of the
vagaries and losses to which it had lately been subjected'.[39]

By the autumn of 1882, Britain was in an even stronger position. Unable to
secure the co-operation of the other powers, Britain had intervened unilaterally
in Egypt to put down a coup d'état staged by Colonel Arabi, an officer in the
Egyptian Army. Though Arabi posed no direct threat to the system of 'dual
control', nationalist riots in June, in which Europeans had been killed, cast
doubt over the security of British investments. Reluctantly, under pressure from
Liberal 'imperialists' like Hartington – secretary of state for India – Gladstone
agreed to send a military force. But while Britain now exercised an
unprecedented amount of influence over Egyptian affairs, it was still impossible
for her to govern the country without the consent of the other European nations
who continued to guarantee the Egyptian loan.[40]

The occupation of Egypt marked a turning-point in British foreign policy, and added a new dimension to the quarantine question. Aggrieved by Britain's unilateral ending of dual control, France took every opportunity to obstruct British initiatives on both the debt commission and the Board of Health. To counter this, Britain was forced to work more closely with Germany, Austro-Hungary and Italy: the nations of the Triple Alliance. The British bombardment of Alexandria also threatened to jeopardise the rapport which the British had established with Muslim leaders in India. Egypt was a predominantly Muslim country, and politically aware Muslims in India took a good deal of interest in the welfare of their co-religionists abroad. Although the Mohamedan Association had recently met in Bombay to celebrate the birthday of Queen Victoria, the British could not count on its unconditional support, since its primary aim was to foster a sense of brotherhood between Muslim peoples.[41] Recognising the implications of the bombardment for Anglo-Muslim relations, the editor of the *Bombay Gazette* condemned the action as being 'without any valid excuse'. A war in Egypt, he warned, 'means unpopularity with the Mussalman subjects of Her Majesty'.[42] Indeed, on a tour of India in 1883–4, the Indian civil servant W. S. Blunt found many Muslims hostile to Gladstone's policy in Egypt. The old British alliance with the Ottomans against Russia had been popular, but the Treaty of Berlin, the British acquisition of Cyprus, her abandonment of Tunis to the French, and the defeat of Arabi had wrought a change in the attitudes of some Muslims towards the British administration.[43] The *Gazette* was equally concerned about the likely effects of the action upon commerce. The risk to steamers using the canal, wrote its shipping correspondent, made business with Europe impracticable. He warned that steamship proprietors might soon choose to return to their old route around the Cape.[44] Europeans clearly perceived the British government's foreign policy to be contrary to their interests in India.

Despite Britain's new position and Granville's overtures to the European powers, 'enormous losses', as the Bombay government described them, continued for several years.[45] The annual imposition of quarantine at Suez during the 'cholera season' had, by 1883, begun to bite deep into the profits of Bombay's mercantile community, and the city's chamber of commerce became more vociferous in its own defence. It criticised the Government of Bombay for not doing enough to deflect international criticism and protested (falsely) that the incidence of cholera in Bombay was no greater than usual.[46] While this was true of the Bombay Presidency (though not for India as a whole) in 1882, when only 7,904 cases occurred, it was not true of 1883, when the number of cases in Bombay rose to 37,934; the highest figure for 6 years.[47] But it was clear that the events of 1882 had hardened attitudes on both sides of the quarantine debate. While Granville had grown more strident in his demands, the French and Turkish governments had grown more intransigent.[48]

All the indications were that the forthcoming sanitary conference at Rome would not be a fruitful one for either the British or Indian governments. Granville had unsuccessfully sought prior assurances that military vessels would be given free passage through the canal providing they did not dock until reaching England.[49] A half-hearted attempt was also made to resolve the pilgrim question, with the British government renewing its demand for withdrawal of quarantine restrictions, and of accommodation charges for poor pilgrims at Kamaran.[50] But the sultan took great exception to Granville's demands, and announced that vessels travelling from India to the Ottoman possessions would henceforth be subject to 10 days quarantine instead of 5. Wyndham, the British chargé d'affaires in Constantinople, was instructed by Granville to continue to press the matter with the sultan, but relations between the two countries had deteriorated since Britain's intervention in Egypt, which was nominally still an Ottoman possession.[51] The sultan may also have expected to gain greater influence in Egypt under Arabi than he had under the system of dual control, since Arabi's nominee as chief minister had been Cherif Pasha, a Turk who had spent many years in the sultan's court.[52] Granville's one success was to secure, for the first and only time, the right of India to send a separate delegation to the conference with full voting rights. Only with this concession was the British government prepared to take part in the proceedings.[53]

The two Indian delegates were Sir Joseph Fayrer and Timothy Lewis: convinced opponents of the Constantinople decision on the communicability of cholera. While Lewis and Fayrer were almost certainly chosen because of the congruence of their views with the political objectives of the Indian adminis- tration, they were not, as we have seen in the preceding chapters, untypical of medical opinion in India. All the medical arguments advanced at international sanitary conferences were, in some degree, articulations of each country's experience of epidemic disease. France seemed to be afflicted with cholera first in her Mediterranean ports, seemingly as a result of commercial exchange with the middle east. This gave rise to the understandable belief that cholera was a disease transmitted by human contact. British epidemiologists were convinced, however, that no single case of cholera had ever reached a British port direct from India, and that the great cholera pandemics had spread overland from Asia to Europe.

Privately, Granville and his colleagues were less than optimistic about the outcome of the conference, as were most commentators in the medical press. A German medical journal declared that 'we do not expect the slightest result from such a conference', while the *BMJ* believed that 'it would settle nothing'.[54] As expected, the conference, which was convened in 1885, proved to be a hotbed of controversy, the chief issue at stake being the nature of quarantine restrictions at Suez against vessels sailing from infected ports. The British and Indian proposal that ships agreeing not to dock before reaching England should be exempted from quarantine was heavily defeated, with only 6 of the 28 delegates voting in its favour.[55] Many nations, particularly France, were genuinely concerned that Britain would use its influence on the Egyptian Board of Health to relax quarantine measures, thought to be the last line of defence against cholera for Mediterranean ports.[56]

The Rome conference concluded with no binding international agreement. Failure to come to terms on the question of the quarantine at Suez was matched by the failure of the delegates to agree on the question of Kamaran. The sultan – angered by Britain's new-found influence in Egypt – blocked British and Indian proposals for a reduction in the length of quarantine at the station. Having been urged, initially against his will, to construct the quarantine stations at Kamaran and El Tor, the sultan was also hoping to recoup something of their cost. Fees for accommodation and the disinfection of ships yielded a substantial income: over 640,000 piastres in 1889. But the sultan was vulnerable to the question of conditions at the stations. Medical officers at the stations urged the sultan, with some success, to reduce the levy for poor pilgrims and to build new, better-ventilated huts.[57] It was in the sultan's own interest to accede to some of these demands, since improvements at Kamaran enabled him to deflect criticism emanating from the British and Indian governments, which claimed that the islands were a danger to health.

With the failure of the Rome conference, the Indian government was forced to reconsider its own sanitary policy with the aim of securing reductions at the next round of sanitary talks. The need for action in regard to the pilgrim traffic was underscored by criticism in the *Times of India* of defective sanitary arrangements for pilgrims in Bombay.[58] The government's first step was to introduce, in 1886, the Bombay Pilgrims Bill, which was enacted later the same year. It placed tighter restrictions on the activities of pilgrim brokers, hitherto notorious for overcrowding their vessels and practising extortion on their passengers.[59] In the coming months, the authorities in Bombay appear to have enforced the act strictly, making an example of any so-called 'brokers' trading without a licence or guilty of fraud. Summing up on the case of one Abdul Karim, convicted under the act on three counts of fraud, the magistrate presiding over the case declared that he would 'deal out such punishment as will be a warning and an example to other brokers similarly inclined. I sentence you in each of these cases to sixteen months imprisonment, that is, four years altogether.'[60] Salvation also arrived in the unlikely form of Thomas Cook and Sons, who agreed in the same year to act as agents for the pilgrim trade in India following a personal request from the new viceroy Lord Dufferin, and Sir Henry Drummond Wolff in Cairo. Cook's were to arrange with railway administrations and steamship proprietors to convey pilgrims to and from the Hedjaz, and to ensure that all the firms with which they did business followed government guidelines on accommodation, food supplies and sanitary conditions.[61] The Bombay government hoped that Cook's high reputation would reassure Muslim leaders and the International Boards that

Bombay was no longer the 'Sanitary Pariah of the East'. The new arrangements were greeted with approval by the *Bombay Gazette*. 'They promise to have good results ... ', its editor wrote, 'the pilgrim traffic is growing yearly in dimensions, and although ... there has been a perceptible change in the manner in which it has been conducted in recent years ... it is still capable of improvement'.

The *Gazette*'s editor pointed out the need for co-operation with the Muslim community if the scheme was to be successful.[62] Other members of the European community in Bombay were less optimistic. A letter addressed to the *Gazette* by one 'Oliver Twist' warned that

> the effect of increasing the space [for each pilgrim on board ships] would be simply that the Hadj would become a more expensive thing than it already is, and philanthropically disposed as Government may be, it has no more right to legislate in that direction than it has to make it law that no-one shall go home except in a first-class P. & O. steamer.[63]

However, the government was determined to press ahead with the new arrangements, and in 1887 consolidated its existing pilgrim legislation in a new Native Passenger Ships Act. In addition to a more thorough inspection of the ship and its passengers before embarkation, the act introduced new regulations making compulsory the provision of special compartments for the sick, an adequate number of latrines, and of cabins exclusively for the preparation of food. Each ship carrying over 100 pilgrims was now required to engage the services of a medical officer, and a penalty of between 10 and 200 Turkish livres was to be levied for each infringement.[64] At the same time, wealthy members of the Muslim community had begun to make a financial contribution to the welfare of pilgrims embarking from Bombay.[65]

Despite the new Pilgrims Act, and Cook's continuing involvement in the pilgrim trade, there occurred no real improvement in conditions on board the majority of vessels. In 1889 a retired Muslim inspector of hospitals, Muhammed Yakub Alikhan, brought to light the overcrowding and intense discomfort experienced by pilgrims on the vessel *Tanjore*. Cook's had sold more tickets for the return journey than there had been accommodation available on board the *Tanjore*.[66] Later the same year, Cook's announced losses, and stated that the arrangement could never be a profitable one. The firm claimed that it had not received the support it had expected from the Muslim community, and agreed to continue the arrangement only if the Indian government agreed to make good any future losses.[67] The government agreed, and made a contribution of £1,000 to cover the shortfall for 1889.[68]

Scandals concerning overcrowding continued, and incurred the hostility of Muslim leaders, but the government continued to defend Cook's and claimed that the accusations made against the firm were groundless. The credibility of the government's position received a severe blow in 1891 after a serious outbreak of cholera occurred on the *SS Deccan*, which had left India for Jeddah. Severe overcrowding below decks and battening down of hatches had facilitated the spread of the disease. The new arrangements seemed to have failed for two reasons. First, the system of inspection of vessels prior to their leaving India was undermined by a lack of trained staff, corruption, and simple incompetence. Likewise, there was no way, under existing arrangements, of preventing ships from picking up extra passengers on the return voyage. Second, the majority of pilgrims, most of whom struggled to meet the cost of the pilgrimage, appear to have resented increased fares more than overcrowding or the lack of sanitary facilities. Sanitation on board pilgrim vessels was primarily the concern of well-to-do Muslims, willing to meet the cost of increased fares and to pay the sanitary levies introduced in some Indian ports.[69]

The British government, however, continued to show little interest in the pilgrim question and to concentrate its energies on the quarantine at Suez. But, by the 1890s, the prospects in this direction were considerably more hopeful than in 1885: there was a growing feeling among the other European governments that quarantine was no longer necessary or desirable. Britain was now also in a position to influence decisions made by the Egyptian Board of Health, having secured its proposed reforms of the board so as to allow more power to Egyptian representatives. According to Adrien Proust, French delegate to the 1892 sanitary conference, 'the Alexandria Council ha[d] nothing international but its name'.[70] One factor contributing to this change in mood was the growing acceptance of the claim, made by the German bacteriologist Robert Koch, to have discovered the cholera bacillus, and of his theory that the disease was transmitted in the water supply. At the Venice conference of 1892, delegates were by no means unanimously agreed upon the validity of Koch's theory, but in 1893, at Dresden, the majority declared themselves in assent, following epidemiological confirmation of the role of the water supply in the Hamburg epidemic the previous year. Of probably more importance, at least in 1892, seems to have been the increasing volume of international shipping which now used the Suez Canal, even though by far the largest proportion was still British.[71] Moreover, it had become clear that quarantine had failed to prevent the spread of cholera into Europe. The Hamburg epidemic was a case in point. At the same time, countries which had no rigid system of quarantine like Britain – which relied on selective medical inspection – had experienced declining mortality from cholera, ostensibly as a consequence of general sanitary reforms.

By the time of the Venice conference in 1892, all the countries represented agreed that vessels should receive different treatment at Suez according to whether they were deemed 'healthy', 'suspect' or 'infected'. France, however, opposed a British proposal that troop-ships be exempt from all restrictions. It is interesting to note that in this matter Britain received the support of the countries of the Triple alliance: Germany, Austro-Hungary, and Italy.[72] For some years

Bismarck had pursued a colonial policy antagonistic to Britain, but after 1885 he had developed an interest in closer co-operation in response to the growth of pan-slavism in eastern Europe. At the same time, Germany's recent acquisition of colonies in East Africa meant that she too had an interest in relaxing restrictions on ships passing through the canal.[73]

The Dresden conference the following year saw further relaxation of the measures at Suez, but none at the quarantine stations in the Red Sea. This reflected both a lack of resolve on the part of the British government, for which the issue was of secondary importance, and the unwillingness of the Turkish authorities to contemplate any such reforms. The Turkish government undoubtedly had genuine concerns about the spread of cholera into its possessions, but it also derived a not insubstantial income from the arrangements, and had a financial interest in their continuance.[74] The pilgrim question figures more prominently on the agenda of the 1894 sanitary conference at Paris, but, far from resolving the issue, it led to yet another direct confrontation between the British and Indian governments. The conference was held just a few months after the worst outbreak of cholera ever recorded at the Hadj: estimates placed the number of dead at over 30,000, out of a total of 200,000 pilgrims. Discussion covered three main areas: precautions to be taken at ports of departure; the sanitary surveillance of pilgrims traversing the Red Sea; and surveillance of shipping in the Persian Gulf – over 90% of which was British. Britain accepted virtually all the terms listed under the first two heads in the hope of exempting its shipping in the Gulf from further restrictions. But, in deference to opinion in India, the British delegation refused to agree to terms requiring pilgrims to be given a minimum space of 21 square feet below decks and to the reintroduction of a 'passport system'.[75]

Despite these concessions, the Indian government – which was no longer permitted to send a separate delegation – was indignant at Britain's acceptance of the rest of the convention. It had not expected Britain to agree to terms which made compulsory the daily medical inspection of pilgrims on vessels leaving infected ports.[76] Such a measure, the government protested, would almost certainly be misconstrued by lower-class Muslims as provocation on the part of the British authorities. 'We are unable to understand', protested the Indian government, 'how the provisions of the Paris Convention, many of which are distinctly opposed to the declared views of the Government of India, were accepted on our behalf by Her Majesty's Government, without any opinion on them having been called for from us'.[77]

The Indian government had no choice other than to incorporate this decision into a new Pilgrims Act, though the introduction of the Bill was delayed until 1895.[78] In order to make the legislation more palatable to the Muslim community, the act, passed later the same year, included a provision that female pilgrims would be inspected only by women doctors, or by special inspectresses under the supervision of a qualified medical officer. But these concessions did little to appease the Muslim press in India, which argued that the increased costs that would attend the improvement of pilgrim vessels would make the passage 'practically prohibitive' to the majority of Muslims. According to the *Moslem Chronicle*, there were 'many among the followers of Islam that set into no account questions of physical discomfort . . . when they have made up their mind to visit the holy shrine of the prophet'. 'To the mass of Mohammedans', it continued,

> particularly the illiterate among them, these restrictions will be construed as an interdict of an annoying, uncalled for and unwarranted nature. It is with special reference to this class of people that we are against the Pilgrim Ships Bill.[79]

No doubt in deference to Muslim feeling on the matter, the Indian government continued to insist that 9 square feet was sufficient space for each pilgrim; contrary to the wishes of the British government which was more urgently seeking a solution to the pilgrim question. These arrangements appear to have been acceptable to some Muslim leaders.[80] But, if we are to believe the *Moslem Chronicle*, the vast majority were outraged by the passage of the act, which had allegedly been rushed through the viceregal council. The *Chronicle* warned of civil disturbance if the act was not repealed:

> It is a known fact that 90 per cent of the pilgrims belong to the straggling classes of cultivators, and mere mendicants. Is Government then prepared to take the very serious risk which a widespread discontent among the most ignorant, the most illiterate and the most fanatic class of Mohammadans is certain to give rise to?

The only way to prevent such an occurrence, it maintained, was for the government to take pilgrims into its confidence and to circulate instructions in the different vernaculars to show that the government had no intention of interfering with the Hadj.[81] In the event, no such unrest occurred, but the act had undoubtedly aroused much ill feeling, which the politically assertive section of Muslim opinion represented by the *Chronicle* did its best to exploit. It thought that 'the Mohammedan community would do well to agitate for more seats on the Imperial Council instead of merely waiting to have their wishes and feelings taken into consideration at the convenient leisure of their rulers'.[82]

The Pilgrims Act did, however, go some way towards restoring international confidence in India, but the Indian government still felt it necessary to sustain pressure on the sultan, and it instituted another inquiry into conditions at Kamaran. Reports were mixed, but the majority supported the government's contention that arrangements there still left much to be desired.[83] Sir Arthur Alban, British ambassador to Turkey, claimed that pilgrims had also been subject to oppression and cruelty in Mecca itself. He called for the expulsion from Mecca of Hassan Dasud, officer in charge of the pilgrim camp, on the grounds of his 'flagrant dishonesty and brutality'.[84] Conditions on board Turkish pilgrim vessels also came under fire. The port surgeon at Aden found the *Abdul Kadir* overcrowded, its 'hospital' badly situated, and its latrine accommodation insufficient. On board the *Sadat* there was no hospital deck and 'some doubt as to whether the medical officer held any qualification'.[85] The Indian government decided to impose a fine of Rs 1,400 on the vessels when they reached Bombay, which it claimed would act as a deterrent to further abuses.[86]

But, despite these efforts to discredit the Turkish authorities, and the Indian government's own attempts at reform, other countries – particularly France – remained adamant that India should agree to a minimum of 16 square feet per pilgrim below decks and to 32 square feet per patient hospital space.[87] Henri Monod, French representative at Dresden and Paris, also launched a concerted attack on sanitary arrangements within India, claiming that they had done nothing to diminish the incidence of cholera there.[88] The pilgrim issue, then, seemed likely to prevent any agreement being reached on the broader question of quarantine at Suez and in the Red Sea. British patience with Indian and French intransigence was beginning to wear thin. In 1896 Dr Dickinson, British delegate to the Constantinople board, reported that 'the Indian authorities persist in reckoning two pilgrims under twelve years of age as one adult pilgrim. I take the liberty, respectfully, to express my regret that [such] a distinction should be made.'[89] Under pressure from other nations, like Austro-Hungary, and with an eye on commercial and strategic interests in the Red Sea, the British foreign secretary attempted to persuade the Indian government to come to terms, but the issue of pilgrim space was temporarily eclipsed by the outbreak of plague in Bombay in 1896.

Plague

The plague, which broke out in Bombay in September 1896, seems to have been imported from Hong Kong, where an epidemic had raged since 1894. It is not proposed to enter into a detailed discussion of the social and political impact of the epidemic in India, but rather to assess its economic impact, and in particular the impact of quarantine restrictions.[90] In the first weeks, the authorities in Bombay did their best to reassure the populace and the international community that the disease was not true plague, but 'bubonic fever' or 'plague of a mild type'. The Bombay corporation's standing committee on health denounced reports to the contrary as 'scaremongering'.[91] By October the committee could no longer deny the existence of full-blown plague in the city, though it was condemned for doing so by the *Gazette*, doughty defender of Bombay's mercantile community:

> Commercial men are greatly afraid lest quarantine should be imposed on vessels leaving Bombay and thus unnecessarily occasion loss and hardship to the labouring class . . . There is a general consensus of opinion that the exaggerated statements of the standing Committee will do great injury to our commerce for some time to come.[92]

Indeed, within a few days quarantine had been imposed against Indian vessels at Suez and at numerous ports around the world, with varying degrees of severity. The quarantine at Suez, however, was no longer an insuperable obstacle to commerce. Under the Venice Convention of 1892, the Egyptian board distinguished between 'infected', 'suspect' and 'healthy' ships, while regulations in force in British ports offered 'practically no hindrance to communication with India'.[93] France, which had hitherto proved inflexible on the quarantine issue, imposed the most severe restrictions against vessels from India. In Marseilles and other Mediterranean ports, steamers from Bombay were prevented from landing their passengers, while, in general, regulations were far tighter than those agreed at Venice and Dresden.[94]

In tandem with Germany and Italy, whose measures were generally less severe, France also imposed a blanket ban on the importation of Indian raw hides (one of the country's chief exports to the West), as these had been deemed susceptible articles by an emergency sanitary conference in Venice in 1897. Other nations usually disinfected only suspect goods, and applied these regulations to those vessels sailing from infected ports. Of all Indian ports, Calcutta was hardest hit by the ban, even though it was virtually unaffected by plague. The city's chamber of commerce protested that the prohibition had occasioned 'grave inconvenience and loss'. The export in hides and skins constituted just over 6% of the total of India's export earnings: out of 21 principal export items, it ranked sixth in importance, having an annual average value of Rs 616 million in 1891–6. Italy, France, and Germany together received over 40% in value terms of India's export of this commodity. Other 'susceptible articles', like raw cotton, formed a greater proportion of India's export earnings, but raw hides were generally regarded as being more likely to harbour plague, and cotton goods were free from similar restrictions.[95]

In Bombay, however, restrictions on India's coastal trade were more harmful to commerce than those imposed in Europe. In order to satisfy the international community that it was taking adequate precautions against the spread of plague to other parts of India, the government was forced to impose full quarantine – rather than medical inspection – at Madras, Karachi, Calcutta, and Rangoon, against ships sailing from Bombay. Together, these ports accounts for nearly one quarter of Bombay's maritime trade.[96]

Disruption of the export trade, together with the flight from Bombay of over 100,000 people, brought the city's commercial life to a standstill. The *Gazette*'s shipping correspondent claimed, in November 1896, that the city's export market was already in a state of 'complete stagnation' and, in December, its editor observed that 'the exodus and the plague scare have had a serious effect in curtailing trade. The share bazaar is closed and foreign business in practically at a standstill.'[97] The situation had worsened, if anything, by January 1897. 'The commerce of this city', declared the *Gazette*, 'is in a more depressed state now than it has been since the share collapse of thirty years ago'.[98]

But in March there were signs of an upturn in Bombay's commercial fortunes following the passage of the Epidemic Diseases Act of 1897. It made provision for a more 'robust' campaign against plague, including segregation of suspects, the medical inspection and detention of railway passengers, house-to-house searches, and so on. A 'Plague Committee', chaired by General Gatacre of the Indian Army, took the reins of Bombay's plague administration from the municipality, and set about applying the new legislation with vigour. While it may have failed to win the confidence of the indigenous population, many of whom reacted angrily against the new measures, Gatacre's committee seems to have reassured the international community that everything possible was being done in Bombay to combat the disease.[99] A second sanitary conference at Venice, held in May 1897, resulted in a further relaxation of measures against India and a modest revival of India's export economy. Regulations against 'susceptible articles', for example, were lifted following scientific advice, based on the researches of the many foreign plague commissions that had visited India in 1897. Hides and skins were now considered safe if disinfected.[100]

The plague epidemic also revived the thorny issue of pilgrimage. At a relatively early stage in the outbreak, the Turkish authorities imposed a quarantine of 15 days against healthy arrivals from India and repulsed any vessels on which plague had occurred. Early in March 1897, further restrictions were enforced prohibiting Indian ships from passing through the Dardanelles, unless they had already been detained for 15 days at a quarantine station.[101] It was clear that, unless action was taken, pilgrims from India would face even more stringent quarantine than in the past. There was even the possibility that Indian pilgrims might be prohibited altogether, which would reflect badly upon the Indian government and authorities in Bombay. They had already had to face criticism from Muslim leaders of their inaction regarding some of the worst slums in the city, in which the disease had taken root.[102] It was also vital not to alienate Muslim leaders at a time when their co-operation was needed in order to secure the success of Gatacre's policy of segregating plague suspects.[103] Many Muslims had already made clear their opposition to this unprecedented degree of state intervention, which touched on some of the most sensitive areas of Islamic culture.

The only course of action left open to the government was to suspend traffic from infected ports and to allow pilgrims to travel from Madras or Karachi instead.[104] The proposal met with an unfavourable reception from the authorities concerned. The municipal corporation of Madras unanimously passed a resolution condemning the Indian government's proposal. It declared the measure 'unwise, unnecessary, and fraught at the present time with serious danger to the health, commerce and well-being of this populous city'.[105] The Madras government argued that the risk of plague spreading to the presidency would be 'greatly increased by the arrival of gangs of pilgrims from Bombay' and urged the Indian government to reconsider. A proposal that Calcutta might be permitted to remain open as a pilgrim port was similarly opposed, creating considerable tension between the city's Muslims and Hindus; many of the latter supporting a blanket ban on the pilgrimage to Mecca (ostensibly on commercial grounds).

The Hindu *Bengalee* newspaper argued that, while religious duty was a good thing, it would be carrying the principle too far to permit the pilgrimage while the plague continued to rage in India.[106] In the Indian legislative council there was considerable sympathy for the Muslim point of view among European members, but Hindu members like Joygobindo Law were vocal in their insistence that the pilgrimage should be stopped altogether. In the opinion of the *Moslem Chronicle*, this was yet another example of the 'sublime disregard which a Hindu is capable of showing to questions of Mohammedan interests when they come up for discussion before the Legislative and Council Boards'.[107]

These disputes between local and central government, and between Muslim and Hindu, drew comment from the secretary of state for India, and once again revealed the conflicting priorities of the British and Indian administrations. Lord Hamilton was under considerable pressure from the Russian and Austro-Hungarian governments to place a ban on all pilgrimage from India, as well as direct pressure from commercial interests in Madras and London.[108] He argued that France had already suspended the pilgrimage from Algeria and it was incumbent on India, as the focus of the epidemic, to do the same.[109]

The viceroy, Elgin, was reluctant to give way: he was confronted directly with the likely public-order implications of any ban, and was concerned not to jeopardise the ongoing policy of Anglo-Muslim collaboration. He protested that a ban on pilgrims leaving Madras was unnecessary, and that it would be 'regarded as interference with the religion of Mohammadans'.[110] Ultimately, Hamilton had to exert his authority over the viceroy, and the 1897 pilgrimage from India was suspended. Elgin's worst fears, however, failed to materialise: there being no perceptible increase in tension between Muslim leaders and the Indian authorities.

In the coming years, however, the gradual relaxation of quarantine restrictions against India was also expressed in a more liberal attitude towards the pilgrimage. The Indian government, under pressure from Britain, made a number of concessions in return for less stringent measures in the Red Sea. In 1909, for example, the Indian government compelled all pilgrim vessels leaving

India to undergo a brief detention at Aden or Perim in return for a reduction in the period of quarantine at Kamaran to 7 days. The efforts of the British delegate to the Ottoman Board of Health secured a further reduction to 5 days in 1910, and in the following year non-pilgrim vessels were subjected to a quarantine of only 10 days from the last port of call. In 1913, quarantine at Kamaran was replaced by a system of medical inspection similar to that in Britain and India.[111]

Conclusion

As an intersection between Indian and imperial affairs, the quarantine debates of the later nineteenth century provide a new avenue through which to explore relations between imperial metropole and colonial periphery. The free passage of ships between Britain and India was high on the agenda of both governments, but equally important to the Government of India was the question of the sanitary regulation of the pilgrimage and its likely effects on Anglo-Muslim relations. The imposition of quarantine against Indian pilgrims and the indictment of the Indian government at international sanitary conferences, for its apparent lack of concern for the health of Indian pilgrims travelling to Mecca, threatened to jeopardise the government's strategy of 'co-operation' with Muslim leaders. A second difficulty lay in the fact that if it were to implement the sanitary controls desired by the European powers and by Muslim leaders, and thus reduce the perceived need for quarantine, the government's actions were likely to be misconstrued by lower-class Muslims as interference in their religious practices and as violations of their personal dignity.

Britain's occupation of Egypt further exposed the cleavage that had emerged between British and Indian interests. The British naval bombardment of Alexandria aroused the indignation of Indian Muslims and, for a time, strained relations between the Indian government and the 'pan-Islamic' Mohamedan Association. For some years afterwards, the occupation of Egypt served to harden attitudes on both sides of the quarantine debate, and especially between Britain and France: there were no constructive international talks on quarantine for nearly a decade. During this period, Britain moved closer to the nations of the Triple Alliance in order to counteract French influence on the Egyptian Board of Health and the commission for the administration of the country's debt. From 1884, Bismarck also developed an interest in closer ties with Britain, and, following the establishment of German protectorates in East Africa, backed British and Indian demands for the free passage of ships through the Suez Canal.

But, if the quarantine issue exposed tensions in relations between rulers and ruled, and within the imperial order, it also revealed rivalry between various indigenous communities. While Muslim leaders claimed to speak for their people as a whole, wealthy Muslims were clearly far more concerned about sanitary conditions on board pilgrim vessels than the majority of pilgrims, for whom the overriding consideration was the cost of the passage. The controversy surrounding the pilgrimage during the plague epidemic also highlighted tension between Hindu and Muslim élites over certain questions of public health. These conflicts, to some extent, reflected sectional economic interests, but, more importantly, growing political rivalry between the leaders of the two communities.

6

Professional visions and political realities, 1896–1914

There have been as many plagues as wars in history; yet always plagues and wars take people equally by surprise. (Albert Camus, *The Plague*)

I call the people every day to be inoculated, but they refuse to come forward. 'Plague doctor', they say, 'now that *you* are here the plague *must* come!', and they laugh at me. They are a backward and ignorant people. (Indian travelling inoculator, quoted in Katherine Mayo's *Mother India*, 1927)

Inspired by public health reforms in the metropolis, and by advances in medical science, sanitary officers formed an outspoken and sometimes influential pressure group within the Indian Medical Service, advocating more extensive financial and legislative intervention in public health. Sanitation, they claimed, was the key to India's development, as well as being a moral obligation on the part of the colonial government. 'Only with the achievement of true hygiene', wrote the sanitary officer, A. E. Grant in 1894, 'would the "Golden Age" sung of by poets and dreamt of by . . . dreamers through countless years' dawn on India.[1] Such views were usually expressed within the context of an authoritarian, paternalistic conception of Britain's role in India, typified by the writings of administrators such as John Strachey and Fitzjames Stephens.[2] The municipalisation of public health under Mayo and Lord Ripon from the 1870s, and the financial stringency of central and provincial administrations, had, in their view, been productive of nothing but confusion and stagnation. What was needed was firm guidance by the government and a willingness to intervene financially in aid of public health.

The plague epidemics of 1896 onwards provided the reform lobby with an unparalleled opportunity to implement its schemes at municipal and local level, as will be discussed in chapters 7 and 8. This chapter reflects on the fortunes of reform-minded medical men in achieving other aspects of their programme: the introduction of more stringent measures for the control of epidemic disease, and the institutional development of medical research. Medical officers, it is argued, were only partially successful in translating their professional rhetoric into reality: India was no 'gigantic laboratory' in which British medical experts were afforded opportunities denied them at home.[3] Rather, the plague epidemic, and the reorientation of medical policy which resulted from it, reveals the colonial state's limited desire and capacity to pursue more vigorous measures.

The medical profession and the plague

Bubonic plague was not, in fact, entirely new to India. There are reports of epidemics having occurred in the seventeenth, and even in the early nineteenth, centuries, and a disease thought to be plague (known locally as *mahamari*) was reported in the remote Himalayan regions of Garwhal and Kankal as late as 1878.[4] Yet, almost without exception, medical men in India had no direct experience of the disease, and had not formed any clear opinions on how best to treat or prevent it should it occur. Thus when plague arrived in Bombay (almost certainly from Hong Kong) there was initially some confusion over the diagnosis of the disease. Although the first cases of plague probably arose as early as August, its existence was not admitted officially until the end of September. But it was not simply medical ignorance that delayed recognition of the disease. The city's authorities and the provincial government shared the fears of Bombay's mercantile community that a damaging quarantine would be imposed against the port if plague was officially acknowledged.[5]

Uncertain of how best to respond to the new threat posed by plague, medical men and colonial administrators reverted to the centuries-old practice of placing plague victims in isolation.[6] The port of Bombay and, before long, Aden and Karachi were placed under quarantine on the orders of the Indian government, in accordance with directives issued by the Egyptian Board of Health in 1882.[7] In Bombay itself, the powers of the 1888 Municipal Act were extended to permit the disinfection of infected dwellings, the destruction of suspect goods, and the removal to hospital of persons suffering from the disease. Infected houses and their occupants could now be placed in isolation for as long as deemed necessary by the newly formed municipal plague committee.

From 1 October the provincial government impressed upon railway companies operating in Bombay the necessity of inspecting their passengers and of preventing persons suspected of having plague from leaving the region. Though the companies were empowered to take such measures under the Railways Act of 1890, inspection was introduced at only one of the two junctions recommended by the government. Railway companies were more concerned about the possibility of unrest at stations, and the disruption of passenger and freight services. Most of these measures were based closely upon recommendations made by Surgeon-General George Bainbridge, head of the

IMS in Bombay. Medical men were also well represented on the plague committee chaired by P. C. H. Snow, ICS, a Bombay municipal commissioner. Four of its 9 members were drawn from the IMS, and another 3 from the city's independent practitioners.[8]

At this early stage, Bainbridge and other medical men in Bombay admitted that they had 'insufficient knowledge' to enable them to deal with plague effectively. Most medical men thought that the disease was 'contagious' in some way, although they differed over how it was conveyed from person to person.[9] Bainbridge's own view was that plague was an 'aerial pulmonary infection', while others felt it might be contracted from inhaling the dust of infected houses, or through inoculation or abrasion of the skin.[10] In the absence of certain knowledge there was general agreement that, for the time being, the best course of action lay in a combination of 'general sanitation and sanitary police'.[11]

This consensus did not last for long: preconceived notions about how plague was spread were modified once medical men in India had the opportunity to observe the disease. Here it is again fruitful to draw a parallel with the 1831–2

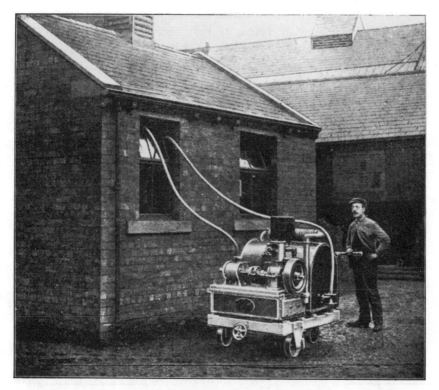

Plate 5   The Clayton 'plague disinfector'

cholera epidemic in Britain, where 'contagionist' doctrine was modified as the disease spread unevenly throughout the country.[12] The spread of plague to other cities and into Bombay's rural hinterland also posed practical barriers to prevention. Medical inspection and cordons sanitaires required large numbers of medical and subordinate personnel if they were to be enforced effectively. Overlapping these considerations were the professional concerns of medical men themselves. As described in chapter 1, there was suspicion in the IMS of bacteriology and recent innovations in medical practice; doubt about the suitability of women and Indians for medical posts; and a long-standing rivalry between the sanitary and medical branches of the service.[13]

Social unrest and the flight of over 100,000 people from Bombay – precipitated by compulsory hospitalisation and the destruction of dwellings – forced Bombay's plague committee to reconsider its policy.[14] By December measures had been made less stringent, though this new policy was not without its critics. The *Bombay Gazette* favoured greater intervention, as there were no indications that mortality from plague was beginning to decrease.[15] Bombay's European community began to demand the compulsory segregation of those who had been in contact with plague victims. 'To leave the matter optional', wrote a correspondent to the *Gazette*, 'is merely to allow the people to govern instead of being governed . . . Kindness and persuasion have done little so far.'[16] Anxious to secure reductions in quarantine at Suez and in European ports, the secretary of state Lord Hamilton echoed these concerns over the effectiveness of measures in Bombay. He questioned the Bombay government's claim that 'wholesale, enforced segregation was not within the practical limits of possibility'. 'The critical state of affairs', protested the governor, was 'not due to the shortcomings of the city's authorities, but to the unreadiness of the inhabitants, their great dislike and distrust of sanitary measures, and their fear of being separated from their families'.[17]

Nevertheless, the secretary of state was determined to press more stringent measures upon the Indian administration. His first move was to engage the services of J. A. Lowson, a Colonial Medical Service officer with experience of plague operations in Hong Kong.[18] Lowson, who was appointed plague commissioner for Bombay, had enlisted the help of the army to enforce hospitalisation and segregation in Hong Kong, and was determined to take an equally 'robust' approach in Bombay.[19] Though the Indian medical establishment considered Lowson a troublesome outsider, it was under considerable pressure from the secretary of state to heed his advice. On Lowson's recommendation the municipal plague committees in Bombay, Poona, Karachi, and Sukkur were replaced with smaller bodies headed by military men, and with only one medical representative. Under the powers granted by the Epidemic Diseases Act of 1897, these committees were empowered to segregate contacts in special camps according to caste and religion, and to inspect and, if necessary, to detain railway passengers suspected of having contracted plague. Europeans were exempted from these provisions.[20]

The new regulations provided the opportunity for medical intervention on an unprecedented scale; an opportunity which was not lost on medical officers and administrators of a more authoritarian bent. Major W. L. Reade, AMS, who had also gained experience of plague in Hong Kong, felt that 'plague operations properly undertaken present some of the best opportunities for riveting our rule in India . . . [and] for showing the superiority of our Western science and thoroughness'.[21] Other reform-minded officials were equally keen to seize the opportunity provided by plague. The *Indian Medical Gazette*, which had long championed the cause of public health in India, felt that 'the authorities in Bombay . . . [had] been slow to recognise the gravity of the situation' and was pleased to see that 'a large number of medical men [had] been deputed to Bombay on special duty, and that encampments were being formed for the purpose of separating the healthy from the sick'.[22]

Plague officers of an authoritarian frame of mind, many of them comparatively young officers of the Sanitary Department, favoured compulsory segregation and cordons sanitaires over voluntary and more general sanitary measures. Their zealous approach probably owed much to their inexperience, but also to their enthusiasm for bacteriological theories and new methods of disease prevention. 'The only effective measure', insisted T. W. Illingworth, deputy sanitary commissioner of Bellary, was the 'segregation of all people in contact with the disease followed by thorough disinfection of their houses'.[23] B. B. Grayfoot, secretary to the surgeon-general of Bombay, also believed that 'in any scheme for controlling an epidemic in a given locality, our attention must be mainly given to the sick man and his surroundings . . . [to] isolation of the sick and segregation of the healthy'.[24]

In rural areas whole villages were sometimes placed in quarantine. S. J. Thomson, sanitary commissioner of the NWP and O believed that cordons were the most effective method of combating plague in rural areas, and placed the small towns of Jawalapur and Kankal under quarantine immediately plague broke out in the neighbouring district of Hurdwar. He continued to enforce segregation of contacts in the district long after the practice had been abandoned in Bombay.[25] Similarly, Deputy Sanitary Commissioner E. Wilkinson strongly favoured the use of cordons sanitaires in his district of the Punjab,[26] while M. J. Mountford, acting collector of Rohri District, had a 'very high opinion of segregation' and dispensed two-week prison sentences to those in breach of the arrangements.[27]

The plague epidemic also provided the testing ground for newer, more specific methods of prevention based on the principles of bacteriology. In October 1896 the Bombay government set up a Plague Research Committee to inquire into the 'nature and history of the disease'. One of those appointed to the committee was the bacteriologist Waldemar Haffkine, who had been despatched to Bombay by the secretary of state. Haffkine – an Armenian Jew – was a controversial figure who had already aroused the suspicion of the Indian authorities during an experimental cholera inoculation programme in 1894.[28] Haffkine's brief in India in 1896 was to investigate the nature of the plague microbe, its mode of spread and the possibility of inoculation against the disease.[29] In December 1896 Haffkine announced that he had devised such a vaccine, raising European hopes of a truly effective method of prevention. 'It is in the highest degree reassuring', wrote the editor of the *Bombay Gazette*, 'to know that in the midst of all the clamour and the futile criticism, science has been silently forging weapons which . . . will defend people from attacks of plague'.[30]

The first positive official response to inoculation came, significantly, from the secretary of state who, in early 1897, suggested that an enquiry be conducted into the feasibility of a programme of inoculation against plague.[31] Following favourable tests in a local prison, Haffkine's inoculation was introduced on an experimental basis into the wider community; first in Bombay, and then into other western-Indian towns. Keen to extend operations further, the secretary of state called in March for weekly reports to be made to him concerning inoculation and the production of vaccine. Hamilton judged progress in this direction to be 'very inadequate', and was equally disappointed with the lack of help afforded to the Frenchman, Yersin, who had been sent by the Institut Pasteur in Paris to Bombay to develop a curative serum for plague.[32]

Though genuine doubts remained over the effectiveness and safety of Haffkine's inoculation, his announcement was greeted with much enthusiasm by a growing minority within the medical services which had been schooled in bacteriology. Here was a means of demonstrating their professional worth and the importance of science in colonial administration. P. H. Benson, sanitary commissioner of Mysore, instituted a programme of inoculation as soon as the city of Bangalore was declared infected, and boasted that it had been more efficiently carried out there than in other cities like Bombay.[33] In the Punjab, Deputy Sanitary Commissioner C. H. James was equally optimistic about the potential of inoculation, and recorded 'excellent results' among those already vaccinated against plague.[34] His colleague, Deputy Sanitary Commissioner W. R. Clarke was similarly impressed by inoculation.[35] It was also an 'open secret that inoculation in the Punjab, where the plague became particularly severe after 1900, was often 'far from voluntary'.[36] But, for the most part, inoculation was introduced with the co-operation of local community leaders, and Indians were often induced to present themselves for inoculation as an alternative to segregation.[37] In other cases these inducements were accompanied by sanctions. In Dharwar District of Bombay Province, for example, uninoculated children were prevented from attending school.[38]

Those who favoured inoculation at an early stage in the epidemic were drawn disproportionately from younger members of the Sanitary Department, most of whom were already familiar with bacteriology from their training under Almroth Wright at Netley. A high percentage of those sanitary officers who had joined the IMS after 1887 had also gained the DPH, which provided instruction in the practical application of bacteriological techniques. They received support for their methods from the fledgling *Journal of Tropical Medicine* in Britain, edited jointly by James Cantlie, RAMC and W. J. Simpson, formerly health officer of Calcutta, and an old ally of Haffkine. 'In the social conditions . . . under which the inhabitants live in a large Indian city', wrote Simpson in 1898, 'it is particularly difficult for . . . sanitary measures . . . to be carried out. There can be little doubt that Haffkine's inoculations are gradually obtaining much favour, not only among the Indian medical profession but also among the general community.'[39]

Yet, in 1898, most IMS officers were unfamiliar with, or displayed little enthusiasm for, these new 'technologies' of prevention; or for the more authoritarian aspects of plague prevention such as the erection of segregation camps. It was almost certainly for this reason that medical men were largely excluded from the reconstituted, more authoritarian, plague committees in 1897. The majority of medical officers accepted the need for some kind of sanitary police, but placed greater emphasis on general sanitary improvements and the evacuation of infected areas. This preoccupation with sanitary conditions was a vestige of the 'environmentalist' framework which dominated medical attitudes to diseases like cholera and malaria until the early 1890s.

In many respects the blend of coercion and sanitation recommended by Surgeon-General Bainbridge to combat plague in 1896 was little different from that advocated against cholera in India prior to 1890. Inoculation, he insisted, should not 'be regarded as a substitute for . . . general sanitary measures; it should be merely auxiliary to them'.[40] Similarly, W. G. King, an officer with over 20 years' experience of medicine in India, warned that inoculation should only be used in addition to general sanitation. 'I have attempted my best', he wrote, 'to struggle against the opinion of those who contend that we should throw up all sanitary measures and simply take to the inoculation syringe'. King was equally opposed to compulsory segregation, preferring a combination of medical inspection and evacuation of infected areas.[41] Captain R. Robertson, a medical officer at Anantapur, also expressed a preference for evacuation as opposed to segregation and cordons sanitaires.[42] The DGIMS, James Cleghorn, similarly believed that the plague was 'only slightly, if at all . . . infectious or contagious in the common acceptance of the terms'.[43] His successor, in 1898, Surgeon-General R. Harvey, shared Cleghorn's view that plague could not flourish other than in insanitary conditions, and that sanitary measures were the 'essential thing' in the fight against plague.[44]

Reluctance to implement inoculation or coercive measures against plague was not simply a function of resistance to bacteriology, but of concern about the possibility of hostile reaction of the kind that had occurred in Poona and Bombay. When compulsory segregation and inoculation were first introduced they invariably met with hostility, or at least a refusal to comply on the part of the indigenous population. In Calcutta, compulsory segregation was 'practically abandoned' after it resulted in a mass exodus from the city,[45] and the plague authorities in Karachi had to promise the city's large Muslim population that no such order would be issued, in an attempt to gain its compliance with other plague regulations.[46] A riot broke out at Gholi in Nasik District of Bombay Province in September 1897 when segregation was introduced, and 18,000 Indians fled Dharwar in fear of inoculation and segregation.[47] Inoculation and segregation impinged on ritual purity and family pride (*izzat*) and, commonly, rumour implicated inoculation in cases of poisoning and deaths from plague.[48]

In their analysis of indigenous responses to plague measures, British administrators and medical men distinguished between Indians of different religions and castes. Reporting a plague riot at Cawnpore, in which six guards at a segregation camp had been killed, the secretary to the government of the North West Provinces wrote that

> in the rural villages . . . the great landlords have hitherto and are still giving the Administration all the assistance it requires in enforcing the plague regulations . . . But in large cities, especially where Mohammedans of the lower orders abound, the question bristles with difficulties, and the Lieutenant-Governor has been from the first apprehensive that panic and disturbance could not always be avoided.[49]

By presenting themselves as intermediaries between the colonial state and the 'rude masses', middle- and upper-class Indians were able to consolidate their hegemony over their less fortunate countrymen.[50] These distinctions are also important in that they reveal the uniqueness of India's experience of plague. Elsewhere in the British Empire, and in the European colonies more generally, there were few attempts to differentiate between, let alone consult, elements of the indigenous population when plague broke out among them. In Cape Colony, the Gold Coast, the German colony of Cameroon, and the French colony of Senegal, segregation was more universal, and justified on more explicitly racial grounds than it ever was in India.[51] British rule in India relied if not on 'collaboration', then on the co-option of indigenous élites, as was shown in chapter 5.

From 1898 to 1900 plague measures in most provinces of India were liberalised as a result of suspicion and hostility among lower-class Indians; and, on a local level, medical officers and administrators began to enter into a dialogue with community leaders about how best to conduct measures against plague. In Satara the effectiveness of plague measures was thought to rest on the 'active and intelligent co-operation of the people themselves'.[52] In rural areas of

Bombay even large-scale evacuation was possible if village headmen were consulted in advance.[53] A voluntary system of segregation was arranged in Karachi, Bellary, and Bombay city, while special 'caste hospitals' were established in Cutch, Ahmedabad, and elsewhere.[54] In Cawnpore there was now much greater sensitivity on the part of the authorities to the treatment of purdah women, and to the value of women as medical personnel.[55] Female medical staff had, in fact, been employed for some time in other districts of India as inoculators and medical inspectresses at railway stations.[56] Similarly, though Indian practitioners of western medicine had played a part in plague operations since the beginning of the epidemic, there was now in some areas acceptance of the need to engage practitioners of traditional Indian medicine. 'If segregation cannot be effected in or near the home . . . ', stated the amended Cawnpore plague regulations of 1900, 'the health officer may require the removal of the sick person to a public hospital for which a *vaid* or *hakim* will be entertained at Government expense to treat those patients who object to treatment by European methods'.[57]

By 1900, given relaxations of international quarantine regulations, the secretary of state no longer insisted that stringent measures be imposed in India. Following the visits of plague commissions from several European countries (including Germany, France, and Russia) there was general agreement that plague was not directly communicable from person to person.[58] The influence of young medical experts, flush with enthusiasm for inoculation and coercive sanitary measures, had been destructive and, in accordance with the recommendations of the Indian Plague Commission which reported in 1900, the Indian government took steps to end any unduly repressive measures still in force in India. The commission was in broad agreement that compulsory segregation should be avoided, that hospitalisation was effective only where there was consultation with the indigenous community, and that evacuation and chemical disinfection were generally beneficial.[59] Haffkine's inoculation was held in high regard, but the commission had reservations about the quality of the vaccine produced to date. Its practical utility was thought to rest on the willingness of the people to submit to it. Inoculation, in the opinion of the commission, should be resorted to whenever possible, but should never be made compulsory.[60] These findings were in accord with the majority of special reports commissioned by the Indian government on the success of inoculation.[61] The results of serum therapy – developed by Yersin and others – in the commission's view had so far proved inconclusive, but trials continued.[62]

In 1900 the Indian government issued a resolution expressing its approval of the report of the plague commission, and resolved that compulsory segregation and corpse inspection, together with other restrictions on population movement, would be abandoned.[63] Mindful of the possibility of a 'second mutiny', the government was anxious to defuse the explosive political situation created by repressive plague measures. In some cities, such as Poona, militant nationalists like B. G. Tilak had channelled hostility against segregation and hospitalisation into a more general protest against British rule.[64] The viceroy, Elgin, was also deeply concerned over reports that Hindus and Muslims had united in opposition to plague measures in several parts of India.[65] The Indian government had always been aware of the dangers of heavy-handed medical intervention, but in 1896–7 had been under considerable pressure from European governments, via the secretary of state, to take drastic measures.

There were also economic reasons for scaling down operations against plague. 'In the present state of the finances', declared the Indian government, 'it is desirable to effect every reduction in the cost of plague measures which can be carried out without loss of efficiency'. Among other savings, the government sought to reduce the number of railway inspection stations.[66] As a consequence, for the first time since 1897, restrictions on internal pilgrimages were lifted. The ban of rail travel to and from infected areas of India had never been a popular measure, and had been heavily criticised by political and religious organisations like the Hardwar Hindu Association, and in the vernacular press.[67] In 1900 pilgrims were permitted to travel to the *Magh Mela*, a Hindu religious festival at Allahabad, without restriction. The lieutenant-governor had decided 'not to take such a step which would offend Hindu susceptibilities throughout the country'.[68]

Within 2 or 3 years of the initial outbreak, medical attention began to shift from the human body to the rat. Medical officers began to notice that rat epizootics frequently preceded outbreaks of plague among humans.[69] By 1900, when the Indian Plague Commission made its report, it 'seemed conclusive that rats in some places, though by no means all . . . [had] been active in dissemi-nating plague'.[70] A growing number of medical officers now saw rat destruction as a key part of their strategy against plague. Reform-minded officers were aware that their attempts to impose a rigid sanitary regime had failed, and that even inoculation had met with a lukewarm response. Seemingly powerless in the face of plague, these medical officers sought a way to regain the initiative, to prove their worth to the colonial government. The rat with its time-honoured association with insanitary conditions provided something tangible around which a campaign for sanitary reform could be mounted. There was a good deal of interest taken by professional journals in the London meeting of a new association for the destruction of rats and in a 'war' against rats in Denmark. There were frequent references to the 'evil role' of the rat and to the 'innate antipathy' felt by human beings towards it.[71]

But by 1907 it was clear that rat destruction was not an effective means of fighting plague. In addition to the sheer scale of the undertaking, the extermi-nation of rats met with opposition from Jains and orthodox Hindus who tolerated all forms of animal life.[72] Nevertheless, because it had become the hub of a more general professional strategy, rat destruction continued in most Indian towns and cities until at least 1910. The Indian government also looked favourably upon rat destruction. In 1907 the viceroy declared that, while complete extermination of rats within a locality was impracticable, such tactics might 'materially diminish' plague within a given area.[73] Rat destruction, by contrast with segregation and even inoculation, was relatively inexpensive and seemed to pose few political problems. Above all it was an art of the possible, even though its actual effects upon the incidence of plague were not beyond criticism.

From 1906, following Liston's confirmation of Simond's theory of 1898, the view that plague might be transmitted by rat fleas was beginning to gain ground in India. Combined with a growing realisation of the ineffectiveness of the rat campaign, this discovery resulted in a more realistic approach to plague prevention, concentrating on the exclusion of rats from commercial and domestic premises. It was thought that such a campaign would have to go hand-in-hand with a programme of popular sanitary education.[74] In addition there was renewed emphasis on inoculation – the only preventive measure that had been shown to be truly effective against plague.[75] There was now some evidence to suggest that inoculation was slowly gaining popularity among the indigenous population.[76]

The plague epidemic provides a vivid illustration of the limits of medical influence upon sanitary policy. At all stages in the fight against plague, medical opinion informed official action, but it was invariably subordinate to the broader economic and political concerns of the colonial regime; especially its fears of civil unrest. Draconian measures against plague were introduced reluctantly by the Indian government, and as a result of international pressure. As soon as this pressure began to wane restrictions on population movement, and other measures, were relaxed. Similarly mounting political unrest in India demonstrated the dangers of heavy-handed interference in the lives of Indians, and plague measures were amended substantially to take account of indigenous sensibilities.

Plague also reveals the two very different conceptions of government, which underlay sanitary policy in India. Like the majority of administrators, most IMS men continued to stress the need for gradualism and general sanitary reforms; younger officers of the sanitary department and military men tended to favour more specific and coercive methods of plague prevention. There had always been a strand of Anglo-Indian opinion which advocated direct rule and more virulent forms of westernisation, but for the 1880s and much of the 1890s this tendency had been held in check; in 1896–1900 it was briefly unleashed. Younger, more assertive medical officers, confident in the powers of western science, were merely its latest incarnation, sharing with previous generations an unquestioning belief in the superiority of western civilisation. More than any other single factor, plague created an awareness in administrative circles of both the potential and the limitations of western science. While it remained wary of interference in the lives of the indigenous population, the government resolved to set medical research in India upon a firmer foundation.

The institutionalisation of tropical medicine

As described in chapter 2, 'tropical medicine' as a relatively distinct body of medical knowledge had been in existence since at least the mid-eighteenth century, but 'tropical medicine' did not become a discipline in the generally accepted sense until the close of the nineteenth century.[77] After 1898 professional journals began to appear, fostering a sense of identity among practitioners of tropical medicine. In 1898 and 1899, in Liverpool and London, the first specialist research and teaching institutions were established, and the first chairs in tropical medicine created. Contemporary practitioners of tropical medicine claimed that this transformation was inevitable given increasing specialisation and the internal dynamism of their subject.[78] Recent studies of tropical medicine, however, have been critical of these teleological accounts. Michael Worboys has shown that its institutionalisation owed more to 'external', political factors than to the accumulation of new knowledge: the London and Liverpool schools of tropical medicine being part of the Colonial Office's policy of 'constructive imperialism'.[79]

But the emergence of tropical medicine as a discipline was not an exclusively metropolitan phenomenon. In India, where the Colonial Office exercised no direct influence upon policy, the discipline emerged in response to pressures generated largely within India itself. Institutionalisation was a consequence of emergency: insufficient knowledge of plague had left the administration almost powerless to combat the disease. Economic and political disruption resulting from plague and plague measures, together with criticism of the government's response to the epidemic, forced the administration to consider more seriously than hitherto the role of medical science in public health policy. Plague was different from other epidemic diseases in India in that it was, to all intents and purposes, an exotic, generating fear and scientific interest on a scale unmatched by malaria and other diseases indigenous to India. Discipline formation also owed much to the professionalising activities of medical practitioners, particularly those who had acquired specialist knowledge in the new sciences of bacteriology and parasitology. In India these specialists had received little official support or recognition, and were regarded with suspicion by their colleagues in the IMS. IMS officers found it difficult to obtain study leave to further their training in laboratory medicine and, as in most tropical colonial countries, laboratory equipment was even more difficult to obtain than in Britain. Until 1900 colonial laboratories were invariably makeshift, ephemeral affairs, and colonial medical researchers complained of isolation from like-minded individuals.[80]

Medical officers complained of a distrust of science in official circles and among members of the medical profession. 'The British race' – claimed A. E. Grant, professor of hygiene at Madras Medical College – 'is avowedly afraid of the world scientific because . . . science is supposed never to pay. Even by many medical officers . . . the pursuit of scientific investigation is looked upon as something quite apart from ordinary teaching and ordinary sanitary work.' In this respect, Britain was compared unfavourably to its European competitors. 'Nothing lately has given the writer greater pleasure', admitted Grant, 'than reading of a review of the Official Catalogue of the German Empire . . . in which is set forth the enormous industries which have grown up in that country as the direct result of scientific investigation'.[81] Others warned of competition closer to home. 'We have allowed a Frenchman to find for us the amoeba of our malarial fevers, and a German the . . . bacillus of cholera which is surely our own disease', complained Dr Crombie, IMS, 'shall we wait till someone comes to discover for us the secrets of the continued fevers which are our daily study, or shall we be up and doing it for ourselves?'[82]

Indeed, controversies over priority for 'discoveries' in the emergent discipline of tropical medicine had distinctly nationalistic overtones. This was especially true of Ross' entanglements with the Italian Batista Grassi over priority in work on the malaria vector.[83] Research-oriented medical men identified their professional goals with concerns over imperial efficiency. 'Scientific medicine', wrote the *Indian Medical Gazette*, was 'necessary to the development of those countries' under British rule.[84] Others, like E. J. Hart, editor of the *BMJ* chose to stress Britain's duty to its imperial subjects. 'It is not right', he protested, 'that we should essay to govern millions and withhold from them the full measure of civilisation. Nor is it seemly that we in England should have to go for so many years to France and Germany for textbooks in a subject in which England should lead the way.' 'The chief want', in Hart's opinion, was that of 'systematic instruction [in tropical medicine] in our medical schools, good textbooks, and insistence by the licensing authorities on a competent knowledge of the subject'.[85]

For reform-minded medical officers like Ronald Ross, British imperialism was first and foremost a civilising force. He believed that the British were 'superior to subject peoples in natural ability, integrity and science . . . They [had] introduced honesty, law, justice, order, roads, posts, railways, irrigation, hospitals . . . and what was necessary for civilisation, a final superior authority.'[86] Ross' 'final superior authority' was Stephen's 'absolute government, founded, not on consent, but on conquest . . . implying at every point the superiority for the conquering race, and having no justification for its existence except that superiority'.[87] Ross, like Stephen, was an exponent of authoritarian imperialism, perhaps reflecting his upbringing as the son of a British Army general in India.

The plague research commissions

It was the outbreak of plague in 1896 that provided the first real opportunity for medical men in India to translate their rhetoric into reality. The formation of the Plague Research Committee at a relatively early stage in the outbreak was an important acknowledgement that medical research had an important part to play in preventive medicine. Though Haffkine and Yersin were sent to Bombay at the behest of the secretary of state for India, their presence in India, and that of the various foreign plague commissions, suggested possibilities for the future development of medical research in India. The research committee, formed on 13 October 1896, comprised Surgeon-Major R. Manser (president), deputed to look into clinical aspects of plague and its treatment; Surgeon-Captain L. F. Childe, its pathology; Dr N. F. Surveyor (the first Indian to be appointed to an official scientific commission), the plague in animals; W. M. Haffkine, the transmission of plague and preventive inoculation; and E. H. Hankin (the United Provinces' bacteriologist and chemical examiner), the vitality and longevity of the plague bacillus under different conditions.[88]

Central to the work of the committee and the plague commission was the question of how plague was spread. In the light of huge epizootics among the rat population, seemingly coincident with outbreaks of the disease among humans, there was much speculation that rats carried the disease. As already stated, lack of agreement on this issue had led to some confusion about how best to prevent plague. Many medical men, like J. Petigara, assistant-surgeon of Broach, had come to believe that rats spread plague directly to humans. Others, like K. B. D. Pestonjee of Surat felt that rats were of little importance in the spread of plague.[89] The majority of medical officers felt that both rats and humans were capable of spreading plague, but there was considerable uncertainty over how the bacillus entered the human body: some thought it was inhaled, others that it entered into the bloodstream through cuts and abrasions.[90]

The German Plague Commission, of which Koch was a member, gave much attention to the question of plague among animals. It concluded that plague did exist among rats and other mammals, and that it might be spread through cannibalism. In its opinion, only small quantities of bacilli were necessary to cause death in rats. By contrast with rats, however, the German commission felt that the susceptibility of domestic animals was very slight. Haffkine also found that plague appeared to have little effect on cattle, horses, and pigs. But monkeys were particularly sensitive to plague, and were used by both the German and Russian commissions in experiments to test inoculation.[91] On the mode of entrance of the bacillus into the human body, H. E. Bitter of the Egyptian commission concluded that infection could take place through the skin, tonsils, the intestinal tract, or the lungs, according to the type of plague in question (bubonic, septicaemic, or pneumonic). Bubonic plague was by far the most common in India. The Russian commission agreed that infection could take place through cuts or abrasions to the skin (usually the feet), even if no local swellings could be found on the body of the victim.[92]

Investigations into the dissemination of plague centred on the question of the longevity of the bacillus outside the human body. The German commission noted that the plague bacillus had a tendency to perish outside the body, pure cultures being extinguished after only 15 minutes' exposure to a temperature of 70 degrees celsius. Plague bacilli were also placed on different materials – earth, wood, wool, cotton, etc. – and tested under different conditions. Under any circumstances, the maximum life of the bacillus was found to be 10 days. The government's bacteriologist, Ernest Hankin, conducted similar experiments, but found that the life of the bacillus never exceeded 6 days, under any condition. These findings were of crucial importance, since they were to form the basis of regulations issued by the 1897 Venice Sanitary Conference regarding the importation of 'susceptible' articles from India. The conference showed caution, accepting the evidence of the German commission.[93]

Equally important were questions of prevention and cure. Research into plague prevention took two directions; the first concerned measures designed to destroy the bacillus outside the human body by disinfection or desiccation. The German commission conducted numerous experiments into the effectiveness of chemical disinfectants like chloride of lime, carbolic acid, and lysol. Hankin pursued a similar line of investigation, concluding that the plague bacillus was somewhat resistant to carbolic acid, but that phenyl, lysol, and certain acids were highly effective.[94] But, while there was broad agreement over the properties of certain disinfectants, the second line of investigation, into the effectiveness of Haffkine's preventive inoculation, was far more controversial. By the end of May 1897, some 7,874 volunteers in Bombay, and 4,352 elsewhere, had been inoculated against plague; apparently with encouraging results. However, a question-mark hung over the reliability of this experiment, as the subsequent history of those inoculated was usually unknown. But the same objection could not apply to Haffkine's trial in Byculla jail, Bombay, where 154 out of 337 prisoners volunteered for inoculation. The readiness of inmates to take part in the experiment probably owed much to the fact that plague had already broken out in the prison. Of those who came forward for inoculation, two subsequently contracted plague, though neither died; among the uninoculated, there were 12 cases, 6 of which were fatal.[95]

On the face of it, these results appeared to provide grounds for mild optimism, but the reaction of scientists gathered in Bombay was mixed, and coloured by considerations which were far from 'purely scientific'. The German commission carried out inoculation experiments of its own, with encouraging results; it also commented favourably on an inoculation trial in Daman district, but found that the immunity conferred by inoculation was limited in duration. After conducting laboratory tests on monkeys, the Russian commission came to a similar conclusion. British medical men were generally not so sympathetic: Rogers and Bitter of the Egyptian commission found little reason for optimism in Haffkine's results. 'The fact that so many thousands of the population of Bombay have been inoculated since the end of January and have not contracted the disease proves nothing', insisted Rogers, 'the same people were presumably exposed to infection from August to the end of January, without being inoculated and without contracting the disease'. The Byculla jail figures were also dismissed by Rogers as inconclusive, without bothering to advance any specific objections.[96]

His assessment was not based solely on scientific criteria (though it might have been objected that the inoculations took place after the epidemic had begun, or that too few prisoners had been inoculated in proportion to the whole) but betrayed a certain amount of personal antipathy toward Haffkine, a laboratory scientist rather than a medical man like himself, as well as concern over the practical implications of over-enthusiasm for the new prophylactic. 'There is always the danger', he warned, "that the enthusiastic advocate for preventive inoculations, more particularly if he have a laboratory and not a medical and sanitary education, should view with indifference if not actually oppose the application of practical sanitary measures'.[97]

Suspicion of foreign laboratory scientists among British-trained doctors was equally evident in attitudes towards serum therapy. During the Hong Kong epidemic, Yersin had experimented with subcutaneous injections of curative serum drawn from horses injected with attenuated cultivations of the bacillus. On the outbreak of plague in Bombay, Yersin visited the city and initiated trials with serum provided by the Pasteur Institute at Nha Thrang, Indo-China. The results were inconclusive, and the reaction of Bombay's medical community – with some justification – almost uniformly hostile. (Though, in Yersin's favour, it should be remembered that the serum had been hurriedly prepared, and that it was weaker than that he had used in Hong Kong.) The best treatment for plague was thought to be 'early and good nursing' and an 'abundance of fresh air'.[98] However, with the arrival of the plague commissions, interest in serum therapy reawakened: the epidemic presented an unparalleled opportunity for bacteriologists, and the discovery of a cure for plague, the guarantee of world-wide renown.

Though he had obtained only moderately favourable results from tests of Yersin's serum, Haffkine was sufficiently encouraged to report that there was a 'possibility of the antitoxic serum rendering service in the treatment of the disease', and to attempt to develop a serum of his own.[99] V. C. Wyssokowitz of the Russian commission was even more sanguine about the prospects of serum therapy. 'En réalité', he claimed, 'le sèrum de Yersin a sauvé un grande nombre d'existences et nous devons très chaleureusement recommender cette méthode de traitement. Le sérum rest d'ailleurs jusqu'ici l'unique remède à employer dans le traitement de la peste.' The only report overtly hostile to serum therapy was again that of Rogers and Bitter of the Egyptian commission, who claimed not only that the results of the tests were inconclusive, but that trials on patients in whom the disease was already well advanced were a waste of time.[100] The results were, and remained, inconclusive, but these initial reactions reveal much about the prevailing anti-laboratory sentiments of an older generation of British-trained medical men.

In keeping with most official medical inquiries in Britain, the Indian Plague Commission, created in 1898, did not itself conduct laboratory investigations into plague, but assessed the evidence presented to it by IMS officers and others on plague duty in India. The commission comprised T. E. Fraser, professor of materia medica at Edinburgh University (president); J. P. Hewett, secretary to the Indian government (Home Department); A. E. Wright, professor of pathology at Netley; A. Cumine, senior collector, Bombay Presidency; M. A. Ruffer, president of the Egyptian Board of health; and C. J. Hallifax, ICS, secretary to the commission. It is notable that no IMS men served on the commission, and understandably this was taken as an affront by the service. The reason for their exclusion seems to be that the Indian government felt that 'differences of opinion between various authorities in India might detract from rather than enhance the value of the Report'.[101]

After 2 years of touring India, and hearing evidence and themselves observing plague measures in operation, the commission concluded that the plague bacillus infected humans by inoculation through the skin and through the nose and throat, but the infection through the alimentary canal was improbable. The theory put forward by the Frenchman Simond, that the bacillus passed into the bloodstream of the victim through the bite of the rat flea was regarded as inconclusive and improbable.[102] Both rats and humans were thought to carry the disease, but it was felt that rats did not often convey the disease over long distances. Certain types of clothing and certain raw materials, especially grain, were thought to harbour plague. No direct connection was established between plague mortality and meterological conditions. Insanitary conditions were also thought to be of only indirect relevance. Overcrowding was an important factor in the spread of the disease, but dirt and sewage did not seem to favour the propagation of the bacillus. Indeed, the commission felt that 'the opinions of plague officers who stress the importance of the connection between sanitary defects and plague were based more on theoretical considerations than on practical experience'.[103]

As regards prevention, the commission concluded that Haffkine's inoculation 'can and does exercise an immune effect' and that no serious ill effects had been produced so far. The results of serum therapy were thought to be inconclusive, but the commission held out hope of improved results in the long run.[104] The commission's conclusions reflected the strong bacteriological bias of two of its members – Wright and Ruffer. The former had been engaged in work on an anti-typhoid vaccine; the latter had been a pupil of Pasteur and Metchnikoff at the Institut Pasteur in Paris, and since 1896 had been professor of pathology at Cairo, where he had conducted research into phagocytosis and dysentery.[105]

Another of the recommendations made by the commission – and which reflected its concern for medical research – was the creation of a network of medical laboratories, to be engaged in investigations into the diagnosis, causation, and treatment of disease, and the effectiveness of prophylactic measures like disinfection. An additional but equally important function was to be the production of vaccines and sera. The commission thought that the laboratories established on an *ad hoc* basis during the epidemic should be made permanent, and that a new central research institute be established at Kasauli, a hill station which from 1900 had been the location of India's first Pasteur Institute.[106]

The Pasteur Institute had been the initiative of several European civilians acting in a non-official capacity. Beginning a fund-raising campaign in 1893, they had secured by the end of 1901, Rs 7,657 in private subscriptions and an Indian government military department grant of Rs 10,291. The Pasteur Institute, modelled on the Institut Pasteur in Paris, was concerned primarily with anti-rabies treatment and the production of anti-rabic vaccines, but also conducted routine bacteriological analyses of water and food items, together with some original research into the nature of disease.[107] Simultaneous with the report of the commission came the Indian government's decision to establish in each British Army command (excepting those in the Punjab and Assam) a bacteriological laboratory with the aim of identifying the chief sanitary problems in military cantonments and of providing assistance to their sanitary officer.[108]

Meanwhile, in Britain, James Cantile and W. J. Simpson, now retired from his post at Calcutta on grounds of ill health, had founded the *Journal of Tropical Medicine*. It was devoted to discussion of the etiology, treatment, and prevention of 'tropical diseases', and to fostering a sense of community between medical men in the tropics; official and non-official alike. In an attempt to secure official sponsorship of tropical medicine, Simpson and Cantlie linked tropical medicine explicitly to questions of imperial and military efficiency; a strategy which proved especially successful during the South African campaign of 1899–1902, amid public concern over levels of disease among British troops.[109] The reforming rhetoric of medical men was soon imbibed by the colonial secretary Joseph Chamberlain, and members of the mercantile community concerned about bankruptcy and indebtedness in the colonies. Some years earlier, with the founding of the Imperial Institute, an applied research organisation, a somewhat more optimistic and expansionist mood had prevailed.[110] Some of this rhetoric had rubbed off on the Indian administration. Concerned that scientific advice was lacking in India, Lord Elgin (viceroy from 1894 to 1899) persuaded the Royal Society, which had a history of involvement in imperial affairs, to establish an Indian Advisory Committee to provide scientific guidance for his government. However, there were no medical representatives on the committee; neither was medicine a priority for the Board of Scientific Advice established, with the same purpose, by Curzon in 1902. Both the Advisory Committee and the BSA favoured research in economic botany and geology.[111]

The trend towards state sponsorship of science provided a climate in which medical research was looked upon with more favour. But the institutionalisation of medical research took place separately, some years after the foundation of the IAC, reflecting its lower priority in the eyes of the Indian administration. The Indian Plague Commission made its recommendations at a time of mounting criticism of the Indian government's record in combating the disease. Simpson, editor of the *Journal of Tropical Medicine*, and an old adversary of the Indian government, was especially critical of its failure to exploit the potential of medical research:

> During the five years in which plague has prevailed in India there has been only one attempt to make anything like a scientific investigation into the subject, and that was in the first months of the plague . . . This apathy is not creditable to the Government which is losing thousands a week of its inhabitants from plague for lack of knowledge concerning the disease.[112]

In response to these pressures, the Curzon administration drew up proposals for a network of medical laboratories in India.[113] Existing laboratories were placed under imperial control and, in 1905, the Central Research Institute (CRI) was established at Kasauli in line with the commission's proposals.[114]

Much of the government's plan for a more extensive network of laboratories remained on paper, but it is unfair to claim that it provided 'no enduring foundation for the growth of medical science' in India.[115] Aside from important individual contributions to medical science by IMS officers, some of the laboratories established at the turn of the century continued to operate after the granting of independence in 1947.[116] Moreover, it is misleading to criticise the Indian government for its 'piecemeal' and 'ad hoc' development of medical research, when these labels, at least before the First World War, could apply equally well to the development of scientific research in Britain.[117] It is also misleading to claim that government chose to 'escape into medical research' as a means of avoiding any further commitment to public health reform.[118] In fact, from 1900 to 1914 the Indian government substantially increased its funding of both public health and medical research. There were, however, significant differences within the medical administration over the role of laboratory research in the broader context of sanitary policy.

Medical research and preventive policy: the case of malaria

Michael Worboys' study of the London and Liverpool schools of tropical medicine depicts two substantially different approaches to tropical medicine. One, espoused by Ronald Ross and the Liverpool school, represented an older, holistic and 'sanitary' tradition, in which laboratory work was integrated into a framework of vigorous practical measures. The other, espoused by Manson and the London school, reflected the Colonial Office's policy of 'deferred development', with its overriding concern with laboratory research and post-graduate teaching.[119] Though by no means static or exclusive, a similar difference in emphasis may be observed among medical officers in India, and is most clearly evident in debates over the prevention of malaria.

Prior to Ross' discovery of the malaria vector there were essentially two methods of preventing the disease: the drainage or avoidance of swampy areas, and the prophylaxis provided by various cinchona preparations, most commonly quinine. By 1900 extensive drainage schemes had been implemented in most of the larger Indian cities and, in 1860, India's first cinchona plantation was established in the Nilgiri Hills in Madras Presidency. Quinine powder manufactured there was not usually sold on the open market, but at a cost to medical departments for distribution among government employees, soldiers, and plantation workers. Quinine was an important 'tool of empire', but it is important not to exaggerate its role in colonial expansion and development.[120] It was not fully effective; it could have unpleasant side effects; it was not always readily available; and cinchona plantations often made considerable financial losses.[121]

Ross' identification of the Anopheles mosquito as the vector of malaria opened new avenues for public health work. Ross was an advocate of mosquito eradication campaigns: the draining of larval breeding ponds, larvicides, and the covering or filling-in of wells. Unable to persuade the government of the utility of these measures and prevented from continuing his research, Ross left India in 1899 a disgruntled and bitter man.[122] Significantly, the first such initiative was a predominantly metropolitan one: Drs R. S. Christophers and J. W. W. Stephens were sent to India by the Royal Society in 1900 in order to conduct experiments in mosquito eradication and other methods of malaria prevention at the military cantonment of Mian Mir in the Punjab. They were assisted in their investigations by Capt. S. P. James of the IMS. Shortly after their arrival a malaria conference, attended by delegates from all over India and from as far afield as West Africa, was convened at Nagpur. Its object was to disseminate up-to-date knowledge on the transmission of malaria, and to discuss the shape which any future preventive measures might take.[123]

With Ross's work still fresh in their minds, there was much talk at Nagpur of the desirability of military-style eradication campaigns like those currently conducted by members of the Liverpool school in Sierra Leone. Malaria work at Mian Mir also concentrated predominantly on the destruction of Anopheles breeding sites. Yet, there were many medical men who expressed doubts over the efficacy of such measures. 'Get rid of puddles by all means', wrote Captain Fearnside, superintendent of the Central Prison, Rajamundra, 'but I doubt whether, even if the whole population of India were put to the work of filling up all the puddles during the rains, the results would justify the expense'. The most effective way of preventing malaria, he believed, was the liberal use of quinine and the segregation of persons suffering from the disease.[124] W. J. Buchanan, shortly to become editor of the *Indian Medical Gazette*, was also convinced that quinine prophylaxis was the best means of preventing malaria in cantonments and prisons.[125]

The limitations of eradication campaigns became more evident following disappointing results at Mian Mir. In his report on malaria operations from 1901 to 1903, S. R. Christophers conceded that 'we have the somewhat startling fact

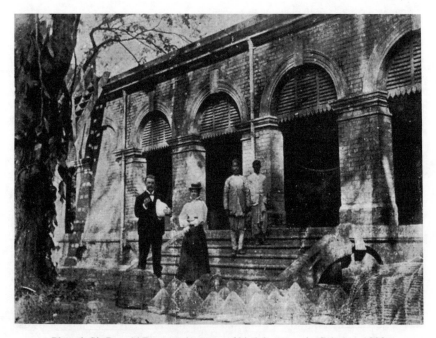

Plate 6 Sir Ronald Ross on the steps of his laboratory in Calcutta, 1898

that in spite of most energetic operations having been carried out continuously for many months, in which the whole of the canals had been cleared, 250 pits filled with earth, and large numbers of other breeding-places destroyed by oil, the reduction of adult Anopheles was at the most very slight'. By 1911 Christophers had come to the conclusion that 'the use of quinine as a prophylactic and as a means of saving the life of actual sufferers must be pushed to the utmost'.[126]

Major Leonard Rogers, IMS, an international authority on malaria, also drew attention to the financial constraints surrounding mosquito eradication. 'It is quite impossible', he argued, 'for the municipalities to find funds for either lining or levelling drains . . . or to keep them continuously kerosened to destroy the larvae, the attempts to do so having [been] abandoned in urban areas of Lower Bengal, while they are still more impossible in rural areas'. Like Fearnside, Rogers was an advocate of quinine prophylaxis and of the segregation of infected persons:

Since it has become known that in highly malarious places a large proportion of the . . . indigenous population harbour malarial parasites . . . from which mosquitoes become infected and carry the disease to Europeans . . . the separation . . . of houses inhabited by European immigrants from native huts by a distance of from one quarter to half a mile has become one of the most important prophylactic measures, which is specially applicable to railway construction and other temporary camps or in planning new towns.[127]

However, there were a good many medical officers who were reluctant to pin their faith on quinine, and a number of these took readily to Ross's method of mosquito eradication. J. A. Turner, health officer of Bombay, boasted that his was the first city in the world where an attempt to combat malaria according to modern knowledge had been made. His plan of attack consisted of general sanitary improvements, drainage, levelling of ground, filling-in of ditches, cleaning of wells, and mosquito extermination.[128] The sanitary commissioner with the Indian government, J. T. W. Leslie, and his successor in 1911 C. P. Lukis, also preferred general sanitary measures to quinine prophylaxis. Commenting on the 'tendency amongst malaria workers to divide into two camps . . . those who advocate anti-mosquito measures and those who pin their faith on quinine prophylaxis', he warned that 'we are perhaps too much inclined to pin our faith entirely on the scientific investigator to the detriment of the practical worker'.[129]

Though Lukis was keen to further the cause of medical research in India – being one of the founding members of the Indian Research Fund Association in 1911 – he was, like Ross, chiefly concerned with its practical application. He was concerned that quinine was not taken up by enough people, though its use had increased since it was first placed on sale to the Indian public in Bengal in

1874 at the price of Rs 1 an ounce. A new process of manufacture developed in Sikkim had made the drug somewhat cheaper, and during epidemics and in very malarious areas it was distributed to Indians free of charge.[130] European soldiers were also reluctant to take quinine regularly because of its nauseating side effects.[131]

Like Ross, Lukis represented an older 'sanitary' tradition, in which medical men combined scientific investigation with their duties as sanitary officers. But Rogers and Christophers held full-time appointments as medical researchers: Rogers as professor of pathology at Madras Medical College and bacteriologist to the Indian government; Christophers as assistant director of the CRI. Rogers and Christophers were more favourably disposed to 'specific' remedies, like quinine, which could be tried and tested under laboratory conditions. There was, however, some common ground between the two camps. Rogers and Christophers, for example, agreed with Ross that some form of segregation of the European and Indian communities was desirable as a preventive against the spread of malaria, yet they were aware that segregation could not be carried out so thoroughly as it had been under Ross in Freetown, Sierra Leone.[132]

The question of quinine prophylaxis was complicated considerably by the controversy which developed around the turn of the century over the etiology of 'blackwater fever' or 'haemoglobinuria'; so called because toxins released into a victim's bloodstream turned his or her urine dark red or 'black'. In retrospect the issue might appear rather arcane, and of little significance outside the pages of the specialist medical journal, but to contemporaries the causation of black-water fever was a matter of profound importance, having direct bearing upon colonial medical policy. One view, the most commonly held among medical men in India, was that blackwater fever was but a variant of malaria. A minority viewpoint, associated with Manson and Sambon at the London School of Tropical Medicine was that it was a disease *sui generis*. The most controversial view, but one which received a good deal of support internationally, was that blackwater fever was a form of quinine poisoning.[133] Though this idea had been in existence for some time, Robert Koch's support for the theory, after 1897, gave it a currency it had not previously enjoyed.[134]

Koch, as Ann Beck has pointed out, 'sometimes permitted his scientific judgement to be obscured by his conviction that Germany depended on emigration for survival as a great power'. In order to encourage German settlement in East Africa, where blackwater fever was prevalent, he was tempted to label blackwater fever as 'nothing but a disease of careless quinine takers'.[135] In other words, the disease was quite preventable and need not pose a barrier to European immigration. However, Koch's assertion seems to have had the opposite effect. Dr Moffat, principal medical officer of Uganda Protectorate observed that many patients in British East Africa would no longer take quinine, and feared that Koch's pronouncement would 'cause much harm'.[136] Colonel

Will, his successor, commented 10 years later that the medical authorities were still in a state of confusion about if and when the drug should be administered, and was himself doubtful of the efficacy of quinine compared to the use of mosquito nets and screens.[137]

In India medical opinion was similarly divided over blackwater fever. Stephens and Christophers maintained that it was simply a complication of malaria, and that quinine prophylaxis, if conducted in a proper manner, was invaluable as a preventive.[138] Leonard Rogers was of the same mind. Reflecting some years later on the blackwater fever controversy, he regretted the 'unfortunate impression created by Koch's theories in many tropical countries', and went on to criticise Manson and others who, while believing haemoglobinuria to be a separate disease, held that quinine excited the condition by inducing a sudden release of toxins from the spleen.[139] Yet there were some IMS officers who felt that the link between blackwater fever and quinine could not be ignored. Of 9 malaria cases treated with large doses of quinine, noted Arthur Powell, an IMS officer in Assam, 7 died, and 2 recovered: the 2 in which quinine treatment had been stopped. 'Till we hear further from Koch', warned Powell, 'his opinion must give us pause'.[140] In his presidential address to Grant College Medical Society, R. N. Khory also expressed his regret that 'the younger members of the profession . . . feel nervous and hesitate in using this important article'.[141] By 1907 medical opinion in India and abroad was moving in support of the 'malaria theory' of blackwater fever. Commentators generally agreed that the writings of Stephens and Christophers represented the latest and most advanced teachings on the subject.[142] However, the connection with quinine could not be denied, and it was now recognised that irregular treatment with the drug could exacerbate malarial symptoms.[143]

At its greatest intensity, the controversy over blackwater fever prejudiced medical men in India and elsewhere in other tropical colonies against the use of quinine, and strengthened the arm of those who continued to advocate more general methods of malaria prevention. Not surprisingly, the principal defenders of the 'malaria theory' of blackwater fever were Rogers, Christophers, and Stephens: the new generation of researchers who had set themselves behind quinine and other specific prophylactic measures. Only grudgingly did they admit that quinine was a complicating factor in the advanced malaria known as haemoglobinuria. Rogers and his colleagues were critical of Manson and the London school for expressing doubts over quinine. Though similar in respect of their full-time professional status as researchers, medical scientists in the colonies were more directly concerned with prevention, and with questions of 'practical imperialism' than their counterparts in the metropolis, for whom recognition among their scientific peers was an overriding concern. As Stephens observed in his *Historical Survey*, 'blackwater fever is perhaps the most important disease, medically and economically, affecting Europeans in the more malarious regions of the tropics. It is the mechanism by which malaria . . . most usually kills.'[144]

Medical desirability and practical limitations were by no means the only determinants of malaria policy in India. Much depended on the willingness of the government to finance malaria schemes, and on the financial and political circumstances affecting municipalities and local boards. After the apparent failure of experiments at Mian Mir and several uncoordinated attempts at mosquito eradication in other parts of India, there was something of a lull in anti-malarial activity. Where preventive measures continued, they had been integrated, and were barely distinct from ordinary sanitary activity. Provincial governments and local and municipal boards were generally reluctant to allot funds for 'special malaria work' or 'experimental demonstrations'.[145]

The first major initiative from the Indian government was its decision to convene an Imperial Malaria Conference at Simla in October 1909. The conference led to the creation of the Central Malaria Committee which was to direct investigations into the epidemiology of the disease and to supervise practical measures conducted by special malaria committees in each province. One of the most important functions of these bodies was thought to be education of the public in methods of malaria prevention; an implicit recognition of the financial and logistical limits to any such programme.[146] The Simla conference also led to the establishment of a new journal concerned with malaria work (*Paludism*), which published the transactions of the central committee. Following the conference, steps were taken to familiarise medical officers with the experimental techniques likely to be needed in any prolonged study of malaria. A course providing instruction in dissection, entomological anatomy, malaria survey work, and so on, was established at the new malaria laboratory at Amritsar. In its first year, the course was attended by 14 medical officers, 6 of whom were indigenous Indians.[147]

The plague epidemic had demonstrated that the use of indigenous agencies, and consultation with local élites, were crucial to the success of public health measures. The inclusion of Indians in research work was an outgrowth of this trend, and a reflection of Morley's decision to increase the recruitment of Indians into the IMS after 1905. Until 1909 anti-malarial operations had been confined almost exclusively to military cantonments and jails, or to the European quarters of Indian cities. Co-operation with the indigenous population was essential if these operations were to be extended, which seemed desirable in view of the fact that Indians were perceived as reservoirs of malarial infection. Government attempted to encourage local and municipal boards to allot more funds for drainage, and to increase the distribution of quinine to the general population.

But attempts to persuade Indians to take quinine as a prophylactic met with mixed success. Dr Amritaraj, health officer of Bangalore, believed the introduction of itinerant dispensaries for the distribution of quinine in Madras Presidency had 'met with scant success'. No attempt had been made to 'explain to the people in a simple and interesting manner the cause of malaria nor was instruction in its prevention given'.[148] Medical officers were themselves uncertain whether quinine should be distributed free of charge, some believing that this should be done only during epidemics. Other measures, like the closing of wells, also proved unpopular with the indigenous population, since wells and tanks had social and often religious significance.[149] Elsewhere drainage operations continued to be hampered by lack of funds, or failed to receive official support because of their implications for economic activity. Agricultural production in most areas of India was heavily dependent on irrigation.[150]

The progress of anti-malarial activity after 1911 was intimately bound up with the development of institutionalised medical research in India. Research into malaria transmission and the effects of quinine prophylaxis had been undertaken for several years at the CRI, under its director Lieutenant-Colonel Semple, RAMC. But malaria work formed only one part of the institute's research programme, which included investigations into dysentery, mala-azar, 'epidemic dropsy', and the effectiveness of various vaccines and sera.[151] However, malaria research was the most important activity of the Indian Research Fund Association, founded in 1912. Its president, Harcourt Butler, was education member of the viceroy's council. Butler was an ambitious man who had harnessed his career to the twin causes of education and sanitary reform. His undoubted energies raised the association to a position of some prominence, from which it was able to attract substantial support in the way of funds and good will.[152]

The IRFA was funded partly by subscription and partly by government. Life members paid a lump sum of Rs 5,000 while temporary members paid Rs 100 annually. Its membership included several prominent Indians; one, Kumar Maharaj Singh, became the association's first secretary.[153] From the Indian government, the association received an annually recurring grant of Rs 5 lakhs.[154] The Finances of the IRFA were sufficient to sustain a periodical – the *Indian Journal of Medical Research* – which was founded in 1913 and edited by the DGIMS and the sanitary commissioner with the Indian government. It took the place of *Paludism* (never a popular publication) and *Scientific Memoirs*, giving the *Indian Journal* official status. However, its pages were open to members of India's non-official medical community.

The sanitary commissioner, the DGIMS, his secretary, the director of the CRI, and the officer in charge of the Malaria Bureau (Central Committee), comprised the other members of the governing body. The governing body, in turn, appointed the Scientific Advisory Board which included three of its own members, plus Christophers, and Ronald Ross as an advisory member. Thus, the very constitution of the IRFA reflected its overriding concern with malaria, now regarded as the most important disease affecting colonial development.[155] Accordingly, the association allotted substantial sums to local governments to carry out surveys of anti-malarial measures; a total of Rs 355,000 in its first year.[156] There was also evidence of an increased willingness on the part of local governments to fund medical research. In 1912 the Bengal government granted a lakh of rupees to enable Rogers to carry out his scheme for the foundation of the School of Tropical Medicine in Calcutta.[157] The Indian government, however, refused an application to help meet recurring expenditure. It also turned down a request from the Bombay government for a grant of 10 lakhs to finance a Bombay School of Tropical Medicine, in accordance with proposals by Major G. Liston, Director of the Plague Research Laboratory.[158] Presumably, only one such institution was deemed necessary.

By identifying themselves with governmental and public concerns, research-oriented medical men managed to create a niche for themselves in the colonial administration, securing full-time posts in a number of research institutes established throughout India. As it became intertwined with the language of imperial efficiency and humanitarian reform, the cause of medical science was taken up by dynamic colonial administrators and prominent Indians, attracting considerable support in the way of private subscriptions and government funds. But India was no 'gigantic laboratory' in which European medical experts were given free rein. Professional objectives succeeded only where they intersected with those of the Indian government. The institutionalisation of tropical medicine came about in response to pressures created by the Indian plague epidemic, and in the wake of international criticism of the government's response to the disease. The same is true of initiatives regarding malaria. Malaria research was given priority because it was thought to be the most important medical barrier to colonial development. By leading the way in malaria research, and by convening international conferences in India, the Indian government sought to enhance its international standing, for malaria was a disease prevalent throughout the colonial tropics. Other diseases, especially those confined to the indigenous population, began to receive more attention after 1900, but attracted far less in the way of government support.

One further point needs to be made concerning the place of medical research in preventive policy in India. The blackwater fever controversy reveals two different (but not exclusive) approaches to malaria control. The first, advocated by Ross, conceived of malaria control in terms of vector eradication and general sanitation; the other placed most emphasis on prophylaxis with quinine. The former had greatest appeal in India, being largely an extension of traditional methods of malaria control. But those who advocated heavy or exclusive reliance on quinine were confined largely to laboratory scientists like Rogers and Stephens, who displayed a predilection for specific measures which could be tried and tested in the laboratory.

7

Public health and local self-government

It is in the municipalities that progress in sanitation must be looked for. (Alfred Lyall, secretary to the Government of India, 1874)[1]

The 1880s saw profound changes in the administration of public health in India. Under Lord Ripon – viceroy from 1880 to 1884 – Gladstonian Liberalism reached its zenith, marked by controversial reforms of the judicial system and the extension of local government. One of the principal motives behind devolution was economic. The reforms of the 1880s did not mark a total break with the past, but accelerated the process of financial and administrative decentralisation set in train by Mayo in the early 1870s. But, whereas Mayo's primary concern was to pass the responsibility for sanitation, road maintenance, and other local services from central to provincial government, Ripon sought, equally, to reform the machinery of local administration. Chief among Ripon's concerns was the lack of indigenous representation on municipal commissions, dominated by 'official', mostly European, nominees. He also aimed to extend representative local government in rural areas, most of which was under the direct control of British district commissioners.

These ideas took shape within the context of growing criticism in British liberal circles of 'paternalistic' government in India, but also bore some relation to practical problems arising from the administration of India. By the late 1860s, it was understood that greater indigenous representation on municipal commissions would be necessary if Indian taxpayers were to shoulder the financial burden of local sanitary works.[2] More generally, administrators had come to recognise that India could be governed only with the co-operation of the Indian people, especially with regard to matters of health and hygiene, which impinged directly on indigenous cultural practices.

Ripon's resolution on local self-government of May 1882 established a majority-elected element on each municipal commission, although provincial governments were left to decide the exact proportion of official to non-official

166

members in municipal bodies under their jurisdiction.[3] Electors constituted only a very small proportion of citizens in each town, comprising Europeans and wealthy Indian ratepayers.[4] Ripon was aware that, in its early stages, the transition to local self-government might prove detrimental to the provision of local services, but saw administrative devolution as the only long-term solution to the problem of how best to govern India. 'It is better to endure the postponement of even really useful measures', he wrote, 'than to check the advance of habits of self-government among the people'.[5] That Indians were ambivalent towards European notions of sanitation and hygiene was already clear from the experience of the provincial capitals, where elected Indian representatives had served on municipal commissions since the early 1870s. In Calcutta, for example, the Municipal Bill of 1871 had been opposed and its enactment delayed for 4 years because of opposition from the Hindu British Indian Association.[6]

Indigenous hostility or indifference towards western notions of public health was only one of several obstacles which stood in the way of administrative decentralisation. Some Europeans viewed moves towards local self-government as an abdication of Britain's responsibility towards its imperial subjects. Many more were perturbed by what seemed to be their loss of authority, particularly after the introduction of the Ilbert Bill in 1883, which granted Indian magistrates the power to try criminal cases against British subjects.[7]

The impact of local self-government upon sanitation in India is still extremely unclear. On the one hand, Hugh Tinker contends that 'only in Bengal was there a real demand for [sanitary] services and some willingness to pay for them. Elsewhere public health services were developed only because officials fostered them.'[8] On the other, Ramasubban claims that the Indian government 'lost the historic moment for initiating sanitary reform' and, at every opportunity, sought to scuttle Indian initiatives on matters of public health.[9] The following analysis evaluates these claims in the light of statistics relating to the income and expenditure of local authorities, and a systematic survey of sanitary reports and government documents. It casts doubt upon Ramasubban's thesis and, in particular, her exaggerated claims for indigenous enthusiasm for public health. It provides some support for Tinker's claim that indigenous resistance was as important as revenue shortages, or the lack of government subsidy, in arresting the development of sanitation in India. The central problem with both approaches is that sanitary progress in India is judged according to standards derived from European experience. Though Tinker's account more accurately reflects the complexity of the situation than does Ramasubban's, neither questions the applicability of western sanitary measures to the Indian context; neither adequately takes into account the actual feelings of indigenous peoples towards these new concepts of hygiene and prevention.

The municipalities

Public health prior to 1882

On the eve of the Ripon reforms, the priority attached to sanitation varied enormously from one municipality to another. In Calcutta, socio-religious barriers and sectional interests stood in the way of reform,[10] while in Bombay City, commercial factors were of paramount importance in shaping the municipality's attitude towards public health. Under pressure from the city's commercial lobby, the municipal commission was anxious to play down the threat from cholera and other epidemic diseases. Since the 1860s, the city had been identified in Europe as the principal source from which cholera spread to the West, and vessels sailing from the port were subject to regular quarantine. Reluctance to acknowledge the incidence of cholera appears to have fostered a certain lethargy regarding sanitation, although a reform-minded minority attempted to goad the corporation into activity.

Most outspoken in condemnation of the municipality was its health officer, Dr Blaney. 'There is not sufficient vigilance', he protested in 1882, against the corporation's failure to take precautions against cholera, 'and if no stimulus be applied, matters will . . . take their course and the city will be overtaken by a great mortality'.[11] The *Bombay Gazette*, champion of the city's commercial lobby, refused to acknowledge that there was any prospect of a cholera epidemic, and defended the record of the corporation on matters of public health. 'During one quarter of last year', it claimed that 'no fewer than 500 persons were removed from buildings in which cholera had shown itself . . . In other cases tiles were taken off infected buildings and holes made in the walls so as to let in light, all walls [were] washed with a solution of carbolic acid and lime, disinfectants were freely used in the homes and in the vicinity.'[12] But it was the want of basic conservancy arrangements that most concerned Dr Blaney and his predecessors.

Opposition to more vigorous sanitary activity came not only from commercial interest groups, but also from prominent members of the indigenous population. In 1869, Bombay's first health officer, John Lumsdaine, felt it necessary to defend his appointment at length in his first annual report, in 1869. His most outspoken opponent was an Indian municipal commissioner – Rao Sahib Vishranth Narayen Mundalik – who argued that 'there can be no doubt whatsoever that we do not require an Executive Officer of Health, which in plain speaking means a Superintendent of Halalcores on 2,000 rupees a month'.[13] Lumsdaine believed that opposition to his appointment was not simply a financial matter, but that it had its roots in traditional Indian notions of hygiene and ritual purity: 'the European was alone eligible' to hold the post of health officer: 'the native may be as good a man, but he is disqualified by caste, deterred by religion. The very nature of the work is such that he cannot undertake it.'[14]

Another obstacle was the unwillingness of the provincial government to involve itself, financially, in the sanitation of the city. In 1867 the sanitary commissioner for Bombay complained that a drainage scheme prepared by the Bombay corporation had been scrapped because the Government of Bombay had decided that 'the onus of producing a financially practicable scheme should ... rest with the municipality ... Government has not proposed that any portion of the cost of such works should fall on the general revenue.'[15] The inadequacy of Bombay's water supply was another frequent cause of complaint, as was the insufficient number of subordinate sanitary staff (road-sweepers, night soil collectors, and so on) employed by the city's municipal commission.[16]

Sanitary conditions were no better in Madras City. The municipal corporation was overburdened with police charges imposed upon it by the presidency government, and had embarked upon a policy of retrenchment in order to reduce its debts. The city's sanitary establishment was reduced at a time when many of its European inhabitants felt that sanitary measures should be stepped up. 'The filthy conditions in which so many streets are found', and the 'nauseous knock-me-down smells that issue from the uncleansed gutters', argued the *Madras Times*, called either for 'greater activity in the Health Department, or for an increase in the number employed in it'.[17] The financial position of the Madras corporation was such that extensions to the city's water supply were delayed, placing it at the mercy of ratepayers who demanded the service they had paid for. In July 1880 the Madras government decided to intervene, in order to prevent the issue of suits against the corporation, allowing it time to complete the water supply scheme.[18] Even advocates of sanitary reform felt that the scheme was 'far too expensive in the existing condition of the municipality'.[19]

The Madras corporation was in no position to borrow more money from government and had little room to increase rates of local taxation, which were already the highest in India.[20] Protests were strongest from the well-to-do Indian residents of the 'Black Town' who, in many cases, had been paying water-rates for 3 years despite not having been connected to the piped supply.[21] Others protested that much of the money taken from them in taxes had been 'squandered and wickedly frittered away', or embezzled by the city's municipal commissioners. Disenchanted ratepayers went to far as to accuse the municipality of favouritism in handing out contracts for public works. In one case it was alleged that the corporation had accepted a tender more expensive than seventeen of the other applications.[22]

Sanitary progress was even slower in the majority of mofussil municipalities. In 1881, no sanitary work of any magnitude was undertaken in the North West Provinces, Berar, Assam, or Madras province. In the other provinces, major sanitary works were confined to a handful of prosperous towns with relatively large European populations. Jubbulapore in the Central Provinces, Lahore in the Punjab, and Dinajpore in Bengal, initiated or completed drainage and water-supply schemes in that year.[23] The cause of sanitary reform in Bengal was aided in 1881 by the government's decision to relieve municipalities of police expenditure. The burden of police charges had been shifted from provincial government onto municipalities in 1867.[24]

Sanitation and self-government

British officials were deeply divided in their attitudes to Ripon's reforms of local government. Senior medical officers, who had backed administrative devolution since the 1870s, declared their enthusiastic support for local self-government. 'The system of local government lately inaugurated', claimed the sanitary commissioner, J. M. Cuningham, 'cannot fail to have a decided effect upon sanitary progress. By giving over these matters to local management, there can be little doubt that the residents will bestir themselves regarding them in a way they have never done hitherto.'[25] He believed that sanitation was an alien system that should not be imposed on the Indian people regardless of their cultural sensibilities. But, like Ripon, Cuningham knew that the success of sanitation would depend equally upon expert guidance and the co-operation of provincial government in implementing and overseeing municipal projects.[26]

Yet many officers of Cuningham's own department did not share his enthusiasm for local self-government; nor, indeed, did many officers of the ICS. Ripon faced protracted resistance from paternalistic administrators like Sir James Fitzjames Stephen and Sir Henry Maine. These men, both formerly legal members of the viceroy's council, campaigned for 'pure and clear intelligence' in government and 'straightforward assertion' of the superiority of the 'conquering race'.[27] The strongest opposition to Ripon came from Bombay, where the Conservative governor-general Sir James Ferguson published a resolution condemning Ripon's proposals as 'unduly radical and premature'.[28] The Bombay government permitted only one-half of municipal commissioners to be elected, the rest being official nominees. In Bengal two-thirds of municipal commissioners were elected, and in Madras and the North West Provinces (NWP), the proportion was three-quarters.[29] It was clear that in Bombay, at least, the newly constituted municipalities would not receive the support from government that Ripon thought necessary for the success of his reforms.

On the eve of the Ripon reforms, municipal allotments to sanitation in all three provinces increased sharply. In Bengal, there was an increase in total sanitary allotments, and in allotments as a percentage of municipal incomes. These increases are expressed graphically in figures 7.1 and 7.2 below, and in tabular form in appendix C. This increase was probably a consequence of the lifting of the very considerable burden of police charges in 1881. The fact that sanitary allotments increased more sharply as an aggregate figure than as a percentage of income suggests that rising municipal incomes may have permitted more money to be spent on local services: municipal incomes in Bengal rose from 2.7 million rupees in 1878–9 to 3.1 million in 1881–2.

Allotments to sanitation in Bombay province also increased between 1879 and 1883, but more unevenly than in Bengal. Here, again, the fate of sanitation appears to have depended on the ability of municipalities to raise sufficient revenue. In Bombay, municipal incomes fell from 2.6 million in 1880 to 2.4 in 1882, rising to 2.9 in 1882. In Madras province the increase in sanitary expenditure was continuous, though less marked than in the other two presidencies, reflecting a slow but steady rise in municipal incomes between 1879 and 1883.

The introduction of local self-government in 1883–4 provided a stimulus to increased expenditure on municipal sanitation; the one important exception being Bombay province.[30] In Bengal, municipal expenditure on sanitation rose markedly, though erratically, from approximately Rs 700,000 in 1880–1 to almost 2.1 million in 1893–4. As a percentage of municipal incomes, sanitary expenditure rose more steadily to reach a plateau of around 40 per cent between

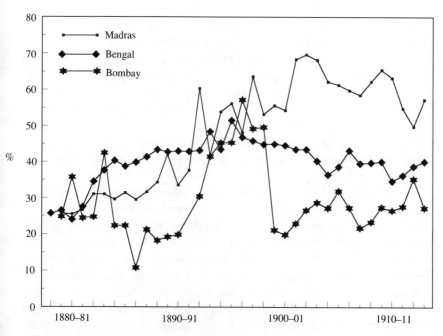

Figure 7.1 Allotments to sanitation as percentage of income: mofussil municipalities

1884–5 and 1893–4. The exceptionally high expenditure on sanitation during 1893–4 may be due in part to large revenue surpluses in that year. The relatively stable proportion of income expended no sanitation between 1884–5 and 1893–4 reflects prevailing attitudes on how best to sanitise Indian cities. The official view, in which most municipal commissioners appear to have concurred, was that large, capital-intensive sanitary programmes were unnecessary and counter-productive. More general and less obtrusive measures, which did not depart radically from existing arrangements, were preferred. Such programmes did not require large injections of capital (their costs being of an annually recurring nature), and were less likely to offend indigenous sensibilities.

The considerable progress in municipal sanitation that occurred in Bengal between 1884–5 and 1893–4 owed much to the underlying stability of municipal incomes. It was not simply that the province was free from famine and serious crop failure during this period, but that the principal sources of municipal income in Bengal were, themselves, linked only indirectly to economic activity. In Bengal, 39 per cent of municipal income was derived from house and land taxes, 28 per cent from water and conservancy rates, and the rest principally from loans. These were forms of fixed taxation and therefore less liable to fluctuations in economic fortunes than other forms of local taxation in India like octroi and terminal tax (taxes on staple goods and imported produce).[31] Another important factor was the Bengal government's comparative readiness to grant loans and make small grants-in-aid available to municipalities for sanitary improvements. In the years immediately following the passage of the Local Government Loans Act of 1879, it lent considerable sums for basic drainage and water-supply schemes.[32] Indeed, municipal sanitation was buoyed up by government loans throughout the 1880s and 90s, but these were conditional on a municipality's previous sanitary record.

Even in Bengal, where sanitary allotments were higher than in other provinces of Indian, municipal commissioners were often reluctant to fund sanitary improvements, sometimes on religious or cultural grounds, but more commonly to save their own pockets and those of their electors. The fact that Indian land-lords dominated municipal commissions in Bengal after 1884 meant that there was considerable hostility to the imposition of the house tax, and that little action was taken in respect of the slums from which those landlords drew their rent.[33]

Indian ratepayers, too, went to great lengths to oppose taxation for sanitary purposes. In 1885 Mohendranath Banerjea and other ratepayers of the Darjeeling municipality petitioned the Bengal government to withhold sanction from the corporations proposal to introduce a water-rate and to increase the existing house rate by one-third. The lieutenant-governor, however, was convinced of the utility of the new tax and permitted the corporation to go ahead with its plans.[34] On other occasions the lieutenant-governor actually made the extension of an elected element under the 1884 Municipal Act conditional upon a municipality's commitment to sanitary works. In the case of Howrah municipality, the granting of an elected element was dependent upon its submitting to the provincial government a scheme for a filtered water supply.[35]

There was, however, some evidence of enthusiasm for sanitary reform among the Indian élite. In 1887, one Bengali bequeathed over a lakh of rupees, while in 1890 Raja Surja Kant donated Rs 112,500 for the building of a waterworks in Mymersingh.[36] Also, once sanitary measures had been introduced in a municipality, indifference or opposition to them generally diminished over time. In 1891, the sanitary commissioner of Bengal noted that many 'prejudices', including those against the trenching of night soil had given way.[37] The following year, he reported that all municipalities under his jurisdiction now trenched their night soil as a matter of course.[38]

Yet the pace of sanitary progress was extremely uneven. Aggregate figures conceal wide variations in municipal sanitary expenditure. In 1893 sanitary allotments varied from a maximum of 82.3 per cent of municipal income in Nasirabad to only 2.2 per cent in Patuakhali.[39] Water purification seems to have been a particularly sensitive issue, since water-supply schemes often interfered with indigenous bathing and cremation rituals; waterworks and filtration plants also entailed considerable expense. In 1891, for instance, the sanitary commissioner of Bengal expressed his displeasure with the failure of municipal commissioners at Monghur to agree to a proposal by the East Indian Railway Company to share the cost of a filtered water-supply to the town.[40]

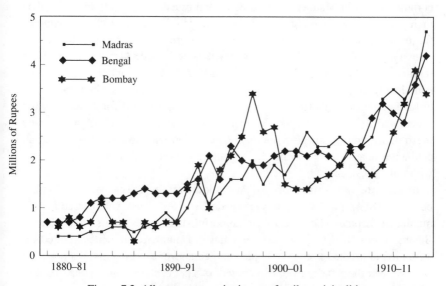

Figure 7.2 Allotments to sanitation: mofussil municipalities

Similarly, the unrest sparked by the building of a waterworks at the sacred city of Benares, in the North West Provinces, provides a dramatic illustration of the cultural limits to sanitary intervention. Proposals to construct a waterworks on the site of an old Hindu temple on the banks of the Ganges caused extensive rioting in the city, led, reputedly, by members of the Gujurati brahmin community. However, it seems likely that the waterworks, an icon of western civilisation, provided the focus for wider social, perhaps political, discontents, and was not in itself the principal 'cause' of the riot.[41]

The introduction of local self-government in Madras initially made little impact on sanitary expenditure in mofussil municipalities. As figures 7.1 and 7.2 show, allotments to sanitation continued to rise at much the same rate as before, and as a percentage of municipal incomes, changed little, with annual figures fluctuating gently around a mean of 33 per cent between 1882 and 1891. Municipal incomes rose steadily from 1.6 million in 1882 to 2.1 in 1890. Thus, while sanitary progress was in no way hampered by the introduction of local self-government, it received no great stimulus either; at least until 1891. As in Bengal, the variables affecting sanitation were threefold: the availability of funds, the attitudes of municipal commissioners, and the level of financial aid from provincial government. Madras was in a comparatively favourable position as regards its principal sources of municipal revenue: the majority of municipal income (46 per cent) was derived from property tax, 14 per cent from water and conservancy rates, and only 10 per cent from trades tax.[42]

This meant that municipal incomes in Madras were relatively stable, being affected only indirectly by fluctuations in economic activity. But municipal commissioners in Madras were no more enthusiastic about public health than their counterparts in Bengal: sanitary officers in southern India complained frequently that municipal sanitary budgets were seldom fully utilised. The sanitary commissioner of Madras noted with concern in 1884 that municipalities regularly failed to make full use of their sanitary allotments, and that government had already taken steps 'to impress upon all municipalities . . . the necessity of utilizing all allotments for sanitary purposes during the year for which they are sanctioned'.[43] Again, in 1886, he expressed consternation at the 'apathy and indifference on the part of municipal boards in utilizing to the fullest extent all available means for removing the insanitary condition of cities and villages' within the presidency.[44]

Indeed, the proportion of sanitary allotments actually spent in Madras between 1882 and 1893 rarely exceeded 60 per cent. The percentage of municipal incomes allocated to sanitation in Madras was also smaller than in Bengal. From 1882 to 1890, the percentage of municipal incomes allotted for sanitation in Madras averaged 31 per cent, and never exceeded 34.3 per cent; in Bengal, over the same period, it averaged 38.8 per cent, reaching a maximum of 43.3 per cent.

Impressionistic evidence also suggests sanitation had made little headway in Madras, even in the presidency capital. In 1884 the *Madras Times* reported that 'the old drains that are still standing are blocked up, so that foul and stinking matter is left there, and mosquitoes breed in large numbers. Besides this, the sands of the beach and the walls of the harbour are used as latrines by the natives.'[45] Five years later, conditions had apparently improved very little. 'At the present time', wrote the editor of the *Times*, 'when showers of rain have helped to stimulate the evils that are submitted to the consideration of the olfactory nerves, we would defy any ordinary mortal to take a stroll about the town or the suburbs without finding plenty of places only too desirous of attention'.[46] In the opinion of most Europeans, Madras was a 'city of foul smells' and its river, the 'silvery Cooum', little short of a 'main drain on a large scale'.[47]

It seems likely that the lower priority attached to sanitation in Madras reflects lower levels of awareness of public health issues among municipal commissioners in the presidency (at least prior to the plague epidemics). However, it remains unclear why municipal commissioners in Madras were slower to take on board western notions of hygiene and sanitation than their counterparts in Bengal. One reason may have been that Calcutta, the capital city, and the locus of British power in India, was the first city to adopt, under European guidance, a western system of public health. Public interest in sanitation is also indicated by the formation of India's first public health society in 1884, which included eight Indian members in the late-1880s.[48] The benefactions of Indian dignitaries also show that these activities had at least some impact on western educated Indians.[49] It was in Bengal, too, that western science made its greatest impact on Indian culture, being actively cultivated by the westernised *bhadralok* community.[50]

Although the extent of Indian enthusiasm for sanitary reform in Bengal was limited to a small western-educated section of the Indian élite, there is even less evidence of indigenous interest in public health in Madras. In fact, in Madras City, there was considerable criticism of the Indian-dominated corporation for its inaction in sanitary matters, albeit largely from disgruntled Europeans. 'The Municipality of Madras', alleged the editor of the *Madras Times*, 'are not equal to the preservation of this city . . . If any native member of the Municipal Council shews [*sic*] a disposition to be useful . . . when the next election in his division takes place, the electors return someone more obsequious. And some are said to enter the Commission because patronage and other advantages attend a seat therein.'[51]

But such criticisms should be viewed within the context of the deeply ingrained European prejudices against Indian life styles and resentment of moves towards local self-government in the 1870s and 80s. Correspondents to English-language newspapers in Madras continually expressed their alarm at 'wretched and unsightly' huts which were considered prejudicial to the health of Europeans.[52] Their frustration at the municipal commission commonly manifested itself in calls for more European executive staff, or for government intervention.[53]

However, the years 1892–3 marked a turning-point in the fortunes of municipal sanitation in Madras, and sanitary expenditure increased sharply during that year. The chief reason for this sudden increase was almost certainly the extension of the Madras Municipal Act to forty more towns in 1890.[54] Prior to that date, the level of sanitary provisions in these towns would have been minimal and, in their first few years, newly established corporations would have spent high proportions of their income in laying the basic foundations of municipal sanitation.

This interpretation is supported by the fact that expenditure on sanitation fell somewhat over the next few years, as fixed costs, such as the construction of latrines, the purchasing of carts, and so on, diminished. Existing municipalities also began to spend more on sanitation at this time. By 1893, the first drainage schemes outside the provincial capital – at Coonoor and Cuddapore – were nearing completion. In the same year, the Government of Madras began to consider the modernisation of the Madras Municipal Act of 1884, so that municipalities would be permitted to raise house taxes and water-rates in order to finance more ambitious sanitary schemes.[55]

Bombay was the exception among the three presidencies in that only there did the introduction of local self-government coincide with a prolonged decrease in sanitary expenditure. Allotments to sanitation fell sharply after 1883, and remained at a low level until the mid-1890s.

To what are we to attribute this decline? One possibility is that municipal corporations had problems in raising funds for sanitary purposes, but on this score the evidence is, at best, ambiguous. On the one hand, aggregate municipal incomes in Bombay rose steadily over this period, from Rs 2.7 million in 1883 to 4.7 million in 1895; on the other, these aggregate figures concealed considerable local variations. In the district of Nasik municipal incomes varied from Rs 40,000 to Rs 1,400; while the aggregate income of municipalities varied considerably from year to year, from Rs 71,920 in 1879, to 55,026 in 1880, to 86,916 in 1881.[56]

Local variations in municipal income are vital when considering sanitary expenditure because, unless a municipality could rely upon a certain minimum income, it was unable to budget for even the most basic sanitary provisions. Individual municipalities in Bombay were more sensitive to fluctuations in economic activity than those in the other two presidencies, since their principal source of revenue was octroi, a tax on the importation of goods. Some 47 per cent of municipal incomes in Bombay was derived from this source, the remainder from water-rates and trades tax. In this respect, Bombay had more in common with the Central Provinces and the Punjab, than with Bengal and Madras. Municipalities in these provinces derived 52 per cent and 90 per cent of their respective revenues from octroi and display marked annual fluctuations in levels of sanitary expenditure.

Octroi was a particularly unpopular form of taxation. As well as providing an unstable basis for municipal revenues, it was evidently a hindrance to free-trade, being actively denounced by British administrators and the indigenous commercial lobby. In 1908, the Punjab Trades Association began a campaign for the abolition of octroi and its replacement with a house tax, such as that which existed in Delhi.[57] Cognizant of the disadvantages of octroi from an administrative point of view, the Punjab government was not unsympathetic to these demands, but prevaricated in the face of opposition from Indian property owners, concerned about its replacement by a house tax. The government favoured a decreased reliance upon octroi, but thought that its total abolition was out of the question.[58]

Similarly, in the United Provinces (formerly, the NWP and Oudh), a committee convened by government to go into the octroi question, suggested its replacement with a graded licence tax on occupations, and on zemindars and other persons of independent means.[59] It concluded that 'octroi is entirely undesirable on many grounds, as a source of municipal income. It is deemed to have all the defects and few of the virtues of indirect taxation, to be a most serious check on trade and prosperity, and to afford opportunities for the oppression of a large class which cannot or will not complain, through inability to express itself or respect for authority and custom.'[60]

Another reason for the decrease in sanitary expenditure following the introduction of local self-government was resistance to western sanitation on the part of municipal commissioners. Sanitary officers in Bombay often claimed that it was not so much lack of money as indigenous customs that stood in the way of sanitary progress.[61] According to T. G. Hewlett, sanitary commissioner of Bombay, the appalling sanitary condition of Nasik was 'an index of the little interest the Municipal Commissioners take in the sanitation of their picturesque city'. What was lacking, in his view, was clear direction and leadership on the part of municipal commissioners, and some means of compelling local authorities to adhere to a basic sanitary standard.[62] The following year he expressed concern that the municipal commissioners at Belgaum had proved 'absolutely incapable of attending to their responsible duties in regard to the sanitation of the town'.[63] Moreover, he had received complaints from some residents of Lonavli about one of the town's own municipal commissioners who had repeatedly flouted sanitary by-laws relating to contamination of the water supply.[64] Summing up the fate of sanitation in the 1880s, in his report of 1891, Hewlett concluded that 'the cause of sanitation has not in any way profited or prospered under local self-government. On the contrary, several towns have of late appeared to me to be growing more apathetic concerning this subject, which does not seem to be popular or fashionable at Congress meetings.'[65]

The prolonged dispute over the drainage of Bombay City provides some support for this view. During the 1880s the sanitary commissioner of Bombay locked horns with the city's municipal commission over his proposals for an underground sewerage scheme, similar to that existing in many European cities. Hindu municipal commissioners appear to have opposed the scheme on financial and socio-religious grounds, and received support from Bombay's health officer Dr Blaney, who thought the scheme unsuited to a tropical climate. Blaney believed that a system of open drains would be more appropriate, claiming it would make the city 'another Hygeia, a sanitary paradise'. The *Bombay Gazette*, however, favoured an underground system, and in 1883 expressed disappointment that a number of Indian municipal commissioners, including the chairman V. N. Mundalik, had supported Blaney in his 'jehad against the new sewerage system'.[66]

In 1885 there was another unsuccessful attempt to lay the scheme before the corporation. 'An agitation was got up at the eleventh hour to resist the proposal', reported the *Gazette*, 'the opposition was unexpectedly strengthened by a rise in the price of materials and in the cost of skilled labour . . . Nothing was done.'[67] Well over a decade elapsed before these differences were finally resolved, the plague epidemics of 1896 onward providing the spur for the scheme's eventual completion. Blaney and Indian commissioners who had opposed the scheme were denounced by the *Gazette* as being partly responsible for the spread of 'bubonic fever' in the city.[68]

But, where municipal commissions had attempted to emulate European sanitary reforms, the results were far from encouraging. The provision of a piped water-supply in Bombay provides one such example. Completed in 1860, the water-supply scheme, which pumped water from tanks in the hills surrounding Bombay, provided very little water per head of population in the city. Even after improvements were made in 1868, the supply was irregular and, in total, equivalent to only 15 gallons of water per person per day. Moreover, there were still problems in securing the purity of the piped supply. One observer commented in 1883 that 'it is a notorious fact that during the hot months of April and May, when the water level reaches low, our drinking water becomes palpably impure to the eye and nauseous to taste, not to speak of its injurious effects on health'.[69]

In the mofussil, the priority attached to sanitation by Indian municipal commissioners varied considerably. In 1889, the Bombay sanitary commissioner praised the Indian chairman of Bulsar municipality for carrying out 'many improvements during the tenure of his office'.[70] But, in the same year, he asserted that sanitation in Dharwar could not be expected to progress 'so long as municipal commissioners continue to use pit privies in their own homes and

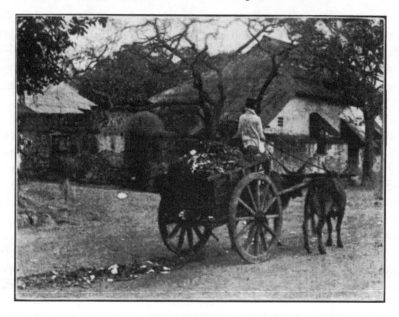

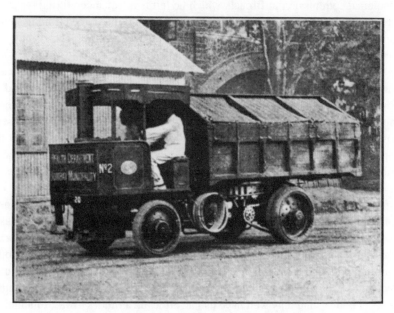

Plate 7 Refuse disposal 'old style' and 'new style' in Bombay

defend the system on the score of its antiquity'.[71] After returning to Dharwar in 1891, the sanitary commissioner was 'not sanguine of the municipality taking the initiative in any improvement bearing on public health. Without guidance and support they are helpless. In my opinion, local self-government is the bane of sanitary progress.'[72] In other areas, as late as the turn of the century, the sanitary commissioner reported opposition to water-rates, ostensibly on religious grounds.[73]

Official reports, in their attempts to differentiate between the performance of municipalities, provide a reasonably accurate picture of indigenous attitudes to sanitation at this time. Sanitary officers were concerned to highlight not only the worst cases of indigenous indifference or 'apathy', but also instances of progress which could be held up as examples to be followed. Moreover, the ambivalent attitude of Indians to municipal sanitation is borne out by existing scholarship on municipal politics in India, and by reports in the indigenous press.[74] The *Hindustani*, for instance, maintained that municipal commissions had been overburdened with the expense of sanitation, and had been compelled to neglect the watering and lighting of streets.[75] Indeed, this preference for 'cosmetic' measures had been a source of constant irritation to British sanitary officers. In 1891, the sanitary commissioner of Bombay expressed his disapproval with the municipal commission in Broach, which he felt had 'squandered [its] means in a reckless and extravagant manner in lighting up [its] roads and cleaning streets to an unnecessary extent whilst [it] grossly neglect[ed] the conservancy and surface cleanliness of the town'.[76]

While indigenous customs and the self-interest of municipal commissioners hampered sanitary progress in Bombay, it is unlikely that the extent of Indian opposition to sanitation was any greater in Bombay than in Bengal, where sanitary expenditure increased following the introduction of local self-government. In Bombay province, the centre of nationalist politics was not the capital but Poona, home of the Deccan Education Society and the Savajanik Sabha. In the 1880s, the Savajanik Sabha came increasingly under the influence of Hindu 'revivalists', most notably Bal Gangalkar Tilak. In the 1890s, and especially after Tilak became leader in 1895, the organisation began to tap a new spirit of Hindu assertiveness evident in Maharashtra since the 1880s. Tilak's own newspaper, *Kesarai*, had played an important part in this upsurge, combining praise of ancient institutions and Hindu culture under British rule. Cultural politics became increasingly important in Bombay after the introduction of local self-government in 1884, with greater indigenous representation on local bodies, and may well have had an effect on attitudes towards municipal sanitation.[77]

Certainly, Poona municipality was notorious for its inactivity on sanitary matters. In 1894 the Bombay sanitary commissioner reported that he had 'made some suggestions to the Health Officer, Dr. Sorab Hormusji . . . but it is not only a waste of money, but a delusion, to employ such a highly qualified Medical Officer unless all his reasonable recommendations are carefully considered and carried out consistently with the means of the Municipality'.[78] However, it is difficult to ascertain how far this revivalist mood had swept other areas of India, or even other parts of western India.

Outside of Bengal, Bombay, and Madras, the development of municipal sanitation proceeded at a more uneven pace. In the Punjab, the implementation of the Ripon reforms coincided with a decrease in municipal expenditure on sanitation, which did not return to pre-1883 levels until 1891.[79] Between 1883 and 1893 the amount spent on sanitation fluctuated significantly, perhaps reflecting reliance on octroi as the principal source of municipal revenue, and local variations in prosperity and attitudes to sanitary reform. In the Central Provinces, returns of municipal expenditure are less complete than for the Punjab, but existing figures suggest a similar pattern of decline after 1883. In 1884, 34 per cent of municipal incomes were allotted to sanitation, but this level was not attained again until 1899.[80] The total amount allotted to sanitation also fell in the decade following the introduction of local self-government. Municipalities in the Central Provinces relied chiefly on octroi for their revenue; 57 per cent of municipal incomes were derived from this source.[81] Octroi's sensitivity to economic conditions may account, in part, for the great variations in total expenditure on sanitation which occurred in the 1880s and 90s.

Sanitary expenditure in the two provinces and in Bombay increased, albeit unevenly, in the early 1890s. But, in all cases, expenditure tailed off slightly in the mid-1890s before rising steeply as municipalities in these regions attempted to combat the spread of plague. Rising sanitary expenditure in the early 1890s follows the strengthening of executive and advisory bodies in the late 1880s, and the growing realisation of the dangers of impure water. The creation of sanitary boards in 1887 was essentially an attempt to address the problem of public health in rural areas, but municipal sanitation also fell within their scope. The boards, which were set up in each province, comprised the local sanitary commissioner, an administrative officer and, later, a sanitary engineer. Their function was to advise municipalities on sanitary matters, and to authorise plans for sanitary projects tendered by municipalities themselves. Municipalities were expected to finance sanitary works from their own revenues, but the salary of the sanitary engineer was defrayed from provincial funds.[82] In an unprecedented move, the Indian government also announced that 'in very exceptional cases, the requirements of which cannot be met from Local or Provincial revenues or by loans . . . [it] would not refuse to consider application from Local Governments in the interests of sanitary improvements of more than local importance'.[83]

As advisers to municipal corporations, sanitary boards were concerned primarily with large sanitary engineering projects. From the late-1880s there was growing concern with the purity of the water supply, following Koch's claim to have isolated the bacterium causing cholera from a water-tank in Calcutta. Existing precautions, like the MacNamara sand-filter which had been used in military cantonments and in some municipalities since 1870, were able to filter most impurities from the water-supply, but not bacteria and other micro-organisms. In response to the findings of bacteriologists like Koch, a new generation of filtration technology was developed at this time using denser filters, like porcelain, capable of preventing the passage of micro-organisms. The new filter used most extensively in British India was the Pasteur–Chamberland device but, towards the end of century, increasing attention was paid to chemical purification, and the development of new substances in addition to potassium permanganate which had been in use for some years.[84]

In the municipalities the concern for water-filtration found expression in the construction of waterworks and the development of sewerage and drainage schemes. Before 1890, such enterprises were confined to the more important cities and a handful of prosperous mofussil municipalities. After 1890, it seems that sanitary engineering became a priority for most of the larger Indian towns, as is illustrated by their greatly increased expenditure on public health.

Capital expenditure on waterworks often added several lakhs of rupees to a municipality's sanitary budget. Expenditure of this magnitude could rarely be defrayed from municipal revenues alone, and was financed chiefly by loans from provincial or, in exceptional circumstances, central government. But, occasionally, municipalities were forced to raise loans on the open market. In 1890, for example, the municipal corporation of Poona borrowed 2 lakhs of rupees for the construction of a water-filtration works while, in the following year, a waterworks was completed at Ahmedabad at a cost of some 6 lakhs of rupees.[85] In this respect Bombay was little different from the other provinces. The marked increase in sanitary expenditure which occurred in Madras in the early 1890s coincided with the extension of the Madras Municipal Act to several new towns, and also with the formation of a sanitary board and the establishment of larger sanitary programmes in several of the mofussil towns.[86] In Bengal a sharp increase in total sanitary expenditure occurred at around the same time, but in percentage terms this increase was not as marked as in Bombay or Madras, reflecting the relatively high level of sanitary expenditure characteristic of Bengal throughout the 1880s. In all three presidencies, there was a slight fall in expenditure in the mid-1890s, perhaps indicating that many of the sanitary schemes initiated in the late-1880s and early-1890s had been completed by this time.

Many large towns still had considerable difficulties in raising revenue for sanitary works. Patna, the most populous municipality in Bengal, excluding Calcutta, was much poorer than many other large towns and was forced to keep taxation levels to a minimum. The sanitary commissioner of Bengal, W. H. Gregg, reported that the commissioners had not been idle in matters of public health, but that any hope of large sanitary works had been abandoned because the money required would divert from the many other and more urgent needs of the town.[87]

In Howrah municipality it was indifference and lack of understanding on the part of the municipal commissioners rather than lack of funds that had retarded sanitary progress. The commissioners, according to Gregg, were businessmen with little knowledge of sanitation and little interest in the health of the town. He wrote of many 'glaring sanitary defects', but it was the state of the city's slum housing that most concerned the sanitary commissioner:

> I have never seen anything so disgustingly filthy in the whole course of my experience as the condition of the drains and the bustee bordering on Dores Road. I had actually to wade through filth ankle deep to get into the heart of the bustee and, when I got there, I found myself in the midst of an atmosphere which nearly overpowered me.[88]

Similar criticisms continued to be levied by Gregg and, in even stronger language, by the Bengal government, prompting a defensive statement from the *Bengalee* – a newspaper representing the professional class in Bengal – to the effect that municipal revenue had increased by 50 per cent since the introduction of local self-government. It claimed that this was proof that municipal commissioners had not neglected their responsibilities, and that they had not been motivated by self-interest.[89] It was a claim which was understandable in the light of repeated and sometimes unjustified European attacks upon Indian municipal commissioners and on the institution of local self-government. But increased tax revenues themselves were no proof of sanitary activity, and were attributable in large part to the incorporation of more towns under the various Municipal Acts. Moreover, there was a kernel of truth in the sometimes exaggerated criticisms of the European press and medical officers. After all, not even the *Bengalee* could deny that Indian commissioners had consistently opposed taxation to fund sanitary improvements in Madras, Bombay, Calcutta, and a host of other Indian cities.

Plague and sanitary reform

Of all the factors affecting municipal sanitation, the coming of plague in 1896 was by far the most important. In the three provinces of Bombay, Bengal, and Madras allotments to sanitation increased dramatically during the early years of the epidemic. In Bombay, where the disease first gained a foothold in India, expenditure rose steeply in 1897 and, although it fell slightly in subsequent years, it remained significantly higher than before 1896–7. A similar rise in expenditure was recorded in Madras, although it was not so great as in Bombay. Although plague had made minor incursions into the north of the province, the prospect of the disease spreading further south was sufficient to provide a spur to sanitary activity. After 1898 expenditure fell, but remained at a higher level than before 1896, although the difference was not as marked as for Bombay, reflecting the comparatively higher level of expenditure in Madras prior to that date. In Bengal, which was also relatively free from plague, expenditure nevertheless increased as preventive measures were instituted. But, again, the increase was not as marked as in Bombay, since municipal sanitation was comparatively well developed in Bengal prior to 1896.

Plague provided the first real opportunity for the wholesale clearance and alteration of indigenous dwellings deemed insanitary by European officials. Under the emergency powers vested in sections 434 and 473 of the Bombay Municipal Act (1888), and similar legislation in other towns, unprecedented numbers of buildings were destroyed and in some cases rebuilt. In one week, at the height of the epidemic in Karachi, 102 dwellings were condemned, 130 were recommended for substantial alteration, and over 4,000 were altered in some minor respect.[90] Plague also provided a stimulus to sanitary work outside the major cities. The political agent of Cutch, in Bombay province, noted in January 1898 that although 'the municipality [was] a very weak one . . . it [had] been strengthened' since the outbreak of plague. There had also been a tightening of sanitary regulations, including the imposition of fines for persons using the streets as latrines.[91] In Ahmedabad plague had induced the municipality to improve the gravely defective water-supply and sewerage systems, although only after much pressure had been brought to bear by the local civil surgeon.[92]

In most cases, the effects of plague on attitudes towards clearance and the sanitary planning of cities were short-lived, but in the larger cities, which had more substantial European populations, the effects were more enduring. In Bombay, the ravages of plague provided the impetus for several ambitious schemes of urban restructuring and for the creation of an improvement trust, funded initially by government, but later by the municipality and from local subscriptions.[93] The trust comprised 4 members nominated by government and 4 elected from the Bombay Chamber of Commerce, the corporation, the Port Trust, and the Millowners Association. The nominated members consisted of the trust's chairman – Mr W. C. Hughes, an engineer – the collector of land revenue for Bombay, and the chairman of the corporation. In short, it reflected European official and commercial interests.[94]

The trust's objectives were fairly loosely defined: it was committed to 'the better ventilation of the densely inhabited parts of the city, the removal of insanitary dwellings, and the prevention of overcrowding'.[95] But, with the exception of a plan to provide model dwellings for 13,500 members of Bombay's 'poorer and working classes', these commitments were interpreted quite narrowly, and almost all of the schemes drawn up by the trust were concerned with the opening-up of congested areas to traffic; measures of obvious benefit to commercial interests represented on the trust.[96] Even the housing scheme failed to match initial expectations, with only 8,000 people being housed by the trust by 1908. Moreover, the rent charged by the trust was prohibitively expensive to the city's poorest inhabitants: the very people who had previously inhabited the slums.[97]

There were, however, some more ambitious proposals for slum clearance in Bombay. In 1905 the city's health officer John Turner argued that 'the undertaking to remove 300,000 people from crowded parts of the city may appear to be gigantic and at first sight impossible . . . There are many difficulties, but all can be overcome: the only way to exterminate plague is to take away its power of attack.'[98] But the municipal commission and the improvement trust remained committed to a system of piecemeal reform, and spoke of the 'hopelessness of wholesale acquisition and demolition'. Such schemes had little chance of success, they protested, unless they came about as a result of initiatives taken by the people themselves.[99]

However, by 1912, town-planning undeniably occupied a position of importance in the minds of sanitary officers, being described in a resolution passed at the All-India Sanitary conference of 1912 as 'the most urgent sanitary need'.[100] Their models for urban planning were predominantly European, being derived from the writings of Ebenezer Howard, from the 'example of Germany' idea publicised by T. C. Horsfall and others, and from the passage in Britain of the 1909 Housing and Town Planning Act. The schemes outlined by sanitary officers were based explicitly on the German principle of 'redistribution' and the English principle of 'betterment'. Betterment required owners of property likely to benefit from any improvement to contribute to its cost; redistribution empowered municipal commissions to alter plots of land and to re-allocate them in order to make an area more suitable for building.[101] By 1912, however, the Bombay improvement trust had, by its own admission, touched only 10 per cent of congested areas, and preferred alteration of existing dwellings to clearance.[102]

It was during his tour of India in 1914 that Patrick Geddes developed his idea of 'conservative pruning', of the gradual restructuring of cities in keeping with their original character. On visiting Madura he recorded that:

One of the poor quarters of this . . . town is at present threatened with 'relief of congestion' . . . We are told that this sweeping and costly plan is not the original one, but is regarded as a moderate and economical substitute for total demolition, that was happily too expensive to obtain the sanction or support of the Government.[103]

The general rise in sanitary expenditure in all three main provinces after 1896 concealed considerable local variation. The sanitary commissioner of Madras complained in 1898 that some municipalities had spent little on sanitation as they had put aside a good portion of their sanitary allotment in order to deal with plague should it appear.[104] In 1900, he feared that Madras had 'lost ground in the general campaign against dirt and disease even if it [had] succeeded, in large measure, in keeping plague itself at bay'.[105] Expenditure on extraordinary measures like the disinfection and ventilation of buildings, evacuation, railway inspection and so on, also detracted from more lasting sanitary improvements in some areas of Bombay province. The sanitary commissioner warned that 'unless Government came to the aid [of municipalities] in relieving them of some portion of [their] debts, sanitary work [would] be at a standstill for years'.[106]

The enormous financial strain caused by plague did eventually induce the Bombay government to assist municipalities in their attempts to combat it. However, municipalities could not rely on regular or generous contributions from government funds. In 1904, the Bombay government considered a plea by the Bombay corporation to be relieved of Rs 1,600,000 plague expenditure as 'unreasonable' given the present deficit in provincial funds.[107] With provincial government finances over-stretched by plague expenditure, the only way in which municipalities could maintain local services was to increase taxation. In Karachi, for example, the water tax was increased by 3 annas per person; this being the 'only means by which the municipality could meet its obligations'.[108]

But government intervention during the plague epidemic established an important precedent for financial support to municipalities in India. From 1903, when the first provincial funds were allocated by the Bombay government for the relief of plague expenditure, the extent of government aid to local bodies for sanitation increased considerably. By 1905, the Indian government, through the agency of provincial governments, contributed a sum equal to one-quarter of the income of local authorities.[109] For much of the late nineteenth century, as Tinker reminds us, government aid to local bodies was severely limited due, in part, to a fall in the price of export goods and the value of silver (to which the rupee was linked) at a time when internal costs were mounting.[110]

The psychological impact of plague, combined with more favourable terms of trade after 1905, had a significant and, in general, a positive effect upon the development of local sanitation in India. From 1908, growing revenue surpluses enabled the government of India to allot annual grants totalling Rs 3 million to provincial governments for sanitary purposes.[111] In 1910–11, a special non-recurring grant of Rs 5.7 million was made, of which 500,000 was intended for the promotion of scientific research and the balance for urban sanitary works. In 1911–12, there was a further grant of Rs 5 million from central government revenues.[112]

Municipal sanitation in all three provinces benefited greatly from these grants.

The effects are most apparent in Bombay, particularly in respect of total allotments to sanitation. The amount allotted to sanitation increased steadily from 1903 to 1906, reflecting steps taken by provincial government to relieve municipalities of plague expenditure, and fell slightly in 1907, as the incidence of plague in the presidency began to decrease. After 1908, following the large increase in government grants, allotments for sanitation increased markedly, peaking at Rs 3.4 million in 1913–14. The same pattern is evident when allotments are considered as a percentage of municipal incomes, but the upward trend is not as marked since it is masked by the receipt of grants for non-sanitary expenditure, particularly for education.[113]

Coincident with plague in northern districts of Madras province, sanitary allotments by municipalities increased from just over Rs 200,000 in 1901–2 to just over 400,000 in 1907–8. Most of this increase came under the head of public works.[114] From 1911, increasing government grants had a marked effect upon levels of sanitary expenditure in Madras. Chiefly as a result of government grants, municipal incomes in Madras rose from around Rs 5.6 million in 1910–11 to 8.3 million in 1913–14. Sanitary allotments rose, though less steeply, from Rs 3.5 million in 1910–11 to 4.8 million in 1913–14. This increase was a direct result of the distribution among municipalities and district boards of grants from central government funds.

In Bengal, government intervention boosted municipal sanitation, with significant increases in allotments to public health after 1908. There was a slight fall in expenditure in 1911–12, but this may simply reflect the reconstitution of Bengal in 1912, when the number of municipal commissions in the province fell from 130 to 111. It may also have been due to the completion, in 1911, of two large sewerage schemes at Darjeeling and Dacca.[115] As in Bombay, the effects of government subsidy are not as marked when allotments are expressed as a percentage of municipal incomes.

There also appears to have been a significant increase in sanitary activity outside of Bengal, Bombay, and Madras at this time. In the Central Provinces, the amount of municipal income devoted to sanitation rose steadily from Rs 301,838 in 1900 to 667,656 in 1909, to 1,328,430 in 1914. There are no details relating to total sanitary allotments for the Punjab, but when expressed as a percentage of municipal incomes it rose from 20 per cent in 1901 to 49 per cent in 1909. Other areas like the United Provinces (formerly, the North West Provinces and Oudh) benefited not only from direct subsidy, but from being relieved of police charges from 1904.[116]

Progress continued unabated until 1914.[117] In 1911, the sanitary commissioner of the United Provinces reported that 'it is yearly becoming apparent that in the larger towns at least, interest in sanitation is growing and the improved health and greater comfort desirable therefrom is more and more recognised by the people'.[118] The same trend was observed by the sanitary commissioner with the Indian government, who noted that 'interest in sanitation has been growing, and a distinct advance has now been possible in consequence of the large and special grants made to the provinces by the Government of India.'[119]

This more vigorous attitude towards public health was not expressed solely in increased expenditure on public works, but also in greater attention to subjects like food adulteration. In 1903, for example, an Indian practitioner Dr Bardi, argued that much of the infant mortality in Bombay could be attributed to impurities in the city's milk supply. 'Sufficient improvement in the state of affairs', he protested, 'could hardly be expected when those guilty of flagrant misdeeds in connection with the milk supply are practically allowed to ply their dangerous trade without any control or checks'.[120]

It is significant that some of the first members of the medical profession to attach real importance to food adulteration were Indian practitioners. For 'modernising' nationalists, it highlighted both the 'backwardness' of their own people and the failure of the British administration to fulfil its 'duty' to its colonial subjects. 'Tuberculosis', declared Dr Sakhar, professor of hygiene and bacteriology at Madras Medical College, 'is very much neglected in the early stages by the patients as well as the medical men in this country'.[121] No doubt this neglect was due to the comparatively low incidence of the disease among Europeans in India, and to the fact that it was a chronic, rather than an epidemic, disease. Unlike plague and cholera, tuberculosis did not cause sudden and extensive disruption of commerce and agriculture.

After the turn of the century, the Indian National Congress was taking a more active part in sanitary debates. After the Morley–Minto reforms of 1909, Congress was better represented on the Indian legislative council, and in 1910 Gokhale and his colleagues took this opportunity to demand that more funds be allotted to provincial governments for sanitary purposes. The move was blocked by British members, who argued that the government 'already borrow[ed] as much as . . . [it] could with safety'.[122]

There were, indeed, many examples of inertia that could be set against the general picture of sanitary progress. In 1907, the sanitary commissioner of Bengal complained that sanitary work in his province had been severely hampered by a lack of 'suitable staff'.[123] The following year, he again claimed that much money had been wasted on defective sanitary works due to 'inefficient supervision', while sanitary activity in many municipalities was still constrained by want of funds.[124] These points were echoed by the sanitary commissioner of Madras in 1909.[125] Lack of interest in sanitation on the part of municipal commissioners was allegedly still a problem in Madras province and in the Central Provinces.[126] Such criticisms were not without foundation, given that the orthodox Hindu press continued to question the value of European health officers and other sanitary staff, and that municipal commissioners continued to oppose increases in taxation for sanitary purposes.[127]

District and local boards

Rural sanitation prior to the Ripon reforms

Prior to the Ripon reforms, the administration of local affairs in rural areas was carried out almost entirely by British district commissioners. Funds for such local works as were carried out in that period were raised from general revenues (rather than taxation specifically for sanitary purposes), with small and occasional contributions from provincial government.[128] The administrative body that carried out sanitary and other local works was the Local Fund Circle. Like municipalities, these authorities suffered greatly from fluctuations in agricultural prosperity,[129] and because of their reliance on the economic fortunes of a particular locality, sanitary activity was sporadic and generally in a 'backward state' compared with municipal towns.[130] The poverty of many rural areas also had a direct bearing on the health of their inhabitants. In 1869, Dr G. Saunders, deputy inspector of hospitals for Bengal, noted that poverty and malnutrition were major causes of ill health in the province, with scurvy and other forms of 'deficiency disease' common among the rural population. Such observations cast doubt on the government's claims to have improved the lot of the Indian peasant, particularly when the state of affairs was attributable to colonial agricultural development. Saunders wrote:

> The governing classes in this country pride themselves on the success which follows on our system of government. . . Our exports increase day by day and year by year. Large quantities of the products of the land are sent across the sea. But it is overlooked that at the same time the price of all articles of food increases; living becomes year by year more difficult for the lower classes; and the labouring class in every agricultural district is worse off than it ever was.[131]

But such strident and far-reaching criticisms were rare, even among Indians, and it was not until the turn of the century that the drain of wealth theory became an important factor in debates over public health.

For much of the 1860s and 1870s the bone of contention was, rather, the high incidence of fever in newly irrigated areas. The zemindars, who had traditionally taken a measure of responsibility for the health of their labourers, refused to pay for the drainage-works that were so obviously required to prevent flooding in low-lying areas. Such works, they argued, were now the responsibility of government, and should be funded out of provincial revenues.[132] Yet British officials in the North West Provinces and other areas steadfastly denied that there was any connection between irrigation and malaria, so the situation had reached an impasse, while in the meantime many thousands died annually in the newly irrigated areas of Bengal, NWP, and the Punjab.[133] As Gopal Chunder Roy, inspector of dispensaries for Burdwan District, Bengal, put it:

Countries that once smiled with peace, health, and prosperity, have been turned
into hot beds of disease, misery, and death. Villages that once rang with the
cheerful, merry tone of the healthful infants, now resound in local wailings and
lamentations . . . The skulls of human beings now strew the fields at every few
yards' distance.[134]

Indeed, as far as many Indians were concerned, the human misery caused by
fever surpassed even that of famine. 'The famine', wrote the *Hindoo Patriot*,
'comes once in ten, twenty, thirty, or fifty years . . . But the attacks of the
epidemic fever are annually recurring . . . If we are talking of an insurance
against famine, why should there not be an insurance against fever'.[135]

The zemindars alleged that new drainage-works had obstructed or disrupted
traditional village drainage schemes: a claim vigorously denied by the
lieutenant-governor of Bengal.[136] But the *Patriot*, which represented *zemindari*
interests, was not alone in its assessment of the fever raging in the Bardwan
District of Bengal. It claimed, correctly, that the majority of medical men in
India concurred in its views on the causation of fever, and was able to cite the
1875 report of the Army Sanitary Commission in its defence.[137] The government's response was to set up a commission of inquiry into the 'Bardwan Fever';
a move which the *Patriot* saw as unnecessary in the light of the medical
consensus surrounding the disease.[138] In its opinion, the commission was a
stalling device, designed to delay action on the part of the government. 'All
schemes of progress, improvement and civilization seem to be a mockery',
protested the *Patriot*, 'when disease and death are rampant in the country without let or hindrance'.[139] The *Patriot* pointed out that 'many millions had been
spent to make barracks healthy for a few thousand soldiers' while 'a thousandth
part of that sum would not have been required for the restoration of the salubrity
of the fever-stricken villages'.[140]

Although this estimate of the money required to drain the areas adversely
affected by irrigation is questionable, the low priority given to the health of
India's rural population was undeniable. Yet the government's policy, even
though it was soon forced to admit the link between poor drainage and fever,[141]
did not change significantly in this respect. In 1880, following the report of the
commission, it passed the Bengal Drainage Act, which did no more than permit
municipalities and district administrations to apply to government for loans in
connection with drainage-works.[142] The lack of any direct financial commitment
on the part of the government meant that the drainage of rural areas improved little in the coming years, and in many areas the incidence of fever actually
increased.[143] Between 1883 and 1887 the number of deaths from fever in Bengal
rose steadily from 900,000 per annum to 1,050,000. 'Deserted villages, ruined
homes and the haggard looks of fever-stricken people' continued to testify to the
dreadful effects of the disease.[144]

The constraints imposed on rural sanitation by lack of funds and the unwillingness of government to intervene were matched by the practical difficulties of enforcing the meagre sanitary regulations which existed at that time. Enforcement was problematic enough in urban areas but vast distances, difficult terrain, and lack of personnel, made the sanitary policing of rural areas almost impossible. Furthermore, the inhabitants of Indian villages, like those in the towns, often found western sanitary regulations incomprehensible or unnecessary. With this in mind, the sanitary commissioner of the North West Provinces and Oudh warned in 1879 of the need for 'caution' in applying sanitary legislation and for ensuring the co-operation of village headmen. 'The people are apathetic at first', he wrote, 'but once a fair start is made, and they get to understand the rules, and to find out how easy it is to comply with them, it is surprising how much can be done with little supervision'.[145] However, it is clear from subsequent reports that this optimism was ill-founded. The scheme, an initiative of the district magistrate Mr McConachey, was extended to only a few villages,[146] and by 1883 'no [sanitary] works of any importance' had yet been undertaken in the NWP.[147]

The year 1880 marked the first attempt anywhere in British India to introduce an element of compulsion into the sanitation of villages. Under the Central Provinces Land revenue Act, village headmen were empowered 'subject to any rules by the chief commissioner, to keep [their] village in good sanitary condition and to report all births and deaths taking place' there. In the same year, 56,000 copies of J. M. Cuningham's *Sanitary Primer*, translated into the vernacular, were distributed in Bengal.[148] But in most provinces, 'no particular attention was paid to the sanitary improvement of villages'.[149] Where sanitary work was undertaken it usually took the form of scavenging and the removal of refuse: allotments made for improvement of the water supply were not always utilised,[150] but as a proportion of sanitary expenditure, the sinking of new wells and improvements to existing ones constituted by far the largest proportion of the local budget. In Bombay province, in 1883, some Rs 148,140 were spent by local fund circles on new wells, out of a total sanitary allotment of 262,194.[151]

The impact of self-government

In place of local fund circles, Ripon's resolution on local self-government established a gradation of local authorities. The smallest, the local board, covered a *tahsil*, or sub-division of a district; it had responsibility for sanitation, education, public works, medical services, and sometimes veterinary work. The largest, the district board, was envisaged as a supervising or co-ordinating body for the local boards. But in all provinces except Assam, Burma, the Central Provinces, and Madras, the district board was entrusted with all funds, and with almost all functions of local government, including the management of local charitable dispensaries – previously in the hands of the local civil surgeon.[152] All these boards were supposed to have a majority-elected element, the power to raise revenue, and to spend it. But, in Bombay and the North West Provinces, local boards initially had only a nominal existence, with provincial government continuing to levy and to disburse land revenues, and with district commissioners exercising great influence over sanitary and other arrangements.[153] The new system came into existence in most provinces in 1885,[154] but existing sanitary legislation, like that in the Central Provinces, remained on the statute books and was eventually extended to other provinces.[155]

It is somewhat harder to gauge the impact of local self-government on sanitary activity in rural areas than in municipalities. Returns of income and expenditure from local boards were not always forthcoming and, in many cases, annual figures for whole provinces are absent, often for many years. However, it is possible to gain an overall impression of how rural sanitation fared in the years after local self-government. The total allotted to sanitation in both Bombay and Madras rose after 1885, reaching its peak in the mid-1890s.[156] As a percentage of local incomes, sanitary expenditure rose steadily in Madras from 1885 to 1890, and remained more or less constant in Bombay until the late-1890s, reflecting a steady rise in local incomes in both provinces. The sharp decline in allotments in Madras in 1890 may be attributed to a large rise in local revenues due to the inclusion of forty new towns into the scheme.[157] No returns of aggregate income or expenditure were received from Bengal until 1888–9.

As in urban areas, rising expenditure on sanitation masked considerable regional variations. In 1886, the sanitary commissioner for the Punjab claimed that 'nothing had been done to improve sanitation in rural areas' in his province and highlighted many 'glaring sanitary defects'.[158] The sanitary commissioner of Berar reported in the same year that 'the sanitary condition of villages still continues in its primitive state and the Sanitary Code, which was issued some time ago, has hitherto been almost a dead letter'. Even in the Central Provinces, the sanitary provisions of the Land Revenue Act still applied to only a few areas.[159]

The obstacles to sanitary improvement in rural areas were, again, the lack of support from provincial government, difficulties in raising sufficient funds from local revenues, and lack of interest among the indigenous population. District boards met infrequently, with zemindar members attending very rarely. Indian landowners viewed the elective principle as a challenge to their traditional authority (already much undermined), and often found themselves unable to follow the unfamiliar procedures of local government.[160] The shortage of funds available for rural sanitation was a frequent cause of complaint among sanitary officials. Summing up the progress of rural sanitation in 1888, the sanitary commissioner with the Indian government recorded that progress had been 'desultory and fitful', and that 'the cause of much of the inaction displayed by local authorities on matters of sanitation has been due to want of funds and to the very inefficient means which have hitherto existed for giving effect to suggested improvements.'[161]

These concerns were shared by the Indian government which, for the first time, in 1887, expressed its willingness to consider grants-in-aid of sanitation to local bodies. Its interest in rural sanitation stemmed, primarily, from the growing realisation that high morbidity and mortality rates among the 'general population' constituted a serious obstacle to economic efficiency. 'After nearly a century of professed village sanitary work', read the government's resolution on the sanitary improvement of towns and villages, 'but little of practical utility has . . . been done for the maintenance of the health of the rural population, on whose working power the prosperity of the country mainly depends'.[162] Others stressed the long-standing concern for the health of military personnel.[163]

During the viceroyalty of the Marquis of Dufferin (December 1884– December 1888), the Indian government was more willing than it had been for some years to consider intervention in matters of public health. In many respects, this was uncharacteristic of the Dufferin administration, which reduced expenditure on most other public works.[164] The government's resolution noted that:

> Some years ago it was generally and correctly felt by Local Governments and Administrators that to press, authoritatively, the subject of sanitary improvement, especially in villages, would be of little avail, and that persuasion and not coercion, was the right plan to follow; it is no less generally felt today that a more forward, though still cautious and tentative policy would now be opportune.[165]

However, there were many who felt that 'such a resolution might have been issued with advantage ten or even twenty years before'. Sanitation, according to the IMS officer H. A. D. Phillips, writing in the *Calcutta Review*, was '*par excellence* a branch of administration in which the state should act in accordance with the ideas of the most advanced and enlightened sections of the community'. Like other paternalistic critics of the Indian government in the 1880s, he dismissed suggestions that sanitary measures should await a higher level of understanding among the rural population:

> Those who know anything of the progress of sanitary reform in England are aware that sanitation was, to a great extent, forced on the people. Even at the present day there are villages in England where sanitary arrangements shock the tourist, and sanitary education is no more advanced than in a Bengal village. Democratic governments have not waited until the people have risen *en masse* and howled for reform: much less should bureaucratic Governments sit with idle hands and await Greek Kalends. These are matters in which it is admittedly the duty of Governments to act in advance of the masses.[166]

The measures proposed by the government would have gone some way to meeting Phillips' expectations, but its new scheme was still heavily dependent on local initiative and local revenues. The chief plank of the new policy was the formation of sanitary boards. The boards were comprised of administrative officers and sanitary specialists, and were supposed to have an executive as well as an advisory function, being granted a budget from provincial funds to disburse on local sanitary works as they saw fit.[167] But in practice sanitary boards did not often acquire these powers until some years after they had been established.

The boards were generally welcomed in the Indian press – particularly as they seemed to offer some hope for areas ravaged by fever – but there was disquiet about their almost exclusively European membership. The *Bengalee* did not object to the formation of sanitary boards *per se*, but to 'the large representation of the official element', which it feared might presage greater interference in local government. 'Any attempt to force sanitary measures on an unwilling people', it warned, 'must lead to failure'.[168]

The other important aspect of the 1887 resolution was the Indian government's declaration that it would, in future, consider making grants to local authorities for sanitary works, where these were of more than local importance. The Indian government also pressed the governments of Bombay and the North West Provinces to empower local boards under their jurisdiction to raise revenue, rather than continue to depend on disbursements from provincial funds.[169] But the extent of financial aid for local sanitation was still extremely limited by comparison with levels of expenditure on other public works, even though these had been declining since 1885. The Indian government was well aware that it invested very little in human capital compared to other colonies; less even than some of the Indian Princely States.[170]

The creation of sanitary boards was followed up in several provinces by the Indian government's passage of a Village Sanitary Act. The Act, passed in 1889, empowered villages to levy a tax in order to raise revenue for sanitary purposes; similar legislation was introduced in Bombay and the Central Provinces in the same year.[171] The Bombay Act provided for a contribution from local boards and from provincial government of two-sixths and one-sixth respectively, the remainder to be raised from the taxation of villagers.[172] Similar legislation was enacted in the North West Provinces in 1890 and in the Punjab in 1891,[173] but no such scheme was inaugurated in Bengal until 1900, and other provinces, like Assam, rejected it as inappropriate for sparsely populated hill and jungle tracts.[174] Even where legislation was introduced it appears to have had little positive effect upon sanitary activity. The results, reported the secretary to the Indian government in 1892, had been 'unsatisfactory';[175] the Bombay Act, for instance, covering only 163 villages.[176]

Indian attitudes to rural sanitation depended to a great extent on whether an individual had received a western education. Modernising 'nationalist' politicians, who had adopted values similar to many reform-minded British officials, were largely in favour of the new measures, but were opposed to further taxation on the grounds that the rural population were too poor.[177] Indigenous representatives on local and district boards were divided on the question of whether to introduce a village sanitary cess. Those in favour argued that it should be introduced gradually, and with the full co-operation of village headmen. Those against stressed the poverty of Indian villagers and the danger that tax-collectors might abuse the powers conferred on them. According to Pandit Jarki Pershad, retired inspector of police and a member of Ahraula local board, Fyzabab division, NWP:

> there [were] very few . . . who [could] pay one anna a month without much inconvenience. The greater part of a village consists of poor labourers who live from hand to mouth. Tax collectors will be a source of trouble to the poor . . . In order to show their authority . . . [they] will tease them to extreme, and the result will be that the inhabitants desert the village.

The raja of Bhanga, another member of the board, also believed that 'no legislation on this subject is desirable at present. The imposition of any house tax on villages is sure to be unpopular, as it cannot fail to be [a] means of oppression.' The mixed response from local boards in Fyzabad District induced the provincial government to amend the legislation to permit its introduction on a more gradual basis and to exempt from taxation those earning less than Rs 60 per annum.[178] A measure of indigenous reticence was the fact that the Village Sanitary Act had been introduced into only 35 villages in the North West Provinces by 1895, 5 years after its passage.[179] Other sanitary measures, particularly those which impinged on Indian landed interests, were also vigorously opposed. The Madras Rivers Conservation Bill of 1884, for example, evoked 'great dissatisfaction among all classes of landed proprietors', in its proposal to restrict cultivation along river banks.[180]

The ambivalent attitude of many Indians to sanitary reform in rural areas suggests that complaints by sanitary officers regarding indigenous indifference towards sanitation were not entirely unfounded. According to the sanitary commissioner of Assam 'much attention has been given to rural sanitation but the chief commissioner points out that little can be done until the people have been educated to appreciate its benefits'.[181] The sanitary commissioner of Bengal also reported that 'the people continue to exhibit the same complacent disregard of most elementary rules of sanitation . . . and the result is that the surroundings of their villages are appallingly filthy . . . Until the purifying of Bengal villages is made a compulsory matter, he continued, 'no advice, however simple and good, will meet with any substantial recognition at the hands of the general public in rural areas'.[182] In the Central Provinces there was apparently little interest in elections to local and district boards, with many seats uncontested or left vacant. Attendance was also sporadic, though it improved after the famines of the late 1890s.[183] However, it is important not to lose sight of the fact that many British officials had their own axe to grind regarding self-government. Many saw the Ripon reforms as undermining their professional authority and as injurious to 'progress'.

Not all sanitary officers attributed the slow advance of sanitation to apathy and indifference on the part of municipal commissioners. There had always been a strand of medical opinion in India that had urged government to take a more active part in matters of public health. In his presidential address to the Indian Medical Congress in 1894, W. G. King, sanitary commissioner for Madras claimed that allegations of indigenous 'prejudice' were often excuses for government inaction:

> Unfortunately for this country it was possible for those responsible for this absence of progress to shelter themselves behind a motto that was so frequently applied to the Sanitary Department that it became a part of the sanitary creed of the day. There were, it was repeatedly stated, prejudices to be overcome; therefore *festina lente* must be the guiding principle . . . There is still enough of the old spirit of *festina lente* prevailing to clog the wheels of progress . . . I maintain that sanitation neither receives its fair share of funds, nor that place in the government of the country it merits.[184]

There was much truth in this statement: between 1889 and 1894, expenditure on public health comprised only 0.15 per cent of the government of India's total expenditure, compared with 4.1 per cent on education.[185] But the blame did not lie entirely with central government. In Bengal, where no village sanitary scheme was introduced until 1900, there was considerable resistance on the part of the provincial government to further expenditure on rural sanitation. The lieutenant-governor claimed that 'it would be wrong to press measures of sanitary reform upon an unwilling and conservative people'.[186] In other areas, like the Punjab, sanitary boards were slow to acquire the control over provincial sanitary budgets that they had been promised. In 1898, the sanitary commissioner of the Punjab recorded that 'no meeting of [the sanitary board] took place during the year, the reason given being that the members, feeling that the Board had no executive power, would meet uselessly'.[187]

Even more important in determining the success of rural sanitary initiatives were general levels of agricultural prosperity. Certain regions, particularly the arid Deccan plateau of central and western India were, in the late-1890s, increasingly subject to famine. But the general economic picture in western India, as for other parts of the subcontinent at this time, is far from clear. In Bombay province, which covered part of the Deccan, revenue assessments rose sharply in the 1870s, creating hardship and discontent in many agricultural areas, culminating in the Deccan Riots of 1875. This prompted the Bombay government to pass the Deccan Agriculturalists Relief Act 4 years later, which aimed to ease rural indebtedness. But the Act appears to have done little to prevent impoverished peasants from falling into the grip of money-lenders, to whom many lost their land. The commercialisation of agriculture during the 1880s, as railways connected an increasing number of agricultural producers with urban markets, resulted in mixed fortunes for rural areas, stimulating production but displacing local trades which could not compete with cheaper imported goods.[188]

In general, agricultural prosperity appears to have risen from 1860–1920, with some set-backs caused by heavy monsoons and plague in the late-nineteenth century.[189] Yet, rising per capital incomes may have reflected the prosperity of richer land-owning peasants, with commercialisation impoverishing those without land.[190] In any case, hardship was sufficiently in evidence during the droughts of the late-nineteenth century to spur the Bombay government to introduce a more flexible system of revenue settlement.[191]

The economic disruption caused by famine and plague in the late-1890s, is clearly reflected in the income and expenditure of district boards. The combined effects of plague and famine temporarily put an end to the limited improvements that had been made in rural sanitation in Bombay. Allotments to sanitation fell sharply in 1898, and remained depressed until 1905–6. These effects are well documented in official reports. 'Owing to the famine and the presence of plague', wrote the sanitary commissioner of Bombay, 'but little progress has been made' in the sanitation of villages.[192] In Berar, another region of western India, 'village sanitation received less attention because of plague and famine relief'.[193] In 1899, plague and famine were accompanied by cholera, a disease often associated with drought;[194] and, the following year, these diseases

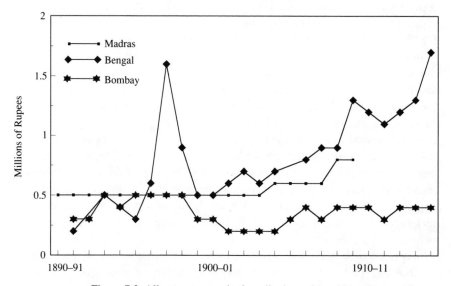

Figure 7.3 Allotments to sanitation: district and local boards

continued to ravage Bombay, while famine severely constricted rural sanitation in the Central Provinces.[195] These conditions persisted in western and central India until 1904–5,[196] and provided ammunition to Indian nationalists such as R. C. Dutt who alleged that colonial rule had resulted in a 'drain of wealth' from India.[197] The mortality crises of the turn of the century also resulted in a more explicit linkage of poverty and ill health, which, with few exceptions, had been ignored or overlooked by the majority of medical officers.[198]

Bengal and Madras, however, were not affected by plague or drought to anything like the extent of Bombay, although famine did cause serious disruption in western Bengal in 1898–9 and in northern Madras between 1900 and 1906.[199] In Madras the total allotted to sanitation fell slightly in 1897, but continued to rise, unevenly, until 1910. As a percentage of local incomes sanitary allotments declined slightly over this period, reflecting a steady rise in local revenue due to increasing government grants for sanitation. But progress was uneven; rising expenditure again concealing considerable regional variations. During this period rural sanitation was at a virtual standstill in many rural districts of Madras.[200]

In Bengal, total expenditure on sanitation rose steeply from 1895 to 1914, with a dramatic increase in expenditure during the early plague years, as private individuals made large donations for sanitary works in the hope that this would protect the presidency against the spread of disease from Bombay.[201] After 1900, a small proportion of this increase would have been due to the inauguration of the 'Patna' village sanitary scheme, which had been introduced into two districts, covering 107 villages by 1904. Under the scheme, members of the district board received notification of villages in an insanitary state, upon which it directed the local board responsible to make the necessary improvements.[202] By 1914, the Patna scheme had been extended to four other districts of Bengal.[203]

In other provinces there was little progress in rural sanitation. The introduction of a system of financial inducements in the Punjab yielded no substantial or lasting improvements.[204] Sanitary activity in the newly constituted provinces of East Bengal and Assam was severely constrained by want of funds.[205] No one method seemed to guarantee sanitary success. Captain Justice, sanitary commissioner for Madras, suggested that 'model villages' be established in each district as an 'object lesson in hygiene', but Major Clemesha, sanitary commissioner for Bengal considered them impracticable, and stressed the need for more education in elementary hygiene.[206] Captain Hutton, sanitary engineer for Madras, drew attention to the limits of sanitary legislation, and underlined the importance of raising public awareness of the dangers of unhygienic practices.[207]

Surgeon-Major McNally, retired sanitary commissioner of Madras condemned the 'partial application of Darwinian principles' that had led to the conclusion that 'sanitation interferes with natural law', and proclaimed that the 'aim of sanitation is to prevent the enfeeblement of individuals by disease' and to 'act positively towards the improvement of the race by improving their surroundings and mode of life'.[208] In 1912 delegates to the All-India Sanitary Conference were virtually unanimous in voicing their concern for the lack of interest in rural as opposed to municipal sanitation.[209] However, outside the Sanitary Department, there were some who felt that the whole question of rural sanitation had been given 'very undue importance' compared with the health of European troops.[210]

Conclusion

Sanitation in India progressed slowly under local self-government. In 1870–9, municipal commissions spent an average of Rs 3 million (some 27 per cent of their total allotment) annually on sanitation; by 1910–19, this had risen to over 9 million (29.5 per cent of municipal budgets).[211] Allotments to sanitation by local and district boards also increased, though generally not as dramatically as in urban areas. At the same time, there was a broadening of sanitary activity, encompassing such matters as urban planning.

Contemporaries were divided over whether they considered this level of

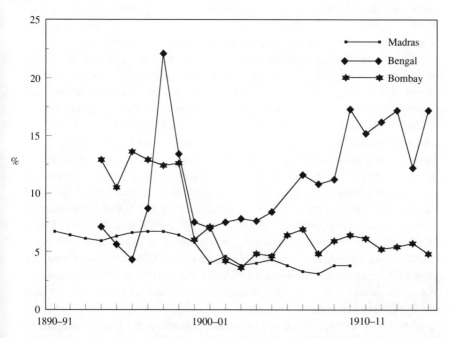

Figure 7.4 Allotments to sanitation as percentage of income: district and local boards

progress satisfactory. Virtually all were agreed that many rural areas had been left untouched, but there was evidence of a certain pride in what had been achieved by some municipal commissions. In 1911, Bombay, formerly 'Sanitary Pariah of the East', was chosen to host the first all-India sanitary conference. Presiding over the conference S. Harcourt Butler (education member of the viceroy's council) described Bombay as a 'great, beautiful and progressive city', a sanitary model for the rest of India. Butler was playing to the audience of civic dignitaries who attended the conference, but also sought to highlight a general trend in which 'old ideas of politics [were] yielding to modern concepts of social duty'.[212]

But there were still those who remained highly critical of public health administration in India. At the conference the following year, Captain Hutton, sanitary engineer for Madras, complained that 'the advance of sanitation in Madras Presidency [was] necessarily slow owing to . . . the reluctance of responsible authorities to provide sufficient funds and the backward condition of the people in understanding sanitary methods'.[213] Indigenous Indian sanitary officials echoed these criticisms.

Rising sanitary expenditure concealed significant regional variations from which it was possible, and legitimate, to draw a number of sometimes conflicting conclusions. In this sense, Tinker's *Foundations of Local Self-Government in India*, which takes into account regional variations, provides a more accurate picture than Ramasubban's sweeping criticism of colonial public health provisions.[214] European comparisons, such as those made by Ramasubban, are misleading since would-be sanitary reformers in India were faced with conflicting cultural values (compounded by political agitation), widespread poverty, and a 'sanitary problem' unparalleled in the western world. Ramasubban also underestimates the extent to which sanitary reform had touched the lives of the rural population in Britain by the turn of the century.

Tinker's account is also more valuable in that it acknowledges the diversity of factors affecting the development of public health. He sees sanitary progress as having been constrained by shortages in local revenue, the government's financial stringency, and by the uncertain attitude towards sanitation displayed by the indigenous population. Ramasubban, however, asserts that the chief constraint upon sanitary activity was the attitude of the colonial government, which, at every opportunity, quashed the reforming initiatives of Indian municipal commissioners. The evidence assembled in this chapter presents a picture more varied, and considerably more complex. In any given area, the development of sanitation depended on a dynamic interaction between government, the local revenue situation, municipal commissions, sanitary officers, and the indigenous population.

Concern to balance central and provincial budgets in the 1870s and 80s, and anxiety about the political consequences of provocation to indigenous customs, served to limit government intervention in public health. In the 1890s the need for strict budgetary controls was underscored by increasingly unfavourable terms of trade which caused internal costs to rise and the value of Indian exports to fall. However, even within these constraints public health was given a low priority by the colonial administration, constituting a much lower proportion of public expenditure than investment in railways and India's economic infrastructure; considerably less, even, than other items of social expenditure such as education. Yet, in the late-1880s, government expenditure on public health began to rise as expenditure on other public works began to fall. In the early-twentieth century, in the wake of the plague epidemic and the government's improving financial situation, spending on public health increased substantially, although it remained a small proportion of the government's total expenditure.

The narrow base of local taxation and fluctuations in economic activity also served to arrest sanitary development; this was particularly true of those provinces, like Bombay and the Punjab, which relied heavily on octroi and other forms of indirect taxation. However, regional differences cannot be attributed solely to variations in prosperity of modes of taxation. The numerous references to the indifference of municipal commissioners towards sanitation which occur in official sanitary reports cannot be dismissed as simply rancour or prejudice on the part of British officials. Indian municipal commissioners often displayed an ambivalent, if not hostile, attitude to western concepts of hygiene and sanitary regulation; reflecting financial self-interest as much as cultural distaste for sanitary measures.

But Indian attitudes towards public health were not uniformly hostile. a minority of western-educated progressives and Indian philanthropists displayed considerable enthusiasm for sanitary reform, and even those who opposed certain proposals that effected their own interests, joined the clamour for more government involvement in public health. These differences in opinion among Indians will be examined more fully in the next chapter.

8

The politics of public health in Calcutta, 1876–1899

Great is sanitation – the greatest work, except discovery . . . that a man can do. But you, O Cleanser will always be a Pariah. Fret not, however, for these dying children shall live, and some day this hideous slum shall become a city of gardens, and it is you who will have done it. (Sir Ronald Ross, *Memoirs*, London, 1923)

The previous chapter gave an overview on the progress of sanitation under local self-government, identifying the various factors affecting its development. This chapter examines more closely the sociopolitical context of public health under local self-government, with reference to British India's metropolis – Calcutta. Public health was the single largest item of municipal expenditure in Calcutta and proved to be the major bone of contention between the city's European inhabitants, the Bengal government, and the Hindu-dominated municipal commission. Sanitary issues also crystallised antagonisms between various sections of Calcutta's western-educated Indian élite, who vied with one another for positions of influence within the municipal corporation. It is argued that the most important features of the politics of public health in Calcutta under local self-government were its domination by Indian property-owning interests, and the opposition of Indian ratepayers to increases in local taxation. These, more than any other factors, prevented the development of an effective machinery of public health in Calcutta prior to 1900.[1] But sanitary progress was also hampered by the prejudices of Calcutta's European population, who, at every opportunity, sought to undermine confidence in the city's corporation.

Public health in Calcutta before 1876

Calcutta was the most important and prosperous city in nineteenth-century British India. Until the transfer of the capital to Delhi in 1911, the city was the seat of administration for the surrounding province of Bengal, and of the Government of India. Situated on India's north-eastern coast, on a branch of the

River Ganges – the Hooghly – Calcutta conducted a flourishing export trade, in jute and other agricultural commodities, with the rest of Asia and Europe. From a small group of villages in the late seventeenth century, it had grown rapidly to a city of over 400,000 persons (excluding its suburbs) by the late 1860s.[2] The comparatively large number of Europeans in the city, and the city's proximity to predominantly Muslim East Bengal, meant that the Hindu population of Calcutta was proportionately smaller than in many other major Indian cities. In 1867 only 60 per cent of its inhabitants were Hindus, while around 30 per cent were Muslim, and the majority of the remainder Christian.[3] Nevertheless, the dominant group among the Indian population of Calcutta was the Hindu *bhadralok* community (literally, 'respectable people'), who claimed, and were accorded, recognition as being superior in social status to their fellows. The *bhadralok* were the descendants of new-rich Hindu landowners who had grown in wealth and influence at the expense of the traditional Muslim and Hindu aristocracy; an aristocracy whose position had been undermined by new forms of land-settlement introduced by the British in the late eighteenth century. There were two distinct estates among the *bhadralok*: the landed notables (*abhijatas*) and ordinary householders (*grihasthas*) – whose western education afforded them access to the learned professions and administrative posts.[4]

It was among the *grihasthas* that European domination of municipal affairs in Calcutta, prior to 1875, was most resented. Between 1794 and 1847, the administration of the city was vested mainly in European justices of the peace. An elected element was introduced in 1848, when a Commission for Improvement took over responsibility for Calcutta's management, but only 3 of its 7 members were Indian.[5] Even these limited gains were lost in the 1850s, when the Bengal government curtailed, and then suspended, the commission's elected government.[6] Distrust of 'non-official' administration increased considerably as a consequence of the mutiny/rebellion of 1857, and in 1863 a new municipal commission was constituted in Calcutta, comprised solely of government-nominated JPs, and with executive power vested in the chairman.[7]

In the 1850s and 60s there was a widespread belief among Europeans that Indians were culturally unfit to be placed in charge of public health.[8] Management of Calcutta's urban environment could be entrusted only to Europeans, although it was readily admitted that their record in the sphere of public health left much to be desired. The dangers of Calcutta's urban environment were already much in evidence in 1803, when the governor-general the Marquess of Wellesley complained of the city's appalling drainage, and lamented the incidence of fever which seemed to attend it. The situation worsened over the coming years, and official concern led to the appointment of a Fever Hospital Commission in 1836, which again recommended urgent action over drainage.[9] Two proposals for drainage schemes made in the 1850s both came to nought because of their alleged impracticability and high cost.[10] The Bengal Municipal

Act of 1848 empowered the Improvement Commission to raise revenue for sanitary works – which it did principally through carriage tax – but the amount generated was inadequate to finance anything more than street-sweeping and the filling-in of stagnant pools. In 1850 the commission regretted that it had 'not been able to carry out any of the great improvements . . . contemplated by Government . . . which would require a much greater expenditure than our limited funds will admit of'.[11] The commission did, however, manage to construct a small number of drains in European quarters of the city; yet, by 1853, the drainage problem was still, apparently, 'the same as it had ever been' and was likely to remain so 'until a proper scheme be devised for a radical reform, and some special funds placed in our hands for carrying such a scheme into execution'.[12]

A more comprehensive scheme was brought before the commissioners in 1855 by the municipal engineer Mr Clark. He proposed a system of combined underground drainage and sewerage, in which five deep receiving sewers would run across Calcutta with their outfall at a salt lake to the west of the city. The plan was heavily criticised in some quarters – particularly by the consortium which planned to reclaim the land under the salt lake – but the commission felt that the proposal was a practical one, and the government had expressed its willingness to grant the commission a loan for the purpose. The scheme, accordingly, went ahead, financed partly by the levy of a new rate, and partly by individual proprietors who paid for the branch drains which connected their premises to the main sewers.[13]

Low demand for private drainage and other financial and practical obstacles meant that the drainage of Calcutta proceeded more slowly than originally envisaged. By 1869 the drainage works were still incomplete, the salt-lake area had yet to be prepared, and a water-closet system (also part of the original plan) had not commenced.[14] Sewage from the city's existing drains continued to flow into the Hooghly, which had become, in the words of the editor of the *Indian Medical Gazette*, the 'reservoir of a deadly poison' – cholera.[15] Until the drainage scheme was finished all that could be done, according to the sanitary commissioner of Bengal, was to improve the existing 'dry-earth' system of sewage disposal and the general conservancy of the city.[16]

The removal of sewage, or 'night-soil' as it was generally referred to, proceeded along lines which would have been familiar to Indians centuries before. All large houses, European and Indian, were provided with a receptacle from which night-soil was collected early in the morning, and taken to large public depots situated throughout the town. At night the contents were removed by bullock cart to the edge of town and thrown into the river. The stench from these carts, as they passed through the city, was nauseating and they were widely regarded as a hazard to health. But the night-soil system served only a small minority of Calcutta's population. The majority had resort only to communal

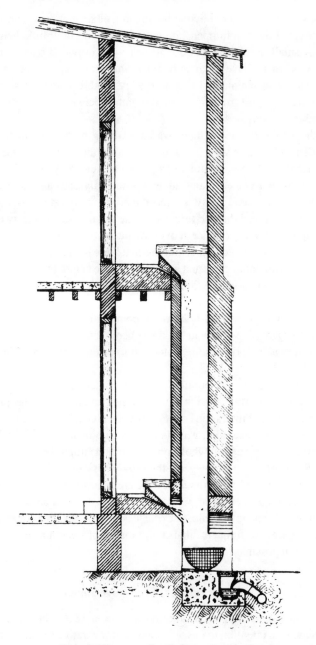

Plate 8 Diagram of an Indian privy

privies, which were shared by the inhabitants of several huts. The sewage from these privies flowed into open 'drains' which were often little better than cess pools. A small number of public latrines were provided by the municipality, but they seem to have been unpopular with the majority of Indians.[17] The commission also maintained a conservancy establishment for street-sweeping and the removal of trade refuse, the latter being charged directly to the proprietors concerned.[18]

By the 1860s, however, there was a growing body of opinion in Calcutta which demanded more specific measures against the spread of epidemic disease. The waterborne theory of cholera causation advanced by John Snow in Britain in the 1850s had gained many adherents in India and, although the majority of medical men found Snow's preoccupation with water too exclusive, the majority were agreed that the time had come to improve the purity of municipal water supplies. By 1867 concern over the purity of Calcutta's water supply was such that the municipal commission raised a large loan of Rs 5,200,000 from the Bengal Government to construct a reservoir in the centre of the city and 67 miles of pipes with pumps where filtered water could be obtained.[19] The cost of the loan was paid back through the levy of a new water-rate, which proved deeply unpopular with the city's *bhadralok* community. A minority of western-educated 'progressives' applauded the scheme, but the majority did not accept the need for such works, and resented the imposition of an additional financial burden.[20]

The other aspects of public health in Calcutta were governed by the Municipal Act of 1863, and were concerned mainly with the prevention of nuisances and the adulteration of food. Anyone who allowed sewer water to flow into the street, for example, was liable to a fine of Rs 10; while the owner of property in a 'filthy and unwholesome condition' might be compelled to pay a fine of Rs 50. But in most respects the provisions of the Act were a dead letter: a policy of 'leniency' was pursued by the commissioners with the complicity of the city's health officer, under which virtually no one was prosecuted for breach of the law, except in the most severe cases. The health officer alleged that breaches were so frequent that they made prosecution of all concerned practically impossible.[21]

The impact of self-government

Such was the state of public health in Calcutta in 1870 when the viceroy Lord Mayo stated his intention to devolve more administrative functions to provincial governments and municipalities.[22] As described in chapter 4, Mayo hoped to encourage local self-government by Indians in existing municipalities – perhaps as a quid pro quo for the higher levels of local taxation that would inevitably follow such a move – and in 1871 a new Municipal Act was passed in Bengal empowering the lieutenant-governor to introduce elections into any municipality at his discretion. The provisions of the Act were extended to Calcutta in 1875, permitting two-thirds of the commission to be elected by the ratepayers.

Not all Indians, however, welcomed the extension of self-government, and in particular of the elective system. The British Indian Association (which represented the *abhijata* community) asked only for a reform of the system of justices to permit more representation of Indian propertied interests. Landed notables and their acolytes – like the editor of the *Hindoo Patriot*, Kristodas Pal – sought to preserve their privileged position on the nominated commission against the increasingly vocal *grihastha* community, who demanded a share of power in the city.[23] These landowners found an ally in the European business-men who had long run Calcutta's municipal affairs in their own interests. The *Patriot* even claimed to detect a 'new spirit of co-operation' between Indians and Europeans.[24]

The main beneficiaries of the Act were western-educated professionals, who had organised themselves independently of the patronage of the landlords in two new groups: the Indian League and the Indian Association, which supplanted the former soon after the reconstitution of the commission.[25] The more orthodox Hindus among the *grihasthas* were represented by the newspaper the *Amrita Bazar Patrika*, and the more 'Anglicised' by the *Bengalee* (edited by Surendranath Banerjea, who was to become an active member of the com-mission). These new organisations found the British Indian Association and the *Hindoo Patriot* wanting in 'national feeling', and were highly critical of the temporary alliance it had forged with Calcutta's European community.[26]

The new commission consisted of 72 members, of whom 24 were appointed by government, and 48 elected for a term of 3 years. In order to secure 'fair' representation of the European community, the Act provided for the election of three commissioners per ward. The first election to the commission took place in 1876: 13,000 of Calcutta's residents were entitled to vote, but only Hindus took much interest in the proceedings. Out of 1,290 Muslims entitled to register as voters, only 239 bothered to do so.[27] The same pattern was repeated in the next election in 1879; the second commission being comprised of 49 Hindus, 17 Europeans, and 5 Muslims. The legal profession was the dominant occupational group among the commissioners, with 18 members; landowners were second with 12 members; and merchants third with 7. The chairman of the commission was a European, W. M. Souttar, and the vice-chairman a Hindu, Sreenath Ghose.[28]

The election of a majority of Hindu members to the commission ruptured the already strained relationship between Calcutta's European residents and the Indian community. Municipal affairs in Calcutta had been becoming increasingly politicised over the previous decade, with Hindu opposition to the water-rate and demands for local self-government.[29] With European representation on the commission now reduced to less than one quarter, the situation had been reversed, with the Hindu commissioners now the scapegoat for the city's ills. The city's health officer, Dr Payne, defended the record of Calcutta's European administration over the years, and proudly displayed statistics showing a marked drop in deaths from cholera in the city from 15.8 per 1,000 in 1866 to 4.3 in 1876. He was less satisfied with the attitude of the new corporation towards sanitation, particularly its reluctance to improve some of the city's worst *bustis* (slum houses).[30] The Army Sanitary Commission in Britain, which took a general interest in matters of Indian public health, also voiced its concern about the state of Calcutta's *bustis*, suggesting that the municipality purchase the land, and sell it at a profit once improvements had been carried out. However, the commission protested that it had no powers of compulsory purchase and that it did not think these necessary.[31] It declared itself perfectly willing to undertake the conservancy and sewerage of these districts provided 'the owners and occupiers are ready to pay for the service'.[32]

Busti reform became a perennial issue of controversy in Calcutta and other Indian cities, touching, as it did, on the economic interests of slum landlords who were well represented on municipal commissions. The *Patriot*, defending the city's *rentier* class, was quick to rebut criticism of the corporation for its inaction over the improvement of *bustis*, claiming that their condition was 'not so bad as in some of the large English towns', and citing the slightly higher death-rate of Liverpool as a case in point.[33] The landlords on the city's *busti* committee and their supporters in the press were implacably opposed to any drastic scheme for the improvement of slum property.[34] They argued strenuously against the wholesale clearances proposed by the health officer – Dr Payne – claiming that piecemeal reform was fairer to both landlords and tenants. The *Hindoo Patriot* wondered whether 'such violent spoliation of property would be sanctioned in England',[35] and alleged that bodies such as the Army Sanitary Commission had no real understanding of the progress that had been made by the corporation.[36]

The drainage of Calcutta was another issue which soon brought European advocates of sanitary reform and the Hindu commissioners into conflict. The mouthpiece of Calcutta's European community – the *Englishman* – condemned the 'factious opposition' of the *Patriot*, and many of the commissioners, to the municipality's new policy of filling in open water-tanks and pools of stagnant water because of their probable connection with cholera.[37] The *Patriot* claimed in its defence that the health officer's campaign against 'foul water' was not based on any scientifically proven theory of cholera transmission, and that such a scheme was impractical because the municipality did not have sufficient funds to carry it out, without increasing taxation.[38]

The issue of taxation was also at the heart of a dispute over the removal of night-soil in Calcutta. The *Patriot* claimed that an 'iniquitous scale of rates' had been charged to householders for this service, and that the establishment was costly, 'bloated', and with little definite work to do.[39] In reality, however, the cost of collecting night-soil was comparatively small, amounting to only 3.4 per cent of the municipality's expenditure in 1876.[40] In fact, Calcutta's finances were far from overstretched. Revenue was very stable compared with many other municipalities – being raised mainly through direct taxation, as opposed to trades tax – and income was usually sufficient to cover expenditure, even though the rate of taxation was among the lowest in British India.[41] The overall prosperity of the city was also increasing, due to a run of good harvests in Bengal and the development of East Bengal and Assam. The value of Calcutta's export trade had increased from Rs 477 million in 1875–6 to Rs 621 million in 1880–1.[42]

The main bone of contention over the funding of municipal improvement in Calcutta was whether sanitary works should be financed by loans, or entirely through taxation. Government loans were not always freely available and were often conditional on the work being commenced at a pre-arranged date, or on a municipality's previous record in public health.[43] In 1886 the Calcutta commissioners complained that government had 'refused to grant loans for improvement, on the policy that local bodies be left to their own resources'. In such circumstances, they were doubtful whether much improvement would be carried out.[44] But such protests had a hollow ring, given the commission's record of resistance to raising revenue through taxation. Calcutta's house rate was still the lowest of any major city in British India, and well below the maximum set by the Government of Bengal.[45] It was against this background, and against the extension of local self-government to other local bodies in the 1880s, that the *Englishman* led aggrieved Europeans in a two-pronged attack on the corporation and on government – both of which appeared to have abdicated all responsibility for public health.

A case which seemed to epitomise Indian 'unfitness' for government, and the reluctance of the authorities to intervene in sanitary matters, was that of Sheikh Darvstoollah against the municipal commission, in which a prosecution was brought against the latter for its failure to remove a public nuisance in the form of a polluted water-tank.[46] The presidency magistrate held that the corporation had done its best to remedy the problem, and that it was not liable to take further action. The outraged editor of the *Englishman* protested that the magistrate had 'failed to grasp the serious nature of the complaint' and that it was impossible to share his 'easy-going views' on the subject. 'If the case has done nothing else', he wrote, 'it has proved how great is the need for a Health Society in Calcutta'.[47]

The society to which he referred was a pressure group, comprised mainly of Europeans, which had been founded in Calcutta in 1884. It had already received considerable publicity in the European press, and in medical journals such as the *Indian Medical Gazette*, whose editor – Kenneth MacLeod – was also chairman of the Health Society.[48] The society represented a substantial element of European society which had been alienated by the Liberal local self-government reforms of the 1870s and 80s. It claimed to act in a spirit of Christian duty and of 'beneficent utilitarianism'. In the words of its president, the Hon. Justice Cunningham, the society had 'enough of apologies, enough of delays, enough of evasion, enough of talk' – the 'day of action' had arrived.[49]

The society drew ammunition for its campaign from a recent report into the sanitary state of Calcutta commissioned by the Bengal government following the report of the German Cholera commission.[50] Although it did acknowledge some improvement in Calcutta's public health, the report indicated that many parts of the city were still in an 'extremely insanitary state'. The administration of public health in Calcutta was 'in a high degree faulty', its statistics 'untrustworthy', and its establishment 'insufficient and without proper supervision'. Moreover, the municipal commissioners had 'deliberately reduced the grant asked for by the executive for sanitary purposes by nearly 3 lakhs sooner than raise the house tax.'[51]

The report was seized upon by the Anglo-Indian press (especially the *Englishman* and the *Pioneer*) as evidence of the failure of local self-government. However, Calcutta's Indian commissioners did not bear the brunt of this onslaught alone; in fact, it was the corporation's liberal chairman Mr Cotton who had become the *bête noir* of authoritarian elements within the Anglo-Indian community. 'Mr. Cotton', wrote the *Bengalee*, 'belongs to that illustrious band of Englishmen who have . . . felt the deepest sympathy with the people'. He had 'rendered a service to the rate-payers of Calcutta which they will not easily forget; and it is time that they should resent the assertions of the *Pioneer* in a practical and substantial manner'. The *Bengalee*, a keen advocate of local self-government, defended the role of the corporation, and argued that although much remained to be done, a good deal had already been achieved in the direction of sanitary reform.[52] The *Hindoo Patriot*, though less enthusiastic about extending Indian representation, nevertheless defended the record of the corporation. The commissioners, it argued, could do nothing without sufficient funds at their disposal. In addition, no Indian witnesses had been called to give evidence to the sanitary commission; a fact which the *Patriot* took to be indicative of the government's hostility to the 'large Babu element' in the municipal commission.[53] It protested that

> those who denounce the native corporators as neglecting sanitary and conservancy works for the purpose of saving their own pockets are either ignorant of the nature of the case, or are deliberately guilty of committing a gross breach of one of the Ten Commandments.[54]

Perhaps the most serious charge made in the report was that the commissioners had not charged the ratepayers of Calcutta up to the maximum permitted by law, prompting the lieutenant-governor of Bengal, Sir Rivers Thompson, to suggest that the corporation be made more accountable to the government. But the *Patriot* pointed out, with some justification, that the corporation's budget, including levels of taxation, had been fixed with the entire approval of the Bengal government.[55]

With the corporation in a vulnerable position, the health society stepped up its agitation in an attempt to embarrass the municipality into action. A correspondent to the *Englishman* claimed that the society's strictures had begun to bear fruit at quite an early stage, and that 'whilst the controversy raged fiercest between the Government and the Municipality, *bustis* were being cleared, and new roads and drains cut through them with an enterprise seldom, if ever, before displayed by the Commissioners in so good a cause'.[56] Protests had also spread to the city's suburbs (shortly to be incorporated within Calcutta City municipality), where 3,000 residents had sent a petition to the Government of Bengal demanding that the suburban municipality be forced to take a more active part in sanitation. According to the *Englishman*, the suburbs had no drainage or water-supply systems, and 'huge open cess-pools' lay 'seething and festering in the sun, filling the surrounding atmosphere with poisonous exhalations'.[57]

Drainage and inadequate conservancy were apparently little better in the city itself. In a lecture to the society on 'Preventable disease in Calcutta', Mr Thomas, a judge of the Small Cause Court, claimed that

> Strong evidence exists in Calcutta which goes to support the doctrine that whatever the nature or cause of cholera may be, filth has much to do with its propagation – filth in air, water and food; filth due to neglected conservancy; filth comprising mainly of the decomposing excreta of men and animals.[58]

The chief defect of Calcutta's drainage system, in the opinion of most observers, was that it combined sewerage with the removal of storm water, causing noxious substances to well up in the city at times of heavy rain. Bad drainage, more than any other factor, was probably responsible for the fact that there had been no improvement in the city's mortality rate, the main component of which was death from fever.[59]

Towards the end of 1885 the health society sought to make public health the main issue at the forthcoming municipal election: 'After keeping up an incessant rattle about cholera, preventable deaths, native apathy . . . and what not . . . it had fully calculated upon an overwhelming majority'.[60] But the society's opponents were equally determined to mobilise an opposition. The *Bengalee* condemned the society as 'the guardian of European and Eurasian interests', and urged Indian rate-payers throughout Calcutta to organise themselves into committees to secure the election of 'the best men'. The health society, it claimed, stood 'discredited in the eyes of the native community for the agitation which some of its leaders set on foot against the Calcutta Corporation'.[61] The results of the election did much to confirm this assertion, the corporation being dominated by Hindu landowners and lawyers as before. The landowning interest, as the *Bengalee* observed, now had 'the largest stake in the town', with twelve representatives in the municipal commission; the legal profession comprising the next largest element with eleven. The remainder comprised doctors, civil servants, merchants, journalists, translators, railway officials, and practitioners of traditional medicine, in that order. After such a result, the *Bengalee* felt that the future of local self-government in Calcutta was assured.[62]

The anti-*babu* rhetoric of the society and its champion the *Englishman* had almost certainly alienated most of the Indian support that it needed to gain a majority in the corporation. Indeed, some months later, the *Patriot* revealed that the society had only 8 Indian members; 2 of whom were western-educated medical practitioners.[63] There was, however, little common cause among the 7 Muslims and 28 Hindus who were elected to the commission; they included

> some Anglicised people who feel disgraced if called Babus and have no sympathy for anything Indian; some candidates for biennial Honorableship [i.e. for seats in the Bengal Legislative Council]; and some applicants for situations for their nephews . . . In the language of the auctioneers, they may be described as a miscellaneous lot – a scratch pack that can never hunt together.[64]

These divisions manifested themselves early in the new commission, when open warfare broke out between the Indian commissioners and the 'Health men and their Babu adherents'. With a good measure of irony, the *Patriot* described the struggle as one between the 'new blood and the old blood retained by the thoughtless electors'. A test resolution on plans to extend the water-supply, which had been outstripped by population growth, failed by two votes, boding ill for the health society and its supporters.[65] The dispute was not so much over whether such works were desirable, but as to how they should be financed. Most Bengali commissioners preferred to raise a loan from government, while the health lobby favoured an increase in the house tax by one-third. The commissioners, in keeping with the interests of their ratepayers, decided to obtain a loan.[66]

Equally controversial was the issue of open-air cremation as practised by Hindus in Calcutta. The health society wished to see restrictions placed on the practice, but with a Hindu majority in the commission there was no real prospect of this happening. Further, the sanitary commissioner of Bengal from 1888 to 1897, Dr W. H. Gregg, could see little wrong in the practice, and argued that there was 'nothing in cremation completely and properly carried out to offend either the sight or one's sense of smell'.[67] Gregg's sympathetic approach won him many friends in the Bengali community. The *Patriot* also praised his defence of the much criticised Indian practice of allowing *pannas* (water-plants) to grow in tanks in the city; Gregg believed that these might even have a purifying effect.[68] He had, in the words of its editor, 'infused fresh blood into the Department of which he is in charge'.[69] He was 'an officer of the modern school, who knows that sanitation to be successful must be based on popular feeling, and that the people must be gradually led along to understand sanitary principles'. In this respect, Gregg stood in marked distinction to his predecessor Dr Lidderdale, who had attempted to coerce Bengali municipal commissioners into submission 'by a process of bullying which he had cultivated to a fine art'. Gregg's approach was, instead, to appeal to indigenous sanitary traditions, and to seek the co-operation of Indian commissioners.[70]

However, the emollient influence of Dr Gregg did little to calm the controversy over sanitation in the Calcutta corporation, which had just acquired a new health officer in the person of Dr W. J. Simpson. From the very beginning, Simpson was identified with the health society and with its supporters in the municipal commission. He had been appointed in preference to two Indian candidates because the European commissioners, to a man, had voted for him, while enough Indians had followed their lead to frustrate the more nationalistic elements within the administration. Surendranath Banerjea wrote in the *Bengalee* of a widespread feeling that 'national interests have been seriously compromised' by the decision, and that there was 'naturally a sense of indignation felt against those commissioners whose action has brought about this result'. He continued:

> If Dr. Simpson has been appointed with the view that the sanitation of Calcutta may be hastened onwards with the speed of the whirlwind, and that the new-fangled ideas of mere theorists may be applied to the conditions of an Eastern city without regard to the wishes or the means of the people, then we have no hesitation in saying that a double injury has been done by the appointment.[71]

In such circumstances it was unlikely that relations between the corporation and its health officer would be cordial or fruitful. Reconciliation was still less likely given Simpson's abrasive personality. Early in his tenure he enraged the city's commissioners by likening the conservancy of Calcutta to that of an African village; conduct which was denounced by the *Bengalee* as 'discourteous and exaggerated'.[72] Simpson also incurred the wrath of his superiors for his criticism of the city's water supply. 'In the riparian districts', he reported, 'the inhabitants have to resort to the river and to the polluted wells in their own houses', while 'the occupants of large bustees have to resort to the nearest filthy tank'. 'In 1884', he continued, 'during the unprecedented outbreak of cholera in Calcutta, the scarcity of water then formed a subject of complaint by some of the Commissioners, but apparently without any effect'. The commissioners naturally resented the implication that they were indifferent to the plight of Calcutta's poorest inhabitants, and claimed that Simpson had ignored the fact that a new pumping station had opened to supply these areas, and that water could now be obtained from every stand-pump for 12 hours per day.[73] The *Bengalee* felt that 'the Commissioners have a right to expect that he will be deferential, and that he will be strictly accurate in his facts'. The *Englishman*, however, claimed Simpson as a 'martyr' to the cause, an irreplaceable asset to a corporation which ill-deserved him.[74]

In 1888, with the passage of the new Calcutta Municipal Act, circumstances appeared to be moving in Simpson's favour. The Act conferred upon the corporation new powers for the removal of *bustis* and compelled it, on pain of interference from provincial government, to fulfil its statutory duties.[75] Simpson was keen to take advantage of this opportunity, but in pursuing it too vigorously he managed to alienate not only the city's Indian commissioners, but also its English chairman, Sir Henry Harrison. The new Municipal Act enabled the corporation to regulate the construction of *bustis* according to sanitary principles, but there were no sections concerning the height of buildings according to the width of streets, or requiring a minimum of airspace between them. The free circulation of air between buildings was, according to Simpson, one of the fundamental principles of sanitation in a tropical climate. Amendment of the Act was, therefore, essential, and particularly since the recent tendency to build slum houses out of brick would make their eventual removal more expensive.[76] Simpson also criticised the corporation for its failure to address the problem of overcrowding in *bustis*, and proposed a scheme for the opening-up of the more crowded parts of the city with eight new roads. Sir Henry took great exception to these remarks, and pointed out that the new Act had only just introduced regulations concerning the overcrowding of dwellings. Simpson had also overlooked the construction of a new road through the previously congested Burma Bazaar, at a cost to the corporation of some Rs 50 lakhs. He considered Simpson's proposal – which had been costed at 150 lakhs – to be totally unrealistic and out of touch with the mood of the corporation.[77] 'Dr. Simpson', he warned

should not allow himself to lose sight of the fact that the Government has resolved to entrust the administration of Calcutta to a body largely composed of Commissioners elected by the rate-payers, of whom nine-tenths are natives of India. The attempt to coerce such a governing body and to compel them to adopt measures diametrically opposed to their own views and those of their constituents, must end in disastrous conflicts. If sanitation is a real boon to the population of a city, it can be made with tact and judgement to appear in that light, and the residents can by degrees be converted from strong opponents to ardent supporters of sound measures of improvement.[78]

But appeals for gradualism went unheeded and the health officer continued his campaign for a tightening of the law regarding slum properties, having the backing of the health society and the tacit support of prominent individuals in the Bengal government. The Municipal Act was, itself, an indication that the government had grown more interventionist of late, and the passage in 1890 of a new provincial law regarding *bustis* was a further setback for Calcutta's *rentier* class. The Act, which required owners of *busti* land to pay rates formerly leviable directly from tenants, apparently entailed 'great hardship upon owners', and was vigorously opposed by Indians in both the legislative council and the corporation.[79] Encouraged by the government's stance, Simpson renewed his demands for more stringent building regulations, which he regarded as 'the most important sanitary measures which it remains to undertake'.[80]

But landowning interests were still dominant in the corporation, and the health officer's proposal was rejected by a 'very large majority' of the commissioners, who argued that the municipality already had sufficient powers under the Act of 1888.[81] By 1894 it became clear to Simpson that there was very little prospect of tightening building regulations further with the municipality as presently constituted.[82] He was by now firmly of opinion that

the consequence of the delegation of power in sanitary matters to local authorities without introducing simultaneously an effective system of authoritative guidance and control, has not been sufficiently realised nor has its paralysing effect been sufficiently appreciated to arouse the Government to action.[83]

The Hindu-dominated commission was also increasingly subject to criticism from another quarter, hitherto largely silent in municipal affairs. Muslim interest in municipal politics had grown steadily in the 1880s, and in the election of 1886 21 per cent more Muslims registered to vote than previously; while, in the same year, the numbers of those registering among the European and Hindu communities fell by 3 per cent and 16 per cent respectively.[84] Muslim participation increased largely in opposition to the 'Babuocracy' in the commission and in the Bengal magistracy, and must be seen against a background of mounting communal tension, exemplified by the cow-killing agitation of the 1890s.[85] Although the number of Muslim commissioners had increased from only 5 in 1876 to 13 (8 of whom were elected) in 1895, the community still felt it was under-represented.[86] 'As it is in the Calcutta Corporation', wrote the editor of the *Moslem Chronicle*, 'so it is everywhere. Whether it is a District Board or a University, the Europeans and the Mohammadans have not the ghost of a chance of election.' He was pleased that his appeal for adequate representation of minorities had received the backing of the *Englishman*, with its 'long record of defending the weak against the unjust attack of the all engrossing Babus'.[87] On matters of public health, alleged the *Chronicle*, the Babu commissioners had been tried and found wanting: the city was a 'veritable hell' and had been made so by the 'indifference and culpable neglect of . . . the Municipal Commissioners'.[88] It agreed with the *Englishman* that the only solution was for the Bengal government to 'interfere with a strong hand' and to force the municipality to take action in sanitary matters.[89]

Calcutta's Hindu commissioners, for their part, had come to the conclusion that the post of health officer was a 'white elephant, maintained at the cost of the ratepayers' blood',[90] while Simpson, like many Muslims, had entered into the demonology of the Bengal nationalist movement. The scale of resentment towards Simpson may be illustrated by the opposition to his deputation (at ratepayers' expense) to the London conference of Hygiene and Demography in 1890. The decision to pay for Simpson's passage – which had been hotly contested within the corporation – was criticised across the board in the Bengali press. The *Bengalee*, the *Amrita Bazar Patrika*, and the *Hindoo Patriot* all objected to the decision on grounds of expense, while the *Indian Daily News* condemned the conference as yet 'another of the pseudo-scientific fads of which the age is prolific'.[91] Simpson was also subject to continual criticism in the corporation for the intemperate language of his official reports, and on one occasion escaped a vote of censure only through the intervention of his erstwhile enemy Sir Henry Harrison, who trod a fine line between the Indian corporators and Calcutta's Anglo-Indian community.[92]

In this atmosphere of mutual distrust and recrimination there was little prospect of any substantial sanitary improvement in Calcutta. The introduction of a piped water-supply in 1869 led to a reduction in Calcutta's crude death-rate from 54.1 per 1,000 in 1865, to only 24.1 in 1873. However, the inability of the city's drainage to cope with this supply and with flooding during the rainy season, meant that malaria and waterborne diseases such as cholera and dysentery began to increase once more, raising the city's death-rate to 36.6 per 1,000 in 1878. Piecemeal improvements to both water-supply and drainage since then had brought the death-rate down to around 27 per 1,000 by 1889, but no substantial reduction could be expected until the fundamental inadequacies of the city's drainage and sewerage systems were addressed.[93] Simpson was determined to remedy the situation and, at his invitation, an eminent English sanitary engineer, Mr Baldwin Latham, spent two weeks in Calcutta inspecting the existing drainage system; his criticisms of which, and proposals for a new drainage scheme, were later submitted in a report to the commission.[94] Baldwin Latham argued that the existing system, which combined drainage with sewerage, was inadequate because the outfall was often blocked by tides at times of heavy rain, causing sewage to well up all over the city.[95] Simpson shared Baldwin Latham's opinion that Calcutta needed separate systems of drainage and sewerage. 'Calcutta', he wrote, 'is an excellent illustration of a town in which, not only the principle of sewerage is wrong, but the original plan defective'.[96] Although the commission considered the report, and accepted many of its criticisms, no action was taken on its recommendations on the grounds that the proposed scheme was too expensive. However, the fact that the scheme carried Simpson's endorsement may well have sealed its fate regardless of its budgetary implications.

Prior to 1896 it seemed that Simpson had little prospect of persuading the municipal commission to take a more active part in sanitary reform, but in that year the situation altered fundamentally with the appearance in Bombay of bubonic plague. The plague, which appears to have arrived in Bombay from Hong Kong in the late summer of 1896, soon took on epidemic proportions, spreading throughout many districts of western India. Its progress was devastating in both human and material terms: by 12 April 1897, plague had claimed 9,640 lives in Bombay city alone,[97] and had brought maritime trade and industrial production in Bombay and Karachi to a standstill.

The immediate reaction of the municipal commission in Calcutta was to take measures to keep plague out of the city, and to equip the Health Department should an outbreak occur. The small sum of Rs 3,000 was placed at the disposal of the health officer for conservancy arrangements, and the Port Commission and the railway authorities were ordered to keep watch over passengers from western India. Rs 68,278 were also made available for an isolation hospital for plague victims. In the event of plague occurring in Calcutta, the emergency provisions of the Municipal Act of 1888 conferred upon the health officer the power to disinfect dwellings, to destroy suspect goods, and to remove persons suffering from the disease to hospital.[98] These precautions, at first, received a guarded welcome in the English-language Bengali press: they did not unduly offend Indian sensibilities, and indigenous personnel had been chosen for the most sensitive task of railway inspection.[99]

But the caution of the municipal commission did not recommend itself to those elements of Calcutta's European community which had long advocated a 'forward' policy in matters of public health. The lieutenant-governor of Bengal claimed that the corporation was dragging its feet over conservancy arrangements in Calcutta, and made a veiled threat that he would have no choice but to intervene if the corporation continued to abdicate its responsibility for sanitation. Rising to the defence of the commissioners, the *Bengalee* claimed that these allegations were totally without foundation, and that any delay in plague precautions was the fault of the executive, which had not been ready with its scheme. Moreover, the health officer's plan for dealing with any outbreak of plague appeared to privilege the more affluent parts of the town, and he had made little provision for the northern areas of the city, the insanitary state of which made them especially vulnerable to epidemic disease.[100]

Thus, the plague scare brought to a head the antagonism and suspicion between the Bengali commissioners and the executive which had been mounting steadily since Simpson's appointment as health officer. The inflammatory statements of government raised the political temperature in Calcutta still further. The *Englishman* could scarcely conceal its delight when reporting in January 1897 that 'the Government of India . . . and the Government of Bengal afford indications of the fact that the Hindu Commissioners must either stop talking or stop being Commissioners', and that the only way to prevent plague in Calcutta was to make sure that the city was 'thoroughly cleansed'. According to its editor, the shilly-shallying of the commissioners, and the 'obstructive' attitude of Banerjea in particular, had given rise to

> a widespread feeling of alarm and distrust, and that feeling, by leading Continental Governments to fear the momentary outbreak of plague in Calcutta, is responsible for the harsh and injurious restrictions which have been imposed universally on the whole shipping of India.[101]

As described in chapter 5, Italy, France, and Germany had placed a blanket ban on raw-hides from India (as well as certain other materials thought susceptible to infection with plague), which were one of India's chief exports to the West. Of all Indian ports, Calcutta was hardest hit by the ban, being the country's chief exporter of hides and skins.

The trade sanctions produced a flood of mail to the *Englishman* condemning the commission's inaction. One correspondent captured the mood of Calcutta's European community when he wrote 'it would be worth while going to any expense to stamp out the disease, and if Municipalities in towns affected are obstructive, it would be best to suspend them, appointing such other men in their place as may be available'. Another urged government to 'take upon themselves what the Corporation fails in energy to perform'.[102] Indeed, in the Bombay Presidency, such measures were already being implemented. On the recommendation of the governor, Lord Sandhurst, the municipal commissions in Bombay and Poona had been suspended and replaced with special Plague Commissions, comprised mainly of military men and civil servants. These commissions, as shown in chapter 6, had implemented a set of draconian anti-plague measures including segregation and house-to-house inspection.

Simpson was fully in favour of introducing such measures should plague break out in Calcutta, but no such outbreak occurred in the critical year of 1897, after which quarantine against India was gradually relaxed. A number of suspect cases occurred, diagnosed mostly by Simpson himself, but these were rejected as bona fide cases by the Bengal Medical Board. Suspicion that Simpson had deliberately mis-diagnosed the cases in order to provoke a plague scare – in support of his plan for drastic sanitary action – was not entirely without foundation.[103] Nevertheless, talk of segregation continued to cause alarm in Calcutta; even after Simpson was forced to retire from his post through ill health in September 1897.[104] In April 1898, shortly after the first confirmed cases of plague in the city, the *Bengalee* warned:

> If segregation is insisted upon, we are afraid there will be concealment of cases. An oriental people with the *zenana* system have a deep-rooted dislike for segregation. Much rather they would die like sheep in their own houses . . . than allow their wives and mothers to be taken to the isolation camps.[105]

Calcutta's new health officer – Dr J. Nield Cook – also had misgivings about the policy advocated by his predecessor. In his opinion, it was 'impossible to carry out a measure like segregation in a large oriental city when the entire population is against it'. He pointed to the fact that segregation had caused great unrest in cities where it had been attempted, and that it had no discernible effect upon plague.[106]

Yet, when plague did break out in Calcutta on 27 April 1898, the mere suspicion that segregation might be introduced caused over 150,000 people to flee the city, and rumours abounded to the effect that the authorities intended to kill persons who were taken to the plague hospital. The exodus prompted the inspector-general of hospitals, Col. T. H. Hendley, to report that all thoughts of segregation should be abandoned, and that the best course was that of evacuating infected areas and disinfecting them. He was also in favour of voluntary inoculation against plague, using the procedure developed in Bombay by the Russian bacteriologist Waldemar Haffkine.[107] The *Bengalee* also believed that 'if the alternatives of inoculation or segregation were proposed, we are sure that in every case inoculation would be preferred, and the people would bless the Government for sparing them the hardships of segregation'.[108]

However, there is little evidence that inoculation was popular with the majority of Calcutta's inhabitants. The sanitary commissioner of Bengal, Major Dyson, believed that the infrequent resort to inoculation may have been a reflection of the comparatively low incidence of plague in the city. Deaths from plague in Calcutta in 1898 numbered only 230, while the following year was 'extremely healthy'.[109] But, in the atmosphere of mutual distrust which existed between Calcutta's European and Indian inhabitants, rumour had it that the authorities meant to poison Indians through inoculation, and rioting broke out in some of the Muslim *bustis*, quickly spreading to some of the surrounding areas. The city was, as the *Bengalee* put it, in a 'state of great excitement, in which scare after scare gave impetus to the exodus movement' and to 'new dangers for the orderly and peace-loving citizens of Calcutta'.[110] Allegations of maltreatment at railway-station plague camps heightened concern over the conduct of the British authorities: Indians had been detained regardless of holding certificates of health, and women were not always examined by female inspectresses, as stipulated in government regulations.[111] The European press served only to fan the flames of civil unrest: in a typically intemperate editorial, the *Englishman* urged Calcutta's police to flog rioters on the spot. By contrast, the *Bengalee*, whose readership stood to lose most – politically and economically – from the rioting, urged the government to show restraint, and persist in its policy of limited intervention.[112]

The plague scare did, however, engender an atmosphere conducive to sanitary reform, and for the first time there was general agreement over the need to institute a new drainage scheme, and for a Building Commission to monitor the construction of new houses in the city. 'It has taken many years to bring about the recognition of the necessity of these measures . . . ', wrote Simpson in 1897, 'the Commissioners are to be congratulated on the advances of the year'.[113] But the sanitary state of Calcutta still left much to be desired. There were frequent and flagrant breaches of municipal by-laws, and there was 'much discussion about the state of Calcutta's streets', which were described by a correspondent to the *Englishman* as 'nothing but a long midden'.[114] These concerns quickly gave rise to demands for more drastic action than that contemplated by the municipality. 'The case of Calcutta', wrote the editor of the *Bengal Times*, 'does not encourage government to entrust sanitation to the tender mercies of self-help'. The recent plague scare had revealed 'loathsome and filthy conditions' which the municipality had failed to prevent.[115]

The appalling sanitary condition of Calcutta was also highlighted by the Sanitary Inspection Committee commissioned by the Bengal Medical Board to tour the city noting sanitary defects. In its report of November 1896, the committee drew attention to the 'complete failure of the Health Department . . . to carry out the ordinary operations of town conservancy', the 'hopelessly insufficient' number of latrines, the deficiency of sewerage and surface drainage, and the 'generally and undeniably filthy condition of the water tanks'.[116] The overcrowding in many districts of Calcutta was equally alarming. Of the 18 wards visited by the inspectors, 14 had a higher population density than London (which then averaged 35,905 per square mile), the average for Calcutta as a whole being 69,200. The three worst wards of the city had a population density of over 100,000 and, the very worst, of 144,640 per square mile. The dwellings themselves equalled even the worst London 'rookeries' for squalor. In one notorious *busti*, the houses were

> built almost back to back. It would nearly be impossible to squeeze between them; sunlight is so far shut out that . . . it is absolutely impossible to do more than grope your way from one part to another within these tenements . . . A heavy sickening odour pervades the whole place; walls and floors alike are damp with contamination from liquid sewage, which lies rotting, and from which there is no escape.

In the opinion of the inspectors, 'no measures short of the compulsory widening of all the roads and lanes' would be of any benefit in the most thickly populated and insanitary areas of town.[117]

The arrival of plague in Calcutta in 1898 prompted more radical suggestions. 'Sooner or later', argued the *Englishman*, the municipality would have to face up to the fact that it must 'sweep the Calcutta bustis away'. It was not merely that these slums were a 'disgrace to a civilised town' but they were also the principal foci of civil unrest:

The worst bustis are those inhabited by lower class Mohammedans. These are a terror not only to the health but to the peace of the city. We question whether any European has ever penetrated into the inner square of some of them, but one can imagine from the outside what the interior must be like.[118]

Impenetrable not only to light and air, but also to the official gaze, Calcutta's slums had become the focus of deep-seated European anxieties, and their eradication a matter of political, as well as sanitary, importance. The dangers represented by *bustis* and their inhabitants were especially evident in Calcutta for, unlike many other Indian cities, where 'the dirty classes' lived at some remove from European quarters, they were scattered throughout the city, directly threatening the lives and property of Europeans and prosperous Indians.[119]

Until the arrival of plague, attempts to improve Calcutta's *bustis* had been piecemeal and had proceeded slowly.[120] The Calcutta Building Commission had drawn up a scheme for driving wide streets through the most congested localities, but its implementation was impeded by lack of funds, leaving a question-mark over the corporation's commitment to sanitary reform.[121] Thus, when plague broke out in Calcutta in 1898, demands for *busti* reform were accompanied by a renewed onslaught against the corporation. Emboldened by incursions on municipal autonomy elsewhere in India, influential sections of the European community began to demand sweeping reforms of the municipal constitution in the name of sanitary reform.

A distinctive feature of this latest wave of agitation was the prominent part played by European commercial interests, concerned at the economic disruption caused by plague. It was alleged that the constitution of the corporation 'practically excluded European men of business from all share in the municipal government of Calcutta'. It was pointed out that under the existing constitution Hindus had significantly more voting power than their numbers in the city warranted, and that this operated to the disadvantage of both Moslems and Europeans. While Hindus constituted 73.3 per cent of those registered to vote, they formed only 69.5 per cent of Calcutta's population. The fact that Hindu ratepayers contributed by far the largest amount to municipal coffers was conveniently overlooked.[122]

The Bengal Chamber of Commerce and the Calcutta Trades Association saw municipal representation as a means of securing the opening-up of congested areas to traffic and trade; in Bombay commercial associations had been instrumental in setting up an Improvement Trust for precisely these reasons.[123]

In Calcutta the European commercial lobby found a champion in the lieutenant-governor of Bengal Sir Alexander Mackenzie – an inveterate critic of the corporation – who seized the opportunity provided by the plague to introduce a bill advocating a much greater degree of executive control over the municipal commission. Mackenzie proposed that a general committee (including representatives of local government and European trading associations) be set up with the power of appointing executive officers independently of the commissioners. In the event of a dispute between the commissioners and the committee over the municipal budget, the latter would refer the matter to the Bengal government, whose decision would be final. The powers of the chairman were also to be greatly increased, while the provincial government would have enhanced powers of intervention in municipal affairs.[124]

These proposals were warmly welcomed by the *Englishman*, which declared that 'those capable of forming an intelligent opinion on the subject were of one mind about the urgent need of Sir Alexander Mackenzie's scheme for placing Calcutta municipal affairs more under European control'.[125] If successful, the bill would 'restore European supremacy' after 'twenty-five years of native mismanagement'.[126] The Calcutta Trades Association also praised the bill, stressing that its early passage would 'at once create a feeling of greater security and confidence and tend to safeguard not only the health of the inhabitants but also the commercial and trading interests of the province'.[127]

Not surprisingly, however, the Calcutta Municipal Bill produced a storm among the city's Indian élite; or at least those sections committed to the extension of local self-government. Surendranath Banerjea denounced the measure as 'retrograde and reactionary' and vigorously opposed the proposal in the Bengal Legislative Council. Indian commercial associations such as the Bengal National Chamber of Commerce also voiced their opposition to the bill, being particularly incensed by their exclusion from any representation on the general committee. To nationalist politicians the bill was but one crest of a 'wave of reaction sweeping across the high places of Government', and was of a piece with other measures such as the recent Sedition and Criminal Procedure acts.[128] However, the bill was welcomed by the patricians of the British Indian Association, and by the Muslim élite, who resented the power and influence which municipal representation had brought the Bengali middle class.[129]

The Bengal government exploited these divisions, claiming that the existing constitution of the municipality did not give fair representation to Moslems and other sections of the Indian community;[130] the *Englishman* claimed that the aristocratic members of the BIA were the true leaders of the Hindu community. But, as the *Bengalee* pointed out, 'the British Indian Association became "true leaders" when they are with the Government and against the community – they are worthless agitators when they side with their own people and protest against the measures of Government'.[131]

Indian opposition to the Municipal Bill consisted largely of public meetings and petitions of protest to the Bengal government. No less than 9 public meetings and 4 ward meetings were held in Calcutta between the end of August 1898 and the middle of March 1899. One indication of the extent of the controversy over the bill was that the measure was debated at Westminster, and widely reported in the British press. Lord George Hamilton the secretary of state for India justified the bill to the House on the grounds that the corporation had neglected its responsibilities for public health, and that the situation had become acute with the arrival of plague in the city.[132] The Bengali corporators were not, however, without support in Britain. A correspondent to the *Manchester Guardian* condemned the bill as a 'sweeping and punitive measure', and dismissed the accusations levelled at the commissioners as groundless.[133]

Most critics of the bill saw the issue of sanitation as a 'mere pretext' for the restoration of European supremacy in municipal affairs. The chief hindrance to sanitary reform in Calcutta, argued the *Bengalee*, was not the attitude of the commissioners, but the city's structural defects which could only be remedied by additional revenue drawn not from property-owners, but from taxes on exported goods such as jute.[134] It had long held that the Calcutta Inspection Report on which many of the allegations against the corporation had been based was in many respects deficient; not least in its tendency to generalise about the health of the city from descriptions of its worst slums.[135] The *Bengalee*'s defence of the corporation's sanitary record, however, was deeply flawed: the report had, in fact, investigated all 24 wards in Calcutta, while an independent report of 1899 appeared to verify many of its findings.[136] Thus, while sanitary reform was a vehicle for ill-concealed European prejudices and political aspirations, there can be no doubt that the sanitary record of the corporation left much to be desired.

The Calcutta Municipal Bill was eventually passed by the Bengal Legislative Council in September 1899. Against a background of mounting hostility in Bengal, and threats to send a municipal delegation to put the case against the measure in Britain, the bill had been rushed through the council at an unprecedented rate.[137] The European commercial lobby, in particular, expressed alarm at the fact that the bill had been made a party issue in Britain, and urged that the matter be quickly resolved.[138] The Calcutta Municipal Act of 1899 was also a more reactionary measure than had been originally envisaged by Mackenzie. Under the stewardship of the new lieutenant-governor Sir John Woodburn, and constant pressure from the *Englishman* and European commercial associations, additional clauses had been added which reduced by half the number of elected commissioners to twenty-five. It was feared that the general committee would find it difficult to oppose a commission over four times its size.[139] The successful passage of the bill, ultimately owed much to the emergency conditions arising from plague, and the resurgence of authoritarian-paternalism under the viceroyalty of Lord Curzon, who had taken up his appointment in 1898. On receiving a deputation from the British India Association, Curzon had stressed that local self-government in India would have to grow 'within safe and well-ascertained limits', and that in some cases, as in Calcutta, this meant 'replacing restrictions which had been too hastily removed'.[140] The Bengal government was, as the *Englishman* put it, relieved to be rid of the 'incubus which has weighed on it so long', while the commercial interests of Calcutta were 'naturally gratified to secure a municipal system in which they have their fair share of influence and representation'.[141] Temporarily, at least, self-government was held in abeyance; in Calcutta's case, representation was not broadened significantly until 1923.

The passage of the Municipal Act came as little surprise to its opponents, because it had for some time been clear that the Bengal government had the unflinching support of the viceroy and the secretary of state. Shortly after the decision was announced, Banerjea and the majority of Bengali commissioners resigned from the corporation *en masse*, and refused to take any further part in municipal affairs. Their lead was followed by the Bengali electorate of Calcutta, which showed little enthusiasm during the seven municipal elections which took place between that date and 1923.[142] This is not to say, however, that the people of Calcutta had lost all interest in the administration of the city. The Indian press voiced popular dissatisfaction with the new regime; with its alleged inefficiency and the additional burdens which it had imposed on the ratepayers.[143] A series of corruption scandals involving municipal contracts also brought the new administration into disrepute, as European business interests in the corporation began to turn their new power to their advantage.[144]

The one significant innovation of the 1899–1923 period was the establishment of an improvement trust in 1912, along the lines of those set up in Bombay and some other Indian cities.[145] The Calcutta Improvement Trust was comprised of a mixture of elected and nominated members. The chairman, Mr C. H. Bompas of the Indian Civil Service, and S. L. Maddox, chairman of the the municipal commission were nominated by government. The nine other trustees were elected variously by the municipal commission, the ward commissioners, the Bengal government, and local commercial associations. Under the Calcutta Improvement Act of 1911, the trust was empowered to acquire land for improvement and to sell it at a profit. The trust also drew income from taxes on local trades and on the transfer of property in Calcutta.[146]

Indian reactions to the trust were ambivalent. While there was support in some quarters for urban improvement, there was opposition to the concentration of power in the chairman of the trust, and to the fact that it had only three Indian members.[147] Still more contentious was the composition of the tribunal appointed to assess land-acquisition cases.[148] It was only after much wrangling that a seat was obtained for one of the elected members of the corporation, and one for the Bengal National Chamber of Commerce.[149] The election by the municipal commission of the 'Peoples' Assessor' to the Improvement Tribunal became a matter of some controversy.[150] The trust gained most of its Indian support from among the mercantile community. The National Chamber of Commerce, the Calcutta Trades Association and the up-country Marwari Association, all saw considerable economic advantage in opening-up congested areas of the city to traffic.[151] However, some Indian traders – particularly those of the bazaars – were antagonistic to the operations of the trust, and claimed that the compensation they received for the loss of land was often inadequate.[152]

The work carried out by the trust in Calcutta, as in Bombay, clearly reflected the commercial interests of its members. The philanthropic language which accompanied the foundation of both the Bombay and Calcutta trusts masked the trustees' real priorities, which were the improvement of the cities' transport networks and the provision of more space for businesses in the heart of the town.[153] In Bombay only 1 of the 4 schemes initially prepared by the trust was concerned with better housing for the 'poorer and working classes',[154] and by 1908 only 8,000 persons had been rehoused out of an original target of 13,500.[155] Similarly, in Calcutta, only 1 of the trust's first 4 schemes involved slum clearance and the building of apartments on the Bombay model, the remainder being concerned solely with the opening-up of *bustis* to traffic. It was also admitted that the rental cost of the apartments (Rs 5 per month) would effectively prevent the poorest and most needy from taking advantage of them.[156] In the following years no more such schemes were planned, with the trust continuing to concentrate on the opening-up of *bustis* for transportation.[157]

Conclusion

The record of the city's European administration stood in stark contrast to the high-flown rhetoric of the health society in the 1890s. In the years immediately following the Municipal Act of 1899, the general death-rate in Calcutta increased from 30 to 43 per thousand, returning to pre-1899 levels only in 1912. Equally, the infant-mortality rate in 1912 was virtually the same as it had been before the restoration of European supremacy in Calcutta.[158] The persistence of high mortality rates in Calcutta undoubtedly reflects factors which were beyond the municipality's capacity to control, but both Indian and European administrations had been guilty of pursuing self-interest to the detriment or neglect of the health of Calcutta's population. To stand any chance of success, a municipal health policy had clearly to secure the confidence of the people. Constructive dialogue between the largely European executive and Indian municipal leaders was clearly possible, and was sometimes achieved, but the prejudices of an influential section of the European community militated against such a resolution in Calcutta.

The controversy over public health in Calcutta was expressive of European grievances concerning their loss of control over local affairs from the 1870s, and of the eclipse of authoritarian paternalism as a guiding principle of government. The plague crisis, and the appointment of Curzon as viceroy in 1898, provided a context in which European control could be reasserted in the name of sanitary progress. Yet sanitation was not simply a pretext for the assault on local self-government. The desire to sanitate Indian cities reflected deep-seated European anxieties about the colonial 'other'. The *bustis* and bazaars of Calcutta, and other Indian towns, were perceived as centres of pestilence and political unrest untamed by decades of colonial administration. Plague brought these anxieties to a head and culminated in demands for the destruction and removal of the city's slum areas, in which both sanitary and political dangers were emphasised.

European antagonism towards the municipal commission placed commissioners on the defensive, and seriously undermined a more constructive approach to sanitation, such as that advocated by the sanitary commissioner, W. S. Gregg or the corporation's chairman, Sir Henry Harrison. Yet, only a minority of Calcutta's Indian élite enthusiastically embraced the cause of sanitary reform. The Health Society attracted only 8 (highly Anglicised) Indian members, while Surendranath Banerjea emphasised the necessity for reforms to keep pace with indigenous sensibilities. But cultural practices were not the greatest barrier to reform in Calcutta. Sanitary reform was opposed largely on economic grounds by the city's *rentier* class, and Indian ratepayers resisted all moves to increase local taxation for sanitary purposes. Given the dominant position of landlords on the municipal commission, and the restraining influence of the ratepaying Calcutta electorate, there was little scope for sanitary reform on the basis of consensus.

Conclusion

In 1901 the director general of the Army Medical Service proudly proclaimed that the British had brought sanitary science to India, stopping the ravages of cholera and 'improving the whole conditions there'[1] – a claim echoed by the majority of those who had served in India as medical officers.[2] Though it was generally acknowledged that much remained to be done, few doubted that British rule had bestowed great and lasting benefits in the field of public health. But, while there were some grounds for self-congratulation, the gap between the rhetoric and reality of colonial medical achievement was unconvincingly wide.

To begin with, British rule had created as many medical problems as it had resolved. The military conquests of the early nineteenth century resulted in the spread of cholera from Lower Bengal to much of the subcontinent, while unregulated urbanisation produced the conditions in which such diseases could thrive. Agricultural development also disrupted traditional systems of drainage, exposing huge tracts of the country to the ravages of malaria and waterborne disease. Following the mortality crises caused by plague and famine around the turn of the twentieth century, death-rates among Indians did begin to decline, but even in the 1930s were much the same as they had been 50 years before.[3] Moreover, as Roger Jeffery has suggested, this improvement was probably due more to rising real incomes and famine subsistence measures than to medical intervention;[4] except in the cases of smallpox and, perhaps, of cholera.[5]

Most recent studies of public health in India have attributed this slow progress to the Eurocentric priorities of the colonial government. What emerged in British India, it is claimed, was a 'distinctly colonial mode of health care' characterised by residential segregation and neglect of the indigenous population.[6] The core of this argument – that colonial medical policy privileged the needs of Europeans and the military – is largely beyond dispute. More questionable is the claim made by Radhika Ramasubban and others that the limited scope of colonial medicine was almost solely a consequence of the parsimony of the British administration, and the indifference of Europeans to the plight of the indigenous population. In

227

such accounts, the potential of indigenous peoples to influence colonial medical policy is generally underestimated,[7] while their role in policy making at district and municipal level has been virtually ignored. There has also been a reluctance to acknowledge important differences of opinion within the colonial administration,[8] and the constraints imposed upon sanitary reform by general levels of prosperity.[9]

In this book I have attempted to give an account of public health in British India which gives proper weight to each of these factors. I have argued that the development of public health is best understood in terms of a dynamic matrix of motives and sectional interests within and between European and Indian communities. These relations have been considered as three connected themes: the role of preventive medicine in the consolidation of colonial rule; its place in debates over how best to govern India; and its importance as a sphere of interaction and conflict between rulers and ruled.

Medicine as a 'tool of empire'

Preventive medicine was, indeed, a 'tool of empire', but its role in the stabilisation of colonial rule in India was more limited than has been suggested by Curtin and others. The most conspicuous success of preventive medicine was in the field of military hygiene, where a battery of sanitary reforms from the mid-1860s, and eventually more specific preventive measures, effected substantial reductions in mortality and sickness among European and Indian troops. However, these achievements should not be exaggerated since, for much of the period 1859 to 1900, admissions to hospital among British soldiers for malaria, typhoid, and venereal disease remained exceedingly high; and considerably higher than among Indian troops. Moreover, during active service, both the British and Indian armies suffered appallingly heavy losses from disease; much heavier than casualties sustained in battle. Thus, while Curtin is correct to identify a decline in mortality among British troops from the middle of the nineteenth century, the effectiveness of the British Army was seriously undermined by disease until the twentieth century. Persistently high morbidity rates also fuelled pessimism about European colonisation of India. Europeans came to regard themselves as exotics, liable to wilt and die if transplanted to Indian soil. Improvements in sanitation did little to alter this perception, or to make service in India more popular with young men and women in Britain.

The concept of medicine as a tool of empire has even less meaning when applied to the relationship between preventive medicine and colonial development. Public health campaigns such as smallpox vaccination may have owed something to general concerns about colonial efficiency, but it is difficult to establish any specifically economic motivation in this period. Labour efficiency was cited as a motive for the establishment of sanitary boards from the late

1880s, but there is little evidence of any concerted effort in this direction in the coming decades. Indeed, agricultural development proceeded with little thought for its medical consequences, and often to the detriment of the labouring population, as the case of fever in Bengal so amply demonstrated. The only unambiguous connections between public health and economic efficiency in this period were experimental anti-cholera inoculation and smallpox vaccination in the Assam tea-gardens, and the growing mercantile interest in slum clearance in some of India's major cities. The improvement trusts, set up in the wake of plague were dominated by European businessmen (later with the addition of some Indian merchants) and concentrated largely on the opening-up of congested areas to traffic and trade.

With the exception of a few research scientists, who benefited from the establishment of research institutes in the early twentieth century, medical men had very limited success in translating their rhetoric of medicine and colonial development into professional gains. The profession ranked low in the Anglo-Indian table of precedence, and insecurity and dissatisfaction were rife throughout this period. The Morley doctrine which stepped up the 'Indianisation' of the IMS in 1905 was the final blow to the service, and marked the beginning of its terminal decline in popularity with medical graduates in Britain.

The other sense in which medicine may be regarded as important in the consolidation of colonial rule is as an instrument of surveillance and 'social control'. So far, writers on medicine in India have been reluctant to make such associations, although David Arnold sees smallpox vaccination as a means by which the British came to 'know' the indigenous population, while Radhika Ramasubban has emphasised the coercive and divisive nature of colonial medical intervention. Although there was, indeed, a desire among military commanders and medical officers to control elements of the indigenous population, this study has shown that it was generally held in check by an administration concerned about the political implications of such measures in the light of the mutiny. The administration feared that interference in indigenous life styles might provoke a popular backlash or jeopardise its relations with indigenous élites.

It is in this light that we must view government directives against the use of cordons sanitaires, the curtailment of the Contagious Diseases Acts, and the permissive nature of most sanitary legislation. Residential segregation, too, was less strictly enforced than in many African countries, and military cantonments continued to play host to large communities of Indian traders, servants, and prostitutes. The only occasion on which the government diverted from its policy of cautious intervention was during the plague emergency of 1896–1900; and then only under heavy pressure from Britain and the European Powers. Generally, the 'civilising impulse' manifested itself in more subtle forms, such as sanitary education and the Dufferin Fund's attempt to penetrate the veil of the *zenana*. But such tactics had little success: even voluntary bodies such as the Dufferin Fund were handicapped by their association with an alien regime, while widespread indifference or hostility towards western sanitary principles severely limited the effectiveness of such measures. If smallpox vaccination and the registration of births and deaths provided a means of 'knowing' the indigenous population, they were a very imperfect means, the accuracy of which was frequently questioned by medical officers.

Visions of empire

There was little consensus among colonial officials concerning the objectives of medical policy in India: official attitudes towards public health were coloured by competing philosophies of government derived partly from European political theory, and partly from the experience of administration in India. At the risk of some oversimplification, there were two broad conceptions of Britain's role in India – authoritarian paternalism, and Liberal decentralism. The former, which had its roots in the 'utilitarian' era of the 1830s, advocated direct government intervention in public health and strong, European executive control of municipal commissions. Notions of colonial responsibility varied considerably among Europeans of this persuasion, but it was here that the 'civilising impulse' was strongest, and where demands for sanitary reform found their fullest expression. These ideas manifested themselves in opposition to local self-government, and in the formation of such bodies as the Calcutta Health Society and the Dufferin Fund. At its best the 'civilising mission' was an expression of genuine humanitarian concern for the plight of indigenous peoples; at its worst, it reflected notions of racial superiority and complete disregard for the sensibilities of the Indian population.

The sentiments expressed by authoritarian paternalists like Ronald Ross and Calcutta's health officer William Simpson had considerable resonance among the Anglo-Indian community, and the reform lobby found powerful champions in such newspapers as the *Englishman* and the *Pioneer*. Yet, in the period 1859–1914, they were unable to exert much influence over sanitary policy. The year 1870 marked a turning-point in the decline of authoritarian paternalism as an active principle in the administration of India. Lord Mayo's resolution on provincial finance of that year set in train a process of decentralisation and local self-government which was greatly accelerated by the Ripon reforms of the 1880s. These reforms, which placed the financial and administrative responsibility for public health with provincial governments and municipalities, reflected the financial dictates of Gladstonian Liberalism, and Liberal distaste for autocratic government. The overriding principle behind public health policy in the 1870s and 80s was that sanitary reforms should proceed gradually and retain the confidence of the people. Any attempt to force public health measures on an unwilling population was seen as counter-productive and politically dangerous.

The importance of such considerations is illustrated by the conflict between the Indian and British governments over the pilgrimage issue. The Indian government's resistance to international sanitary regulations concerning the pilgrimage – in the face of opposition from Britain and despite the economic advantages of a settlement to the quarantine issue – demonstrates the high importance attached to good relations with Muslim leaders, who had been cultivated as a counter-weight to the assertive Hindu middle class. Resistance to directives from Britain also occurred in several other branches of sanitary policy, most notably in response to the insistence of the Army Sanitary Commission on tighter sanitary policing in and around military stations.

However, authoritarian elements within the Anglo-Indian community could not always be held in check. At the close of the nineteenth century, under intense pressure from Britain and the European Powers, the colonial administration was forced to introduce draconian anti-plague measures. During these years, European control was gradually re-exerted over municipal affairs in the name of sanitary progress, while medical officers were afforded an opportunity to experiment with new technologies of prevention – particularly inoculation against plague. With the lifting of the severest quarantine restrictions against India in 1898, and in the wake of violent protests against plague measures, regulations were relaxed considerably. However, a precedent for greater government involvement in public health had been established, and grants in aid of sanitation at district and municipal level increased substantially in the 1900s, marking a move away from the financial stringency of the 1870s and 80s.

In disagreements over public health in India, and between the Indian government and foreign powers, medical theory and medical experts played a crucial role. Medical experts were carefully selected and employed by the Indian government to provide theoretical justifications for its sanitary policy, and especially its opposition to quarantine and cordons sanitaires. This is most clearly demonstrated by the government's choice of delegates to international sanitary conferences, and by its attempts to stifle discussions of cholera theory in official reports. As is illustrated by the case of Dr DeRenzy, the government was prepared to discipline those officers who persistently criticised official medical doctrine. In its opposition to quarantine and to proposals that the government fund large sanitary engineering projects, the atmospheric theory of cholera transmission associated with Dr Bryden was maintained as official doctrine in the face of growing internal dissent and international ridicule. Only slowly, following international acceptance of Koch's cholera bacillus in the early 1890s, did the government's position begin to shift in line with medical opinion outside India.

Indian attitudes and responses

No clear pattern emerges in Indian responses to western hygiene and public health measures: attitudes varied considerably over time and between different sections of the indigenous population. However, one or two generalisations can be made. Firstly, suspicion of, or resistance to, western sanitary measures tended to diminish over time; secondly, those measures whose effects were most readily apparent, like smallpox vaccination, tended to be the most popular. However, given the unreliability of official statistics, and marked regional variations, it is important not to overstate the popularity of smallpox vaccination, or to underestimate the cultural and logistical obstacles which continued to work against such measures. The trust of the indigenous population, if it was won at all, was won only slowly, through co-operation with community leaders and with due regard to Indian sensibilities. But even the limited successes of smallpox vaccination proved something of an exception to the general rule. The testimonies of both Europeans and Indians indicate that hostility or indifference towards sanitary regulations persisted in most areas of India throughout this period.

True enthusiasm for sanitary reform was confined to a western-educated urban minority, whose commitment was sometimes spurious given the wide-spread reluctance among Indian property owners to countenance increases in rates and domestic taxation to finance sanitary reform. Moreover, Indian advocates of sanitary reform like Surendranath Banerjea, constantly stressed the need for gradualism, and for public health to progress hand-in-hand with the education of the people. For this reason, and given European resentment of Indian influence in municipal affairs, Indian reformers had little in common with the most vigorous exponents of public health among the European community; although they enjoyed good relations with medical officers who shared their belief in gradualism.

Active opposition to public health measures had two dimensions. The first was popular resistance to coercive sanitary measures, and was most clearly evident during the plague epidemics of 1896 onwards. Here, terror at the prospect of isolation and segregation, fuelled by political agitation, culminated in a mass exodus from several cities, rioting, industrial unrest, and even assassination. The fear and economic disruption caused by these events was an important factor in the liberalisation of plague measures from 1898, and demonstrates that the government's anxieties over medical intervention were well founded. The second form of Indian resistance to western sanitary measures manifested itself at municipal level, in ratepayers' opposition to taxation for sanitary purposes, and to by-laws which adversely affected Indian economic interests. The latter dimension is clearly illustrated in the case of Calcutta, where the Indian *rentier* class dominated the municipal commission from 1876 to 1899.

In league with Indian ratepayers, slum landlords on the commission thwarted the activities of the predominantly European health society, and succeeded in opposing a range of sanitary initiatives, including regulations to prevent the overcrowding of rented properties.

Epilogue

The First World War did not, in itself, mark a turning-point in the development of public health in British India. It did, however, cause considerable disruption of medical services since medical officers were sent abroad to serve with the Indian Army in the Middle East, Africa, and Europe. At the outbreak of the war, there were a total of 748 IMS officers in India, but only 56 were permitted to remain there for its duration.[10] Yet, as in Britain, the war saw an extension of initiatives concerning maternal and children's health.[11] Indian troops also returned with new aspirations concerning democratic reform and better social provisions such as health care. The Montagu–Chelmsford reforms of 1919, which made provincial governments responsible to a majority of elected representatives, and the increasing 'Indianisation' of the IMS after the war, offered the prospect of realising such aspirations.

But, while government expenditure on health increased in the interwar years, provincial governments continued to operate within strict financial limits, and particularly during the depression of the early 1930s.[12] Equally, the commitment of many Indian politicians to sanitary reform remained dubious, with a marked preference for expenditure on education. Medical research was also curtailed in this period. The report of the Inchcape Commission in 1923 led to drastic reductions in research personnel and in the amount of money allocated to medical research.[13] Although death-rates from such diseases as smallpox and cholera continued to decline, there was much truth in R. Palme Dutt's comment of 1940 that 'provision for the most elementary needs of public hygiene, sanitation or health is so low, in respect of the working masses in the towns or in the villages, as to be practically non-existent'.[14]

But one final question remains: was the slow progress of public health in India inevitable given practical constraints on reform, or were there other options which might realistically have been pursued by the colonial authorities? Ramasubban, for instance, is critical of the government's failure to initiate a programme of sanitary reform on European lines.[15] David Arnold also implies the need for greater government involvement in public health, and is critical of the transfer of sanitation to financially ill-equipped and inexperienced munici-palities.[16] Roger Jeffery, however, remains 'uncertain how much difference would have been made by any conceivable historically available alternative', and stresses the financial, practical, and administrative constraints on health policies in India.[17]

Jeffery is undoubtedly correct to draw attention to these practical difficulties. As chapter 7 of this study has shown, sanitary progress depended heavily on the state of local revenues and systems of taxation. There were also considerable logistical and technical problems in mounting such operations as smallpox vaccination and anti-plague inoculation. In this sense, and given widespread indigenous suspicion of colonial medical intervention, any vigorous programme of sanitary reform, such as that advocated by Ramasubban, seems unrealistic. Also, given the political and practical necessity of co-operation with Indian élites – in public health as in other areas of administration – it is difficult to see how government could have done other than devolve such matters to local authorities. It is true, as David Arnold contends, that this 'municipalisation' was driven partly by financial considerations, but it was also, especially in the 1880s, a recognition of political realities.

This is not to say, however, that alternative approaches did not exist. It was clear that many municipalities and local boards were unable to raise sufficient revenue for vital sanitary reforms, and that government aid was urgently necessary. The government's reluctance to promote drainage in fever-stricken areas of Bengal is one of the more glaring examples of its weak commitment to the health of the Indian people. A more concerted effort by government to assist struggling local authorities would undoubtedly have done much to improve the situation here and elsewhere in India. Yet much also depended on indigenous peoples themselves, and particularly the example set by community leaders. In this respect local élites often left much to be desired, as the case of Calcutta demonstrates.

In sum, improvements in public health depended on active co-operation between colonial officials and indigenous peoples, and this necessitated gradualism and sensitivity to Indian interests. It also required direction and, more especially, financial aid from central and provincial government. But neither the government nor key sections of the indigenous population displayed the kind of commitment necessary to the progress of sanitation. Arguably, such co-operation was impossible in a colonial situation in which notions of racial superiority, and cultural distance, made difficult constructive relations between rulers and ruled, and in which government priorities would always favour the former.

Appendix A

The Indian Medical Service

Highest qualifications held by IMS officers, 1851–1914

Year of entry	Single licence	Double licence	MB/MD	Post-grad.	FRCP/ FRCS	BA/MA
1851–5	26 (44.1)	17 (28.8)	16 (27.1)	8 (13.6)	3 (5.1)	0
1856–60	26 (45.6)	18 (31.6)	13 (22.8)	2 (3.5)	1	2
1861–5	2 (28.6)	3 (42.9)	2 (28.6)	3 (42.9)	0	0
1866–70	0	26 (49.1)	25 (47.2)	7 (13.2)	3 (5.7)	5 (9.4)
1871–5	0	11 (61.1)	5 (27.8)	1 (5.6)	1	0
1876–80	0	28 (60.9)	18 (39.1)	5 (10.9)	4 (8.7)	1
1881–5	0	9 (52.9)	8 (47.1)	5 (29.4)	0	3 (17.6)
1886–90	0	9 (36.0)	16 (64.0)	10 (40.0)	2 (8.0)	4 (16.0)
1891–5	0	10 (45.5)	12 (54.5)	1 (4.5)	4 (18.2)	3 (13.6)
1896–1900	0	48 (32.7)	99 (67.3)	67 (45.6)	31 (21.1)	31 (21.1)
1901–5	0	74 (32.3)	156 (67.7)	86 (37.6)	49 (21.4)	45 (19.7)
1906–10	1	49 (26.8)	133 (72.7)	76 (41.5)	25 (13.7)	42 (23.0)
1911–14	1	37 (33.3)	73 (65.8)	32 (28.8)	12 (10.8)	22 (19.8)

Figures in parentheses denote the proportion of IMS officers holding a particular qualification. Note that recruits sometimes held more than one of the qualifications listed above.
Source: Crawford's *Roll of the Indian Medical Service*: IOR: L/MIL/9/413–18, 'Papers of surgeons selected by the Board of Examiners 1882–94'; L/MIL/9/419–27, 'Papers of candidates selected for the IMS 1895–1914'; L/MIL/9/428–9, 'Registers of IMS candidates'.

Highest qualifications held by IMS officers appointed to full-time sanitary posts

Year of entry	Single licence	Double licence	MB/MD	Post-grad.	FRCP/FRCS	BA/MA
1851–5	3 (30.0)	4 (40.0)	3 (30.0)	1 (10.0)	1 (10.0)	2 (20.0)
1856–60	0	3 (50.0)	3 (50.0)	0	0	0
1861–5	1 (11.1)	7 (77.8)	1 (11.1)	3 (33.3)	0	0
1866–70	0	10 (52.6)	9 (47.4)	13 (68.4)	2 (10.5)	2 (10.5)
1871–5	0	3 (30.0)	7 (70.0)	6 (60.0)	2 (20.0)	0
1876–80	0	3 (20.0)	12 (80.0)	13 (86.7)	2 (13.3)	3 (20.0)
1881–5	0	2 (20.0)	8 (80.0)	8 (80.0)	2 (20.0)	3 (30.0)
1886–90	0	9 (34.6)	17 (54.6)	25 (96.2)	1 (3.8)	3 (11.5)
1891–5	0	7 (50.0)	7 (50.0)	14 (100.0)	2 (14.3)	2 (14.3)
1896–1900	0	10 (43.5)	13 (56.5)	22 (95.7)	2 (8.7)	2 (8.7)
1901–5	0	8 (24.2)	25 (75.8)	32 (97.0)	0	0
1906–10	0	4 (18.8)	18 (81.8)	22 (100.0)	4 (18.2)	2 (9.1)
1911–14	0	6 (42.9)	8 (57.1)	14 (100.0)	1 (7.1)	3 (21.4)

Notes and sources as previous table.

IMS recruits 1837–1914: occupation of father

Occupation	1855–84	1885–96	1897–1914
Medical practitioner	89 (18.2)	45 (16.6)	52 (16.9)
Clergyman	59 (12.0)	29 (10.7)	29 (9.4)
Armed services	32 (6.5)	24 (8.9)	12 (3.9)
Teacher/academic	11 (2.2)	8 (2.9)	16 (5.2)
Lawyer	25 (5.1)	9 (3.3)	16 (5.2)
Civil servant	45 (9.9)	33 (12.2)	2 (0.6)
Businessman/merchant	35 (7.1)	32 (11.8)	34 (11.0)
Tradesman/labourer	42 (8.6)	18 (6.6)	11 (3.6)
Gentleman/esquire	31 (6.3)	9 (3.3)	6 (1.9)
Landowner	2 (0.4)	5 (1.8)	2 (0.6)
Kt., MP, peer	0	0	1
Planter	5 (1.0)	5 (1.8)	3 (1.0)
Farmer	19 (3.9)	12 (4.4)	8 (2.6)
New professions	44 (9.0)	30 (11.1)	45 (14.6)
Miscellaneous	1	1	6
Indians	50 (10.2)	11 (4.1)	65 (21.1)
Total known	490	271	308

'New professions' include accountancy, engineering, dentistry, banking, and management. Indians are classed separately since no details regarding their circumstances of birth are available in recruitment records.
Sources: as previous tables.

Senior Medical officers

Examining physicians and surgeons to the EIC

John Hunter   1793–1809
William Dick   1809–18
W. F. Chambers   1818–35
J. R. Hume   1835–45
John Scott   1843–59
J. R. Martin   1859–64

Presidents of the India Office Medical Board

J. R. Martin   1864–74
J. Fayrer   1874–95
W. R. Hooper   1895–1903
A. M. Branfoot   1904–13
R. H. Charles   1913–23

Surgeons-general and directors-general of the IMS (university attended)

J. C. Brown   1871–5   (Edinburgh)   Bengal Service
J. F. Beatson   1875–80   (Glasgow)   Bengal Service
J. M. Cuningham   1880–4   (Edinburgh)   Bengal Service
B. Simpson   1885–90   (Trinity, Dublin)   Bengal Service
W. R. Rice   1890–5   (Queens, Ireland)   Bengal Service
J. Cleghorn   1895–7   (Edinburgh, Vienna)   Bengal Service
R. Harvey   1898–1901   (Aberdeen)   Bengal Service
B. Franklin   1901–6   (University College, London)   Bengal Service
G. Bomford   1906–11   (King's College, London)   Bengal Service
C. P. Lukis   1911–18   (London)   Bengal Service

Sanitary commissioners with the Government of India

J. M. Cuningham   1868–84
B. Simpson   1885–90
W. R. Rice   1890–5
J. Cleghorn   1895–7
R. Harvey   1898–1901
B. Franklin   1901–3
J. T. W. Leslie   1903–9   (Aberdeen, Oxford)   Bengal Service
J. C. Robertson   1911–13   (Glasgow)   Bengal Service
W. W. Clemesha   1914–15   (London)   Bengal Service

Provincial sanitary commissioners

Assam

1876	W. H. Audley
1877	A. C. C. DeRenzy
1880	J. J. Clarke
1884	A. Eteson
1888	C. P. Costello
1893	W. P. Warburton
1894	A. Stephen
1898	C. W. Carr-Calthrop
1903	D. Wilkie
1912	R. N. Campbell
1914	H. E. Banatlava

Bengal

1870	D. B. Smith
1872	C. J. Jackson
1874	J. M. Coates
1875	R. Harvey
1876	J. M. Coates
1877	R. Harvey
1878	J. M. Coates
1880	R. Lidderdale
1882	F. W. A. DeFabeck
1883	R. Lidderdale
1888	W. H. Gregg
1897	H. J. Dyson
1902	F. C. Clarkson
1904	W. W. Clemesha
1906	F. C. Clarkson
1909	W. W. Clemesha

Bihar and Orissa

1912	E. C. Hare

Bombay

1870	T. G. Hewlett
1878	J. Lumsdaine

1883   T. G. Hewlett
1887   C. W. MacCrury
1892   J. W. Clarkson
1898   A. W. F. Street
1899   J. W. Clarkson
1903   O. H. Channer
1906   T. E. Dyson
1911   H. A. Forbes-Knapton
1912   T. E. Dyson
1914   F. H. G. Hutchinson

Burma

1870   J. McNeale-Donnelly
1875   W. P. Kelly
1879   J. M. Joseph
1881   W. Pearl
1882   D. Sinclair
1891   P. W. Dalzell
1893   D. Sinclair
1895   G. T. Thomas
1896   D. Sinclair
1899   C. C. Little
1904   R. Macrae
1905   W. G. King
1907   C. E. Williams
1910   J. A. Harriss
1911   C. E. Williams

Central Provinces

1869   S. C. Townsend
1872   J. Brake
1873   S. C. Townsend
1876   J. F. Barter
1880   W. Watson
1881   J. H. Lock
1888   G. C. Chesnage
1890   J. G. Pilcher
1891   W. B. Center
1893   G. C. Ross
1895   J. H. Newman

1896   G. Hutcheson
1899   A. Scott-Reid
1901   W. A. Quayle
1902   M. D. Moriarty
1905   P. A. Weir
1907   A. M. Crofts
1908   P. A. Weir
1909   T. G. N. Stokes

Madras

1868   J. L. Ranking
1870   W. R. Cornish
1875   H. King
1876   W. R. Cornish
1879   M. C. Furnell
1884   G. Bidie
1885   W. Farqhaur
1856   J. A. Laing
1893   W. G. King
1905   H. Thomson
1907   W. W. Clemesha
1909   H. Thomson
1910   W. A. Justice
1914   H. Thomson

Punjab

1868   A. C. C. DeRenzy
1876   H. W. Bellew
1886   A. Stephen
1888   W. A. C. Roe
1890   A. Stephen
1894   W. A. C. Rice
1898   C. J. Bamber
1907   E. Wilkinson
1909   C. J. Bamber
1910   E. Wilkinson
1912   S. Browning-Smith

North West Provinces and Oudh

1868   C. Plank
1886   J. Richardson
1890   G. Hutcheson
1895   J. J. Thomson
1896   G. M. J. Giles
1901   J. Chaytor-White
1902   S. J. Thomson
1908   J. Chaytor-White
1910   J. C. Robertson
1912   J. A. Harriss

Appendix B

Military sanitary expenditure

Expenditure on military sanitation: all-India

Year	Expenditure	Year	Expenditure
1874–5	9 242 085	1894–5	8 665 922
1875–6	725 917	1895–6	8 901 312
1876–7	7 022 292	1896–7	8 140 534
1877–8	7 213 653	1897–8	8 583 112
1878–9	5 458 719	1898–9	9 926 242
1879–80	5 653 961	1899–1900	
1880–1	6 262 426	1900–1	
1881–2	4 847 971	1901–2	
1882–3	6 735 325	1902–3	13 253 283
1883–4	5 750 030	1903–4	12 588 420
1884–5	5 790 488	1904–5	8 030 768
1885–6	6 456 710	1905–6	8 326 534
1886–7	5 974 683	1906–7	
1887–8	5 613 362	1907–8	
1888–9	6 074 202	1908–9	8 310 027
1889–90	9 102 988	1909–10	
1890–1	9 832 152	1910–11	8 704 100
1891–2	9 068 203	1911–12	8 617 716
1892–3	8 593 935	1912–13	9 609 218
1893–4	7 402 741	1913–14	8 572 630

Source: Reports of the Sanitary Commissioner with the Government of India (1875–1914).

Appendix C

Public health and local self-government

Allotments to sanitation: Bengal mofussil municipal committees

Year	Income	Allotment	% of income
1878–9	2 679 328	688 587	25.7
1879–80	2 604 545	690 204	26.5
1880–1	2 791 209	669 890	24.0
1881–2	3 106 731	853 087	32.0
1882–3	3 328 762	1 148 423	34.5
1883–4	3 263 614	1 232 651	37.6
1884–5	3 041 223	1 225 613	40.3
1885–6	3 084 571	1 193 729	38.7
1886–7	3 263 614	1 298 918	39.8
1887–8	3 291 448	1 359 368	41.3
1888–9	2 955 158	1 279 583	43.3
1889–90	3 138 641	1 340 299	42.7
1890–1	3 120 971	1 338 897	42.9
1891–2	3 451 618	1 477 293	42.8
1892–3	3 739 825	1 611 864	43.1
1893–4	4 314 317	2 088 129	48.4
1894–5	3 732 074	1 619 720	43.4
1895–6	4 553 651	· 2 345 130	51.5
1896–7	4 349 548	2 035 588	46.8
1897–8	4 264 986	1 953 363	45.8
1898–9	4 247 310	1 902 794	44.8
1899–1900	4 684 589	2 103 380	44.9
1900–1	4 977 650	2 215 054	44.5
1901–2	5 162 352	2 240 460	43.4
1902–3	4 950 383	2 128 665	43.4
1903–4	5 498 182	2 210 269	40.2
1904–5	5 777 295	2 102 935	36.4
1905–6	4 967 128	1 917 311	38.6
1906–7	5 262 176	2 267 997	43.1
1907–8	5 747 680	2 270 334	39.5
1908–9	7 373 133	2 927 134	39.7
1909–10	8 082 914	3 233 166	40.0
1910–11	8 766 333	3 033 151	34.6
1911–12	7 808 730	2 826 760	36.2
1912–13	9 322 039	3 609 497	38.7
1913–14	10 528 748	4 211 499	40.0

Source: Reports of the Sanitary Commissioner to the Government of Bengal (1879–1914).

Appendix C

Allotments to sanitation: Madras mofussil municipal committees

Year	Income	Allotment	% of income
1878–9	1 406 670	361 514	25.7
1880–1	1 508 723	384 724	25.5
1881–2	1 473 234	393 353	26.7
1882–3	1 596 920	456 766	31.0
1883–4	1 720 210	495 536	31.0
1884–5	1 927 462	571 199	33.2
1885–6	1 879 490	590 160	31.4
1886–7	1 856 720	547 795	34.9
1887–8	1 961 390	619 774	31.6
1888–9	1 988 130	681 294	34.3
1889–90	2 042 070	857 328	32.1
1890–1	2 117 640	709 092	33.5
1891–2	2 652 995	997 380	37.6
1892–3	2 551 800	1 539 485	60.3
1893–4	2 747 600	1 145 366	41.7
1894–5	2 526 060	1 362 785	53.9
1895–6	2 886 470	1 623 540	56.2
1896–7	3 325 370	1 600 203	48.1
1897–8	3 228 120	2 052 273	63.6
1898–9	2 956 220	1 571 540	55.4
1899–1900	3 498 110	1 943 601	55.6
1900–1	3 205 747	1 740 791	54.3
1901–2	3 066 534	2 085 338	68.0
1902–3	3 776 753	2 634 042	69.7
1903–4	3 301 052	2 258 194	68.2
1904–5	3 778 848	2 350 207	62.2
1905–6	4 090 055	2 505 689	61.3
1906–7	3 834 977	2 293 131	59.8
1907–8	3 904 647	2 285 782	58.5
1908–9	4 052 060	2 521 557	62.2
1909–10	5 000 060	3 276 761	65.5
1910–11	5 588 983	3 531 567	63.2
1911–12	6 087 697	3 337 180	54.8
1912–13	7 301 330	3 640 065	49.8
1913–14	8 266 411	4 729 529	57.2

Allotment figures after 1901–2 are calculated on a slightly different basis from those prior to that date. After 1901–2, they include public works in total, as opposed to sanitary projects only, slightly inflating the amount apparently allotted to sanitation. Use of figures under this more general heading has been unavoidable, since, after 1900, the *General Municipal Review* provides the only source from which figures relating to sanitary allotments can be obtained.

Sources: Reports of the Sanitary Commissioner for the Government of Madras (1879–1914); and *General Municipal Review, Madras* (1900–1915).

Allotments to sanitation: Bombay mofussil municipal committees

Year	Income	Allotment	% of income
1879–80	2 555 796	632 905	24.8
1880–1	2 132 772	763 117	35.7
1881–2	2 403 286	585 800	24.4
1882–3	2 919 425	722 280	24.7
1883–4	2 710 952	1 148 903	42.4
1884–5	2 966 624	660 806	22.1
1885–6	3 070 624	683 668	22.3
1886–7	3 132 776	338 763	10.8
1887–8	3 479 558	736 449	21.2
1888–9	3 486 667	635 497	18.2
1889–90	3 595 909	691 307	19.2
1890–1	3 519 221	699 612	19.8
1891–2	3 507 678	1 369 288	39.0
1892–3		1 905 531	
1893–4	3 394 824	1 031 861	30.3
1894–5	4 474 809	1 852 570	41.4
1895–6	4 749 303	2 150 827	45.3
1896–7	5 522 074	2 501 157	45.3
1897–8	5 892 572	3 370 551	57.2
1898–9	5 326 199	2 620 490	49.2
1899–1900	5 526 695	2 743 860	49.6
1900–1	6 895 003	1 457 687	21.1
1901–2	7 198 403	1 427 509	19.8
1902–3	6 223 667	1 422 475	22.9
1903–4	5 984 404	1 590 634	26.6
1904–5	6 109 925	1 755 477	28.7
1905–6	6 849 925	1 862 875	27.2
1906–7	6 998 933	2 235 477	31.9
1907–8	7 132 476	1 947 918	27.3
1908–9	7 992 502	1 735 771	21.7
1909–10	8 151 611	1 900 737	23.3
1910–11	9 202 824	2 518 218	27.8
1911–12	9 716 431	2 570 603	26.5
1912–13	11 636 120	3 215 211	27.6
1913–14	10 975 326	3 861 355	35.2
1914–15	12 573 669	3 425 979	27.2

Source: Reports of the Sanitary Commissioner to the Government of Bombay (1880–1915).

Allotments to sanitation: Bombay local and district boards

Year	Income	Allotment	% of income
1891–2	2 498 312	332 227	13.3
1892–3		286 907	
1893–4	4 008 855	517 870	12.9
1894–5	4 113 115	432 920	10.5
1895–6	3 806 842	516 698	13.6
1896–7	4 005 823	517 870	11.8
1897–8	4 145 747	516 221	12.4
1898–9	3 842 185	482 465	12.6
1899–1900	5 727 491	342 207	6.0
1900–1	4 542 921	322 449	7.1
1901–2	4 084 873	173 488	7.1
1902–3	4 438 842	161 172	3.6
1903–4	4 896 941	235 775	4.6
1904–5	4 800 157	223 093	4.6
1905–6	4 384 296	279 666	6.4
1906–7	5 685 096	394 875	6.9
1907–8	6 358 510	307 778	4.8
1908–9	6 406 055	375 426	5.9
1909–10	6 497 809	416 058	6.4
1910–11	6 878 715	422 849	6.1
1911–12	6 832 039	352 902	5.2
1912–13	7 177 471	390 378	5.4
1913–14	7 634 897	433 611	5.7
1914–15	7 848 589	373 558	4.8

Figures relating to income and allotments do not always appear in the former series of reports, and the latter series begins only in 1890.

Sources Reports of the Sanitary Commissioner to the Government of Bombay (1880–1914); *Reports on the Administration of the Local Boards in the Bombay Presidency* (1890–1914).

Allotments to sanitation: Madras local and district boards

Year	Income	Allotment	% of income
1889–90	1 492 763	563 332	37.7
1890–1	8 113 429	541 254	6.7
1891–2	8 304 687	529 091	6.4
1892–3	7 904 903	482 499	6.1
1893–4	7 893 344	462 908	5.9
1894–5	7 583 700	475 148	6.3
1895–6	7 547 420	498 029	6.6
1896–7	7 967 830	532 977	6.7
1897–8	7 910 730	526 972	6.7
1898–9	7 962 700	513 766	6.4
1899–1900	8 614 840	501 311	5.8
1900–1	12 020 070	477 867	4.0
1901–2	10 831 015	499 429	4.6
1902–3	13 272 804	509 050	3.8
1903–4	13 593 767	550 614	4.0
1904–5	13 690 290	583 104	4.3
1905–6	15 949 167	601 023	3.8
1906–7	17 360 405	582 436	3.3
1907–8	19 657 628	613 507	3.1
1908–9	20 812 941	794 112	3.8
1909–10	21 022 316	792 960	3.8

Figures for 1910–14 are not available from either source. Record V/24/310 containing this information is missing from the India Office Records, and information concerning sanitary allotments ceases to appear in Madras sanitary reports after 1900.

Sources: Reports of the Sanitary Commissioner to the Government of Madras (1879–1901); General Local Fund Review, Madras (1900–1910).

Allotments to sanitation: Bengal local and district boards

Year	Income	Allotment	% of income
1891–2	6 213 324	200 362	32.2
1892–3	7 193 805		
1893–4	6 685 552	474 325	7.1
1894–5	6 674 986	371 184	5.6
1895–6	6 770 986	292 787	4.3
1896–7	7 274 232	636 143	8.7
1897–8	7 105 065	1 567 741	22.1
1898–9	6 690 172	894 450	13.4
1899–1900	7 279 076	549 386	7.5
1900–1	7 050 196	496 957	7.0
1901–2	8 065 037	605 194	7.5
1902–3	9 217 377	722 249	7.8
1903–4	8 402 888	639 175	7.6
1904–5	7 962 577	667 692	8.4
1905–6	6 893 342		
1906–7	7 208 880	839 839	11.6
1907–8	7 938 862	856 196	10.8
1908–9	7 876 020	882 909	11.2
1909–10	7 493 721	1 295 431	17.3
1910–11	7 809 239	1 188 448	15.2
1911–12	6 729 752	1 090 363	16.2
1912–13	7 170 761	1 230 769	17.2
1913–14	10 730 770	1 314 368	12.2
1914–15	10 047 964	1 728 946	17.2

Figures relating to allotments have been extracted from the former, and income, the latter. Gaps in figures relating to allotments cannot be filled from District Board reports since sanitary expenditure occurred under a variety of heads, including 'medical', 'civil works", and 'miscellaneous'.
Sources: Reports of the Sanitary Commissioner for the Government of Bombay (1892–1915); *Reports on the Working of District Boards in Bengal* (1892–1915).

Notes

Introduction

1 P. D. Curtin, '"The White Man's Grave": image and reality, 1750–1850', *Journal of British Studies*, 1 (1961), 94–110; *The Image of Africa. British Ideas and Action, 1780–1850* (Madison, Wisc., 1964).

2 P. D. Curtin, *Death by Migration. Europe's Encounter with the Tropical World in the Nineteenth Century* (Cambridge, 1989). On the human costs of empire, see also D. Geggus, 'Yellow fever in the 1790s: the British Army in occupied Saint Dominique', *Medical History*, 23 (1979), 38–58; P. Burroughs, 'The human cost of imperial defence in the early Victorian age', *Victorian Studies*, 24 (1980).

3 D. R. Headrick, *The Tools of Empire: Technology and European Imperialism in the Nineteenth Century* (Oxford, 1981).

4 D. Arnold, 'Introduction', in Arnold (ed.), *Imperial Medicine and Indigenous Societies* (Manchester, 1988), pp. 10–11.

5 For the limitations of French military medicine in Algeria before the 1860s see A. Marcovich, 'French colonial medicine and colonial rule: Algeria and Indochina', in R. MacLeod and M. Lewis (eds.), *Disease, Medicine, and Empire. Perspectives on Western Medicine and the Experience of European Expansion* (London, 1988), pp. 103–18.

6 On Dutch colonial medicine see G. M. van Heteren, A. de Knecht-van Eekelen and M. J. D. Poulissen (eds.), *Dutch Medicine in the Malay Archipelago 1816–1942* (Amsterdam, 1989).

7 L. Stewart, 'The edge of utility: slaves and smallpox in the early eighteenth century', *Medical History*, 29 (1985), 54–70; R. B. Sheridan, *Doctors and Slaves: A Medical and Demographic History of Slavery in the British West Indies 1680–1834* (Cambridge, 1985).

8 See M. Worboys, 'The emergence of tropical medicine: a study in the establishment of a new scientific speciality', in G. Lemaine et al. (eds.), *Perspectives on the Emergence of Scientific Disciplines* (The Hague, 1977), pp. 76–98; E. J. Hart, 'An address to the medical profession in India, its position and its work', *BMJ* (1894), 1469–74.

9 M. Worboys, 'Manson, Ross and colonial medical policy: tropical medicine in London and Liverpool, 1899–1914', in MacLeod and Lewis (eds.), *Disease, Medicine, and Empire*, pp. 21–37.

249

10 A. Balfour and H. H. Scott, *Health Problems of the Empire* (London, 1924).

11 M. W. Swanson, 'The sanitation syndrome: bubonic plague and urban native policy in the Cape Colony, 1900–1909', *Journal of African History*, 18 (1977), 387–410.

12 P. D. Curtin, 'Medical knowledge and urban planning in tropical Africa', *American Historical Review*, 90 (1985), 594–613; D. Headrick, 'Cities, sanitation and segregation' in his *The Tentacles of Progress. Technology Transfer in the Age of Imperialism, 1850–1940* (Oxford, 1988).

13 R. Ramasubban, *Public Health and Medical Research in India: Their Origins Under the Impact of British Rule* (Stockholm, 1982).

14 S. Marks and N. Anderson, 'Typhus and social control: South Africa: 1917–1950', in MacLeod and Lewis (eds.), *Disease, Medicine, and Empire*, pp. 257–83.

15 R. C. Ileto, 'Cholera and the origins of the American sanitary order in the Philippines', in Arnold (ed.), *Imperial Medicine*, pp. 125–48.

16 M. Lyons, *The Colonial Disease. A Social History of Sleeping Sickness in Northern Zaire, 1900–1940* (Cambridge, 1992).

17 David Arnold suggests that this was one of the motive forces behind smallpox vaccination campaigns in British India. See 'Smallpox and colonial medicine in nineteenth-century India', in Arnold (ed.), *Imperial Medicine*, pp. 45–65.

18 M. Vaughan, *Curing their Ills. Colonial Power and African Illness* (Cambridge and Oxford, 1991).

19 Ramasubban, *Public Health and Medical Research in India*; 'Imperial health in British India, 1857–1900', in R. MacLeod and M. Lewis (eds.), *Disease, Medicine, and Empire*, pp. 38–60.

20 This argument was originally stated in my 'Towards a sanitary Utopia? Professional visions and public health in India, 1880–1914', *South Asian Research*, 10 (1990), 19–40.

21 M. Harrison, 'Quarantine, pilgrimage, and colonial trade: India 1866–1900', *Indian Economic and Social History Review*, 29 (1992), 117–44.

22 I. J. Catanach, 'Poona politicians and the plague', *South Asia*, 7 (1984), 1–18; D. Arnold, 'Touching the body: perspectives on the Indian plague, 1896–1900', in R. Guha (ed.), *Subaltern Studies V* (New Delhi, 1987), pp. 55–90.

23 See for example: R. Jeffery, *The Politics of Health in India* (Berkeley, 1988), pp. 42–58; P. Bala, *Imperialism and Medicine in Bengal: A Socio-Historical Perspective* (New Delhi, 1991).

1 The Indian medical service

1 On 'professional imperialism' (the process by which professional knowledge acquires a superiority over other forms) see E. Freidson, *Profession of Medicine: A Study of the Sociology of Applied Knowledge* (New York, 1970); T. Johnson, *Professions and Power* (London, 1972); I. Illich, *Limits to Medicine: Medical Nemesis: The Expropriation of Health* (London, 1976). On professions as a vehicle of social mobility, and links between the sociology of the professions and class theory see: J. Parry and N. Parry, *The Rise of the Medical Profession: A Study of Collective Social Mobility* (London, 1976); M. S. Larson, *The Rise of Professionalism: A Sociological Analysis* (Berkeley, 1977).

2 For example: I. Inkster, '"Marginal men": aspects of the social role of the medical community in Sheffield, 1790–1850', in D. Richards and J. Woodward (eds.), *Health Care and Popular Medicine in Nineteenth Century England* (London, 1977), pp. 128–52; M. J. Peterson, *The Medical Profession in Mid-Victorian London* (Berkeley, 1978); 'Gentlemen and medical men: the problem of professional recruitment', *Bull. Hist. Med.*, 58 (1984), 457–73; I. Loudon, *Medical Care and the General Practitioner, 1750–1850* (Oxford, 1986); W. Bynum and R. Porter (eds.), *Medical Fringe and Medical Orthodoxy 1750–1850* (London, 1987); H. Marland, *Medicine and Society in Wakefield and Huddersfield 1780–1870* (Cambridge, 1987).

3 W. B. Baetson, 'Indian Medical Service: past and present'; Crawford, *Indian Medical Service*; D. MacDonald, *Surgeons Twoe and a Barber: Being Some Account of the Life and Work of the Indian Medical Service (1600–1947)* (London, 1950); Sir N. Cantlie, *A History of the Army Medical Department*, 2 vols. (London, 1974).

4 J. L. Brand, *Doctors and the State: The Medical Profession and Government Action in Public Health, 1870–1912* (Baltimore, 1965); M. A. Crowther, 'Paupers or patients? Obstacles to professionalization in the Poor Law Medical Services before 1914', *J. Hist. Med.*, 29 (1984), 33–54; D. E. Watkins, 'The English Revolution in Social Medicine, 1889–1911' (University of London PhD. thesis, 1984). On Indian services see: E. Blunt, *The Indian Civil Service* (London, 1937); B. Spangenberg, *British Bureaucracy in India. Status, Policy and the ICS in the late 19th Century* (Delhi, 1976); T. A. Heathcote, *The Indian Army: The Garrison of British Imperial India, 1822–1922* (London, 1974); D. Arnold, *Police Power and Colonial Rule. Madras 1859–1947* (Delhi, 1986).

5 Crawford, *Indian Medical Service*, I, pp. 1–6; W. B. Baetson, 'Indian Medical Service: past and present', *Asiatic Quarterly Review*, 14 (1902), 272–320; MacDonald, *Surgeons Twoe* (London, 1950).

6 The founding and expansion of hospitals in British India is discussed in M. Harrison, 'Medicine in India: a historical survey', in *Fidea Research Foundation Award Lecture Series*, 7 (New York, forthcoming).

7 Crawford, *Indian Medical Service*, II, pp. 243–57.

8 *Ibid.*, II, pp. 117–25.

9 *Gazette of India*, 2 March 1864, pp. 84–6; *Memorandum On Measures Adopted for Sanitary Improvements in India up to the end of 1867* (London, 1868).

10 Ramasubban, 'Imperial health', p. 41.

11 IOR P/434/43 (nos. 1–8), 'Duties to be discharged by the sanitary commissioners with the local governments and administrations in the Bengal Presidency, 19 September 1868.

12 Peterson, *Medical Profession*, p. 38.

13 I. Waddington, 'General practitioners and consultants in early nineteenth-century England: the sociology of an intra-professional conflict', in Woodward and Richards (eds.), *Health Care and Popular Medicine*, pp. 164–88; Crowther, 'Paupers or patients?'; Brand, *Doctors and the State*, pp. 85–106.

14 Crawford, *Indian Medical Service*, II, p. 326.

15 *IMG* (May 1897), 301. IMS officers wishing to obtain further qualifications had to make use of whatever time they were granted in furlough. Only in 1913 was extra furlough granted specifically for study leave: *JTM* (September 1913), 280.

16 *IPC*, II, p. 11.
17 *IMG* (September 1876), 243; see also (June 1876), 163.
18 *IMG* (May 1877), 131.
19 *IMG* (June 1906), 143; see also D. G. Crawford, 'The Medical Services in 1905', reprinted from *IMG* (March 1905); WIHM, Crawford Collection.
20 Peterson, *Medical Profession*, p. 125.
21 Arnold, *Police Power*, p. 73.
22 Crawford, *Indian Medical Service*, I, p. 386. In addition to their 'pay grade', all IMS officers received an award of at least Rs 150 per month when on military service.
23 J. A. Turner and B. K. Goldsmith, *Sanitation in India* (Bombay, 1922), p. 6.
24 *JTM* (September 1907), 305.
25 NAI. GOI (Medical), sec. to Punjab govt. to sec. to GOI, submitting letter from commissioner and supt., Jullunder Div., 17 December 1900.
26 NAI. GOI (Medical), sec. to Punjab govt. to sec. to GOI (Home Dept.), 9 October 1902.
27 *IMG* (October 1913), p. 339; B. R. Tomlinson, *The Political Economy of the Raj 1914–1947* (London, 1979), pp. 17–19.
28 Second- and third-class grades received considerably less: Rs 10–25 and Rs 5–20 per month, respectively. Crawford, *Indian Medical Service*, II, pp. 117–20.
29 *JTM* (November 1906), 320.
30 *JTM* (January 1907), 26.
31 *JTM* (November 1908), 329.
32 Crawford, *Indian Medical Service*, II, p. 121.
33 *IMG* (October 1865), 342.
34 *IMG* (June 1872), 37–8.
35 *IMG* (December 1909), 462.
36 *IMG* (January 1912), 23, 27.
37 *Madras Times*, 1 July 1880.
38 *JTM* (February 1906), 39.
39 Ross, *Memoirs*, p. 44.
40 For example: R. J. Blackham, *Scalpel, Sword and Stretcher; Forty Years of Work and Play* (London, 1931).
41 W. Harvey, 'The Indian Medical Services as a career', reprinted from *Dollar Magazine*, 1906?; WIHM, Crawford Collection.
42 European perceptions of the Indian climate are discussed at length in chapter 2.
43 Crawford, *Roll of the Indian Medical Service*, p. 653.
44 WIHM, RAMC 397: Hall papers, ERR 2/14 – confidential reports on medical officers.
45 WIHM, RAMC 351: Thomas Wood's diaries and notebooks, 1861 and 1867; entry of 29 January 1867.
46 WIHM, RAMC 953: unpublished autobiography of Capt. William Morrison, 1860–95.
47 *East India Register and Directory for 1842* (London, 1842), p. 121.
48 *JTM* (December 1910).
49 J. Cantlie, 'Tropical life as it affects life assurance', *JTM* (January 1911).
50 Peterson, *Medical Profession*, pp. 52–3, 67.

51 *IMG* (May 1868), 111.

52 *IMG* (June 1868), 119.

53 *IMG* (March 1869), 59.

54 *IPHMJ* (September 1909), 90.

55 Peterson, *Medical Profession*, pp. 34–6.

56 *IMG* (May 1865), 124.

57 Jeffery, *Politics of India*, pp. 50–8.

58 G. C. Roy, *The Causes, Symptoms and Treatment of Burdwan Fever, or the Epidemic Fever of Lower Bengal* (London, 1876), pp. 151-2. Roy had been educated in Glasgow and London, where he obtained an MD degree and an FRCS respectively. He was a convert to Christianity, and believed fully in the superiority of western medicine over traditional Indian practices.

59 *IMG* (August 1887); *Hindoo Patriot*, 8 August 1887. The *Patriot* was prepared to support the campaign against 'quacks, charlatans and empirics' on the condition that indigenous medical practitioners would also be registered under the proposed legislation.

60 *JTM* (February 1899), 192.

61 *IMG* (March 1912), 109.

62 B. D. Metcalfe, 'Nationalist Muslims in British India: the case of Hakim Ajmal Khan', *Mod. Asian Stud.*, 19 (1985), 8–9.

63 NAI. GOI Home (Medical) Sarat Chandra Ghose to viceroy, enclosing letter from sec. to GOBe., 2 March 1900. See also S. M. Bhardwaj, 'Homeopathy in India', in G. R. Gupta (ed.), *The Social and Cultural Context of Medicine in India* (New Delhi, 1981).

64 NAI. GOI Home (Medical), sec. to GOI (Home Dept.) to sec. to Punjab govt., no. 8, 19 July 1913.

65 See chapter 4, and J. C. Hume, 'Rival traditions: western medicine and *Yuna-i Tibb* in the Punjab, 1849–1889', *Bull. Hist. Med.*, 51 (1977), 214–31. In response to a barrage of complaints from the medical profession, the employment of specially trained *hakims* was discontinued in the Punjab in 1886.

66 *IMG* (January 1912), 21–3; (March 1912), 109; (January 1914), 30; NAI. GOI Home (Medical) nos. 45–6, May 1914, the Madras Medical Registration Laws, 1914; no. 50, January 1914, 'Memorial of the All-Indian Ayurvedic and Unani Tibbi Conference against the Medical Registration Act of 1912'.

67 Crawford, *Indian Medical Service*, I, pp. 527–9.

68 *Qualifications and Examination of Candidates for Commissions in the Medical Services of the British and Indian Armies* (London, 1860).

69 The sources for this data are IOR. L/MIL/9/413–18, 'Papers of surgeons selected by the Board of Examiners 1882–94'; L/MIL/9/419–27, 'Papers of candidates selected by the Board of Examiners for the IMS 1895–1914'; L/MIL/9/428–29, registers of IMS candidates. This data is presented in appendix A.

70 Between 1851 and 1871 an average of 30 per cent of IMS recruits held medical degrees (MBs and MDs) while the percentage of the medical profession so qualified in Wakefield and Huddersfield was slightly lower at 25 per cent.

71 Crawford, *Indian Medical Service*, II, p. 325.

72 Marland, *Medicine and Society*, pp. 270–1; Watkins, 'English revolution', p. 74.

73 FRCSs and FRCPs comprised on average 19.7 per cent of IMS officers between 1865 and 1896, 11.7 per cent of British MOsH from 1857 to 1887, and 7.6 per cent of registered practitioners in Wakefield.

74 Turner and Goldsmith, *Sanitation in India*, p. 6.

75 *IMG* (September 1871), 185–9.

76 *IMG* (May 1871), 97.

77 *IMG* (June 1871), 123.

78 *IMG* (June 1871), 123.

79 *IMG* (December 1908), 402.

80 MacDonald, *Surgeons Twoe*, pp. 221, 223–4.

81 Jeffery, 'Recognising India's doctors', p. 310.

82 *IMG* (October 1913), 396–9.

83 Sources: IOR. L/MIL/9/413–18; L/MIL/9/419–27; L/MIL/9/428–29. These data are presented in appendix A.

84 Source: Crawford, *Roll of the Indian Medical Service*.

85 Source: Crawford, *Roll of the Indian Medical Service*.

86 Spangenberg, *British Bureaucracy in India*, pp. 79–92.

87 See appendix A – Senior Medical Officers.

88 Peterson, *Medical Profession*, pp. 66, 80, 125.

89 Jeffery, 'Recognising India's doctors', pp. 305–9.

90 E. Freidson, 'The theory of professions: state of the art', in R. Dingwall and P. Lewis (eds.), *The Sociology of the Professions. Lawyers, Doctors, and Others* (London, 1985), pp. 19–35.

91 Spangenberg, *British Bureaucracy in India*, pp. 14–51.

92 *IMG* (September 1871), 188; see also (September 1867), 129.

93 Arnold, *Police Power*, pp. 73–4.

94 Peterson, *Medical Profession*, pp. 198-201; 'Gentlemen and medical men'.

95 The sources for figure 1.3 are Crawford's *Roll*, for the period 1837–96, and Surgeons' Records IOL. L/MIL/9/413–27, for 1897–1914. These data are presented in appendix A. Indians are classed separately since no details regarding their birth are available in recruitment records.

96 See G. Crossick (ed.), *The Lower Middle Class in Britain 1870–1914* (London, 1977).

97 Heathcote, *Indian Army*, p. 139.

98 Crawford, *Roll of the Indian Medical Service*.

99 Peterson, *Medical Profession*, p. 125; N. D. Lankford, 'The Victorian medical profession and military practice: army doctors and national origins', *Bull. Hist. Med.*, 54 (1980), 511–28.

100 Arnold, *Police Power*, p. 74.

101 Jeffery, 'Recognising India's doctors', p. 310.

102 Source: Crawford, *Roll of the Indian Medical Service*.

103 G. Johnson, *Provincial Politics and Indian Nationalism: Bombay and the Indian National Congress, 1880–1915* (Cambridge, 1973), pp. 118–50; M. N. Das, *India Under Morley and Minto. The Politics Behind Revolution, Repression and Reforms* (London, 1964).

104 Jeffery, 'Recognising India's doctors', p. 311.

105 Arnold, *Police Power*.

106 B. B. Misra, *The Indian Middle Classes. Their Growth in Modern Times* (London, 1961).
107 For example, *Bengalee*, 28 May 1887.
108 Spangenberg, *British Bureaucracy in India*, pp. 1–9.
109 Ballhatchet, *Race, Sex and Class Under the Raj*, pp. 99–100.
110 Arnold, *Police Power*, p. 82.
111 Quoted in Ballhatchet, *Race, Sex and Class*, pp. 103–7.
112 *IMG* (May 1913), 193.
113 Crawford, *Roll*, p. 205.
114 *BMJ* (1874), 511. Chakravarty was representative of Indian medical graduates prior to the first world war inasmuch as the majority were Christian or Parsi, rather than Hindu or Muslim. See Jeffery, *Politics of Health*, p. 84.
115 Turner and Goldsmith, *Sanitation in India*, p. 5.
116 *JTM* (July 1909), 198.
117 Jeffery, *Politics of Health*, pp. 84–6.

2 Tropical hygiene: disease theory and prevention in nineteenth-century India

1 The core of this chapter was originally conceived as a critical response to the prevalent notion that 'colonial science' was dependent on, and subservient to, European scientific authority; and to accounts of tropical medicine which locate its emergence in the late nineteenth century (e.g. M. Worboys, 'Science and British colonial imperialism, 1895–1940' (University of Sussex DPhil thesis, 1979)). These aspects are discussed more fully in M. Harrison, 'Tropical medicine in nineteenth-century India', *British Journal for the History of Science* (1992), 25, 299–318. My objectives in this chapter are somewhat different, and relate more to the cultural significance of tropical hygiene, and in particular its role in the creation of the 'colonial subject'.
2 C. Curtis, *An Account of the Diseases in India, as they appeared in the English fleet, and in the Naval Hospital at Madras, in 1782 and 1783; with Observations on Ulcers, and the Hospital Sores of that Country* (Edinburgh, 1807), p. xvi.
3 Paisley to Curtis, February 1774, cited *ibid.*, p. 86.
4 *Ibid.*, p. 90.
5 George Ballingall, *Practical Observations on Fever, Dysentery, and Liver Complaints, as they occur amongst the European Troops in India* (Edinburgh, 1818), p. 40.
6 *Ibid.*, pp. 41, 81.
7 J. Lind, *Essay on the Diseases Incidental to Europeans in Hot Climates* (London, 1768), p. 44.
8 J. Clark, *Observations of the Diseases which prevail in Long Voyages to Hot Countries, particularly those in the East Indies; and on the same Diseases as they appear in Britain* (London, 1809), pp. 78, 84.
9 *Ibid.*, p. 81.
10 It was, perhaps, the increasing frequency and extent of Europe's encounter with the tropical world which led to a revival of interest in the Hippocratic corpus in the second through to the fifth decades of the eighteenth century. For the Hippocratic

tradition and its influence on eighteenth-century climatic theory see: J. Dedieu, *Montesquieu et la Traditional Politique Anglais en France; les Sources Anglais de l'Esprit des Lois* (Paris, 1909), pp. 205–7.

11 Montesquieu's notion of climatic influence as expressed in *De l'Esprit des Lois* was not consistently deterministic although it was sufficiently strong to enable him to explain different cultural, political and religious traditions in such terms. Count Buffon, in his *Histoire Naturelle, Générale et Particulière* (1749–1804) employed a similar climatic theory in his explanation of variation in the natural world, including the physical characteristics of humans. Although Montesquieu and Buffon were not without their critics, their work was in a very real sense 'the repository of the age', as well as being enormously influential on subsequent generations of scholars. For an extensive discussion of these theories see C. J. Glacken, *Traces on the Rhodian Shore. Nature and Culture in Western Thought from Ancient Times to the End of the Eighteenth Century* (Berkeley, 1967), pp. 565–610; see also W. Anderson, 'Climates of opinion: acclimatization in nineteenth-century France and England', *Victorian Studies*, 35 (1992), 135–57.

12 See for example *The Travels of Mizra Abu Talibkhan* (1810), discussed in T. Raychaudhuri, 'Europe in India's xenology: the nineteenth-century record', *Past and Present*, 137 (1992), pp. 159–60.

13 Lind, *Diseases Incidental to Europeans*, pp. 171–2.

14 J. Hunter, *Observations on the Diseases of the Army in Jamaica and on the best means of Preserving the Health of Europeans in the Climate* (London, 1788), p. 24; and 'Disputation on the varieties of man', inaugural dissertation to the fellows of the Royal Society, 1775.

15 W. Falconer, *Remarks on the Influence of Climate, Situation, Nature of Country, Population, Nature of Food, and Way of Life, on the Disposition and Temper, Manners and Behaviour, Intellects, Laws and Customs, Forms of Government, and Religion, of Mankind* (London, 1781), p. 2.

16 Clark, *Diseases which prevail in Long Voyages*, p. 345.

17 Ballingall, *Practical Observations on Fever*, pp. 3–6.

18 Curtis, *An Account of the Diseases in India*, pp. 280–1. Curtis did not, however, believe that all Europeans were equally adaptable to tropical climates. They were more or less fitted according to certain 'idiosyncrasies of habit' and physical characteristics, with persons of sanguine temperament and swarthy complexion being the most easily acclimatised (p. xxiv).

19 A. Burt, *A Tract on the Biliary Complaints of Europeans in Hot Climates; Founded on Observations in Bengal; and consequently designed to be particularly useful to those in that Country* (Calcutta, 1785), pp. 9–10, 14.

20 See P. D. Gaitonde, *Portuguese Pioneers in India: Spotlight on Medicine* (London, 1983); T. J. S. Patterson, 'The relationship of European and Indian practitioners of medicine from the sixteenth century', in G. J. Meulenbeld and D. D. Wujastyk (eds.), *Studies in Indian Medical History* (Groningen, 1987), pp. 119–29.

21 On 'orientalism' in India see S. N. Mukherjee, *Sir William Jones* (London, 1968); D. Kopf, *British Orientalism and the Bengal Renaissance* (Berkeley, 1969); P. J. Marshall (ed.), *The Discovery of Hinduism in the Eighteenth Century* (Cambridge, 1970); G. Viswanathan, *Masks of Conquest* (New York, 1989).

22 See B. S. Cohn, 'The command of language and the language of command', in

R. Guha (ed.), *Subaltern Studies IV* (Oxford, 1985), pp. 276–329; E. Said, *Orientalism* (New York, 1979).

23 Mukherjee, *William Jones*, pp. 14–16.

24 On indigenous Indian medical traditions see O. P. Jaggi, *Indian System of Medicine* (New Delhi, 1973); A. L. Basham, 'The practice of medicine in ancient and medieval India', and J. C. Burgel, 'Secular and religious features of medieval Arabic medicine', in C. Leslie (ed.), *Asian Medical Systems: A Comparative Study* (Berkeley, 1976), pp. 18–43 and 44–59 respectively; Poonam Bala, *Imperialism and Medicine in Bengal: A Socio-Historical Perspective* (New Delhi, 1991), pp. 23–39.

25 For an informative account of medical botany in British India see R. Desmond, *The European Discovery of the Indian Flora* (Oxford, 1992).

26 Whitelaw Ainslie, *Materia Indica; or some Account of those Articles which are employed by the Hindoos, and other Eastern Nations, in their Medicine, Arts, and Agriculture* (London: Longman, 1826), p. xxxv.

27 *Ibid.*, p. 499; see also J. F. Royle's *An Essay on the Antiquity of Hindoo Medicine* (London, 1837).

28 G. Playfair, *The Taleef Shereef, or Indian Materia Medica* (Calcutta, 1832).

29 James Johnson, *The Influence of Tropical Climates, more especially of the Climate of India, on European Constitutions; and the Principal Effects and Diseases thereby induced, their Prevention and Removal, and the means of Preserving Health in Hot Climates, rendered obvious to Europeans of every capacity* (London, 1815), pp. 416–37. *Dictionary of National Biography* (hereafter *DNB*): James Johnson (1777–1845). Born in County Derry, Ireland, Johnson moved to Co Antrim at the age of 15 to take up an apprenticeship with a surgeon apothecary, and resided there for 2 years. After spending a further 2 years as an apothecary's assistant in Belfast, he moved to London to study for a qualification in surgery, which he obtained in 1798. Immediately afterwards, Johnson gained employment as a surgeon's mate on a naval vessel, and sailed to Newfoundland and Nova Scotia. In 1800 Johnson took part in an expedition to Egypt, and in 1803 sailed for India where he remained until 1806. On returning to England, he continued to serve in the Royal Navy until 1814, when he left with a high reputation to set up a practice in London.

30 *Ibid.*, pp. 456–7.

31 H. H. Wilson, 'Kushta, or leprosy; as known to the Hindus', *Trans. Medical and Physical Society of Calcutta*, 1 (3 May 1823), 2–3. On Wilson's scholarship see O. P. Kejariwal, *The Asiatic Society of Bengal and the Discovery of India's Past 1784–1838* (New Delhi, 1988), pp. 118–61.

32 *Ibid.*, pp. 4–5. On the persistence of this notion see *Leprosy in India: Report of the Leprosy Commission in India 1890–91* (Calcutta, 1892).

33 C. Maclean, *Results of an Investigation respecting Epidemic and Pestilential Diseases; including Researches in the Levant concerning Plague*, 2 vols. (London, 1817). Maclean was also an exponent of Brunonian therapeutic ideas, placing him in opposition to the Cullonian mainstream of medical opinion in Britain. See M. Barfoot, 'Brunonianism under the bed: an alternative to university medicine in Edinburgh in the 1780s', in W. Bynum and R. Porter (eds.), *Brunonianism in Britain and Europe* (*Medical History*, Supplement 8, London, 1988), pp. 23–4.

34 *DNB*. Charles Maclean (1788–1824) began his medical career as a surgeon on an East-Indiaman, but in 1792 settled in Bengal, where he took charge of a European

hospital in Calcutta. On Maclean's political radicalism see R. Cooter, 'Anti-contagionism and History's medical record', in P. Wright and A. Treacher (eds.), *The Problem of Medical Knowledge* (Edinburgh, 1982), pp. 96–7.

35 Johnson, *Influence of Tropical Climates*, pp. ix, 27, 94.

36 *Ibid.*, p. 88. The notion of lunar influence on the causation and course of fevers was not uncommon in India, and owed as much to conversations with Indian practitioners as to observation. See, for example, Francis Balfour, *Treatise on the Influence of the Moon in Fevers* (Calcutta, 1784).

37 James Johnson, *The Economy of Health, or The Stream of Human Life from the Cradle to the Grave, with Reflections, Moral, Physical and Philosophical on the Successive Phases of Human Existence* (London, 1837).

38 M. Durey, *Return of the Plague: British Society and the Cholera 1831–2* (Dublin, 1979), pp. 105–18. Several other texts, specifically on cholera, were written by Indian medical officers especially for a European audience. See for example: James Annesley, *Sketches of the Most Prevalent Diseases of India* (London, 1831); James Kennedy, *The History of the Contagious Cholera; with Facts Explanatory of its Origin and Laws, and of a Rational Method of Cure* (London, 1831).

39 Throughout the 1830s mortality among British troops in Bengal averaged around 70 per 1,000 per annum – never falling below 60 per 1,000, while over the same period in Britain the mortality rate for soldiers never exceeded 20 per 1,000. In the coming decades mortality among British troops in all parts of India increased considerably, falling below 40 per 1,000 only in the 1850s. See Curtin, *Death by Migration*, p. 24. For subsequent mortality/morbidity rates among British troops see the following chapter.

40 Johnson, *Influence of Tropical Climates*, pp. x, 2.

41 *Ibid.*, pp. 3–4.

42 Kennedy, *History of the Contagious Cholera*, pp. 2–3.

43 T. Araud, 'General and medical topography of Meerut', *Trans. Calcutta Medical and Physical Society*, 1 (4 September 1824), 292–8.

44 D. S. Young, 'An account of the general and medical topography of the Neelgerries', *Trans. Calcutta Medical and Physical Society*, 4 (7 July 1827), p. 55.

45 J. Grierson, 'On the endemic fever of Arracan, with a sketch of the medical topography of that country', *Trans. Calcutta Medical and Physical Society*, 2 (5 March 1825), 209.

46 Young, 'Medical topography of the Neelgerries', p. 45.

47 *Ibid.*, p. 53.

48 D. Kennedy, 'Guardians of Edenic sanctuaries: Paharis, Lepchas, and Todas in the British mind', *South Asia*, 14 (1991), 77.

49 See the description of the Khasia tribe of the Jyntia Hills in north-eastern India in J. H. Thornton, *Memoirs of Seven Campaigns. A Record of Thirty-Five Years' Service in the Indian Medical Department in India, China, Egypt, and the Sudan* (London, 1895), p. 130.

50 W. Twining, *Clinical Illustrations of the More Important Diseases of Bengal with the Result of an Inquiry into their Pathology and Treatment* (Calcutta, 1835).

51 J. Thomson, *A Treatise on the Diseases of Negroes as they occur in the Island of Jamaica, with Observations on the Country Remedies* (Kingston, 1820), pp. 35, 16.

52 *DNB*. James Ranald Martin (1793–1874) was the son of a minister on the Isle of Skye. He was admitted as a student to St George's Hospital, London in 1813 and became a member of the Royal College of Surgeons in 1817, whereupon he joined the Bengal Medical Service. After 3 years in Orissa as a military surgeon, Martin began civil practice in Calcutta, leaving India in 1843 to become president of the East India Company's Medical Board. In the same year, he became a Fellow of the Royal College of Surgeons, and was elected a Fellow of the Royal Society in 1845. Martin was knighted in 1860 and served on the Army Sanitary Commission established in 1857.

53 J. R. Martin, *Notes on the Medical Topography of Calcutta* (Calcutta, 1837), p. 45.

54 *Ibid.*, p. 43.

55 See G. D. Bearce, *British Attitudes Towards India, 1784–1858* (London, 1982).

56 *Ibid.*, pp. 24, 27–8.

57 *Ibid.*, pp. 43, 45, 52.

58 J. R. Martin, *The Influence of Tropical Climates on European Constitutions, including Practical Observations on the Nature and Treatment of the Diseases of Europeans on their Return from Tropical Climates* (London, 1856), p. 35.

59 J. Jeffreys, *The British Army in India: Its Preservation by an Appropriate Clothing, Housing, Locating, Recreative Employment, and Hopeful Encouragement of the Troops* (London, 1858), pp. 1–3.

60 *Ibid.*, p. 14.

61 *Ibid.*, p. 15.

62 *JTM* editorial (December 1909), 354; J. Cantlie, 'Tropical life as it affects life insurance', *JTM* (January 1911), 35–41.

63 WIHM. RAMC 177: Sir Joseph Fayrer's newspaper cuttings, 1876–98.

64 R. S. Mair, *Medical Guide for Anglo-Indians* (London, 1874), pp. 3, 20.

65 *SCGI* (1890), pp. 56–7 and (1889), p. 14.

66 E. J. Tilt, *Health in India for British Women* (London, 1875), pp. 20, 63, 72.

67 *SCGI* (1890), 58 and (1899), 61.

68 M. M. Kaye (ed.), *The Golden Calm. An English Lady's Life in Mogul Delhi* (Exeter, 1980), p. 49.

69 *SCGI* (1890), 58.

70 *SCGI* (1885), 193.

71 C. A. Gordon, *Army Hygiene* (London, 1866), p. 352.

72 J. Fayrer, *European Child Life in Bengal* (London, 1873), pp. 30–1.

73 See D. N. Livingstone, 'Human acclimatization': perspectives on a contested field of inquiry in science, medicine and geography', *History of Science*, 25 (1982), 359–94; J. S. Ewart, 'The colonisation of the sub-Himalayas and Neilgherries, with remarks on the management of European children in India', *Trans. Epid. Soc.*, 3 (1883–4), 96–117.

74 W. Moore, 'The constitutional requirements for tropical climates, with special reference to temperaments', *Trans. Epid. Soc.*, 4 (1884–5), pp. 37–8, 46, 48. See also Moore's 'Is the colonisation of tropical Africa by Europeans possible', *Trans. Epid. Soc.*, 10 (1890–1), 27–45. According to Moore, 'the Anglo-Saxon race, excepting probably the Jews, are perhaps better fitted to brave extremes of climate than any other section of mankind' (p. 29). An optimistic note about colonisation – though

confining its attention to the hill stations of India – is struck in J. Chesson's *Report on the Hill-Station of Panchgunny, near Mahableshwar* (Bombay, 1862).

75 The parasitologist L. W. Sambon and Robert Koch were two of the foremost exponents of this view. See also Livingstone, 'Human acclimatization', p. 369.

76 *Englishman*, 26 January 1899.

77 M. Pelling, *Cholera, Fever and English Medicine* (Oxford, 1978), pp. 113–45. See also J. B. Morrell, 'The chemist breeders: the research schools of Liebig and Thomas Thompson', *Ambix*, 19 (1972), 1–46.

78 See, for example, *Reports of the Sanitary Commissioner with the Government of India*.

79 J. Snow, *On the Mode of Communication of Cholera* (London, 1855), 2nd edn. and *On Continuous Molecular Changes, More Particularly in the Relation to Epidemic Diseases* (London, 1853); A. P. Stewart and E. Jenkins, *The Medical and Legal Aspects of Sanitary Reform, 1866–69* (London, 1869), p. 10.

80 Watkins, 'Revolution in social medicine', pp. 347–54; Curtin, *Death by Migration*, pp. 59, 105.

81 E. A. Parkes, *Manual of Practical Hygiene. Prepared Especially for Use in the Medical Service of the British Army* (London, 1864), pp. xvi, 437. Edmund Alexander Parkes (1819–1876), was educated at Christ's Hospital School London, and University College London. Graduated MB and admitted MRCS in 1840. In 1842 Parkes joined the AMS and served for 3 years in India, gaining experience of dysentery, hepatitis, and cholera. In 1845, Parkes retired from the army and went into private practice in London. In 1846 he graduated MD from London University, with a thesis on dysentery and Indian hepatitis. From 1852–5 Parkes edited the *Medico-Chirurgical Review*, and in 1860 was appointed professor of hygiene at the newly founded Army Medical School, Chatham. The school was transferred to Netley in 1863. At Netley, Parkes carried out important research in several branches of medicine and imparted his views to successive generations of IMS, AMS, and NMS recruits. See also Pelling, *Cholera, Fever, and English Medicine*, pp. 70–4.

82 Parkes, *Practical Hygiene*, pp. 431, 437.

83 *Ibid.*, pp. 21–2, 36, 47–8, 158, 432. However, acceptance of specific modes of putrefaction did not necessarily entail the implementation of more specific preventive measures. As Christopher Hamlin has put it, 'The zymotic analogy made it plausible to think of the entire insanitary environment as contributing . . . [to epidemic disease], while the perpetual threat to health of putrefaction was the basis on which Simon and his medical inspectors harried local officials into removing filth': C. Hamlin, 'Providence and putrefaction: Victorian sanitarians and the natural theology of health and disease', in P. Branglinger (ed.), *Energy and Entropy. Science and Culture in Victorian Britain* (Bloomington, Ind., 1990), pp. 93–123.

84 Parkes, *Practical Hygiene*, p. xvi.

85 *Ibid.*, pp. 132–6. A small minority continued to believe that the Hindu diet was best suited to life in tropical climates. See G. H. Fink, 'Food of the natives of India', *JTM* (October 1906), 310–12.

86 *IMG* (April 1868), p. 87.

87 *DNB*; obituary, *Trans. Epid. Soc.*, 26 (1906–7), 78–9. Sir Joseph Fayrer (1824–1907), born Plymouth, the son of a commander in the Royal Navy. After a brief study of engineering, Fayrer made a voyage to the West Indies and South

America as a midshipman on a West Indian steampacket. In 1843 he sailed with his father to Bermuda, where his experience of an outbreak of yellow fever inclined him towards medicine. After entering Charing Cross Hospital in 1844, Fayrer was admitted MRCS in 1847 and gained a commission in the medical service of the Royal Navy. Soon afterwards, Fayrer resigned his commission to travel around Europe in the company of Lord Mount-Edgcumbe. He ended his tour at Rome, where he resumed his study of medicine and, in 1849, obtained its MD degree. In 1850 Fayrer left Europe to take up the post of assistant surgeon in the Bengal Medical Service, where he busied himself in medical and cultural activities, becoming president of the Asiatic Society of Bengal in 1867. He was instrumental in founding a zoological society and the zoological gardens in Calcutta. In 1869 Fayrer became personal surgeon to the new viceroy Lord Mayo but, in 1872, returned to Britain because of ill health, whereupon he was appointed president of the India Office Medical Board. Fayrer was widely respected in Britain, becoming personal physician to the Prince of Wales and president of the Epidemiological Society in 1879. He was made Companion of the Order of the Star of India in 1868 and a baronet in 1896. A prolific writer on medicine, climatology, and venomous snakes, Fayrer was one of the last exponents of the 'universalistic' approach to medicine which typified the IMS in the first half of the nineteenth century.

88 J. Fayrer, *The Natural History and Epidemiology of Cholera* (London, 1888), p. 6.

89 J. Fayrer, *Preservation of Health in India* (London, 1894), p. 9.

90 Fayrer, *Epidemology of Cholera*, pp. 52–3.

91 *Ibid.*, p. 36.

92 H. H. Bellew, *The Nature, Causes, and Treatment of Cholera* (London, 1887), p. 19. By this time, both ozonic and electrical theories were out of vogue in Britain: see Pelling, *Cholera, Fever, and English Medicine*, p. 148.

93 W. Guyer Hunter, 'The origin of the cholera epidemic of 1883 in Egypt', *Trans. Epid. Soc.*, 3 (1883–4), 51. See also, C. A. Gordon, 'Experiences in relation to cholera in India from 1842 to 1879', in *Trans. Epid. Soc.*, 15 (1895–6), 48–67.

94 *SCGI* (1877), 24.

95 T. G. Hewlett, *Report on Enteric Fever* (Bombay, 1883), pp. 1–7.

96 Hewlett, *Enteric Fever*, p. 157. See also *SCGI* (1877), 24.

97 Examples of the dominant view include: Général Duvivier, *Solution de la Question de l'Algérie* (Paris, 1841), p. 14; J. A. N. Perier, *De l'Hygiène en Algérie* (Paris, 1847), p. 133; A. Chantemesse and E. Mosny (eds.), *Traité d'Hygiène. Etiologie et Prophylaxie des Maladies Transmissibles par la Peau et les Muqueses Externes* (Paris, 1911), p. 258. An exception is W. J. Eames, 'Chill and malaria', *BMJ* (January 1875), 109.

98 E. Sergent and L. Parrot, *La Découverte de Laveran* (Paris, 1931).

99 Ross, *Memoirs* (London, 1923), p. 126. G. Harrison asserts that in India, in the 1880s and 90s, Laveran's discovery was 'either ignored, explained away, or rejected as simply beyond belief': *Mosquitoes, Malaria and Man* (London, 1978), p. 12.

100 *BMJ* (December 1894), 1472. One of the few exceptions was the confirmation of Laveran's discovery by Henry Van Dyke Carter, IMS: Harrison, *Mosquitoes, Malaria and Man*, p. 16.

101 See, for example, *Report on the Stations of Ootacamund and Coonoor* (1865), p. 1.

102 *SCGI* (1892), 24. See also, J. P. Goubert, *The Conquest of Water. The Advent of Health in the Industrial Age* (Oxford and Cambridge, 1989), pp. 48–51.

103 *SCGI* (1894), 25.

104 In his address to the Medical Society of London in 1901, A. Crombie stated that 'climate as climate takes but a small part of the etiology of disease among European immigrants to the tropics': *JTM* (December 1901), 418. The exceptions included sunstroke (or 'heat apoplexy'), tropical neurasthenia, and 'Delhi boil'. See D. Kennedy, 'The perils of the midday sun: climatic anxieties in the colonial tropics', in J. M. MacKenzie (ed.), *Imperialism and the Natural World*, 118–40; A. C. C. DeRenzy, 'The prevention of heat apoplexy', *Trans. Epid. Soc.*, 4 (1884–5), 63–71; F. Pearse, 'Prickly heat'', *JTM* (June 1899), 297–8.

105 *SCGI* (1897), 26; (1898), 26; *BMJ* (January 1898), 1620; (June 1898), 1521; (November 1899), 1376; *Lancet*, June 1899, p. 1501; *IMG* (November 1899), 403.

106 C. A. Chambers, 'Enteric fever in Indians, with special reference to its occurrence in the Indian Army', *JTM* (September 1913), 280–2.

107 E.g. W. R. Cornish, *Reports on the Nature of Food of the Inhabitants of the Madras Presidency and the Dietaries of Prisoners in Zillah Jails* (Madras, 1863); D. M. McCoy, 'Investigations on Bengali jail dietaries with some observations on the physical development and well-being of the people of Bengal', *Sci. Mems.*, 37 (1910), 1–226.

108 *SCGI* (1898), 26. See also, *IMG* (August 1899), 293.

109 R. Pringle, 'Enteric fever in India: its increase, causes, remedies, and probable consequences', *Trans. Epid. Soc.*, 9 (1889–90), 111–32; H. Skey Muir, 'On the cause of enteric fever in India', *Trans. Epid. Soc.*, 10 (1890–1), 22–6.

3 The foundations of public health in India: crisis and constraint

1 A. R. Skelley, *The Victorian Army at Home: The Recruitment and Terms and Conditions of the British Regular, 1859–1899* (London, 1977), p. 22.

2 C. Hibbert, *The Great Mutiny: India 1857* (London, 1978), pp. 196–7, 202, 231, 256, 288; Sir Joseph Fayrer, *Recollections of My Life* (Edinburgh, 1890), p. 174.

3 Jeffreys, *The British Army in India*, p. ix.

4 The members of the commission were Richard Airey (quarter-master-general and president), Douglas Galton (asst. under-secretary for war), John Sutherland, T. G. Logan (inspector-general of hospitals), Edward Belfield (deputy director of works, War Office), Proby T. Cantley (member of the Council of India), James Ranald Martin (inspector-general of hospitals and president of the India Office Medical Board), Robert Rawlinson (Local Government Act Office), and J. J. Frederick (secretary).

5 *Report of the Commissioners Appointed to Enquire into the Sanitary State of the Army in India, Parliamentary Papers*, I and II (1868).

6 Jeffreys, *The British Army in India*, pp. 155–7.

7 *SCGI* (1870), 1.

8 C. A. Gordon, *Army Hygiene* (London, 1866), p. 322.

9 F. Nightingale, *Observations on the Evidence contained in the Stational Reports submitted to her by the Royal Commission on the Sanitary State of the Army in India* (London, 1863), p. 69.

10 Jeffreys, *The British Army in India*, p. 59.

11 C. A. Gordon, *Army Hygiene*, p. 367.

12 E. C. Freeman, *The Sanitation of British Troops in India* (London, 1899), pp. 94, 97.

13 Nightingale, *Observations*, p. 37.

14 Parkes, *Practical Hygiene*, pp. 132, 136–52, 158.

15 Gordon, *Army Hygiene*, pp. 39, 42.

16 *Ibid.*, p. 38.

17 Caldwell, *Military Hygiene* (London, 1905), p. 51.

18 Freeman, *The Sanitation of British Troops in India*, p. 52.

19 Jeffreys, *The British Army in India*, p. 19.

20 Nightingale, *Observations*, pp. 31–2.

21 Gordon, *Army Hygiene*, pp. 25–6, 30.

22 I.e. 6 years service with the colours instead of 12, followed by 6 years in the reserve.

23 Roberts, *Enteric Fever in India*, p. 6.

24 J. Cole, *Notes on Hygiene with Hints on Self-Discipline for Young Soldiers in India* (London, 1882), pp. 1, 10.

25 Roberts, *Enteric Fever in India*, p. 11. From 1903–6 the incidence of drunkenness convictions amounted to only 12 per cent of the British Army in India; the lowest previous figure being 33 per cent in 1871–5.

26 WIHM, RAMC 397/ERR 1–1/1: barrack reports of Sir John Hall, 1852.

27 See Anne Summer's critique of the 'Nightingale myth' in her *Angels and Citizens: British Women as Military Nurses 1854–1914* (London, 1988), pp. 13–23. Also, Sir John Hall, *Observations of the Report of the Sanitary Commissioners in the Crimea, during the Years 1855 and 1856* (London, 1857), p. 4.

28 C. A. Gordon, *Army Hygiene*, p. 354.

29 *Parliamentary Papers*, xix (3184), pp. iii–iv.

30 *Principles of Construction for Barracks for Single and Married Men: Remarks of the Army Sanitary Commission* (London, 1864), p. 5.

31 *Ibid.*, p. 9.

32 Clark, *Observations on the Hygiene of the Army in India*, pp. 29–31.

33 *Procs. of the Sanitary Commission for Bengal* (1865), 64.

34 *Memorandum on Measures adopted for Sanitary Improvements in India up to the end of 1867* (London, 1868).

35 J. L. Ranking, *Report on the Military Sanitation in the Presidency of Madras* (Madras, 1868), p. 12.

36 *SCGI* (1867), 148, 191; (1868), 73.

37 Nightingale, *Observations*, p. 72.

38 *Ibid.*, p. 11; Ranking, *Military Sanitation*, p. 29.

39 See appendix B: allotments to military sanitation.

40 Nightingale, *Observations*, pp. 5–6.

41 *SCGI* (1870), 8; (1872), 193–4.

42 *SCGI* (1875), 119–20.

43 *SCGI* (1876), 129; IOR P/1003 GOI (Sanitary), memo of Army Sanitary Commission on the report of the sanitary commissioner with the Indian government for 1875.

44 IOR P/1003 GOI (Sanitary) no. 177, general order by commander-in-chief, 30 July 1877.

45 Thornton, *Memories of Seven Campaigns* (London, 1895), pp. 148, 309.

46 See appendix B.

47 See *Reports of the Chemical Analyzer to the Government of Bombay* (1876–90) and *SCGI* (1896), 23.

48 *SCGI* (1895), 193.

49 Nightingale, *Observations*, p. 10.

50 Ranking, *Military Sanitation*, p. 5.

51 Caldwell, *Military Hygiene*, p. 57.

52 *Ibid.*, p. 58.

53 *SCGI* (1907), 13–16.

54 *SCGI* (1904), 21.

55 Freeman, *The Sanitation of British Troops in India*, p. 17.

56 Caldwell, *Military Hygiene*, pp. 42–3.

57 *Ibid.*, p. 43.

58 E. Roberts, *Enteric Fever in India, and other Tropical and Sub-Tropical Regions: A Study in Epidemiology and Military Hygiene* (London, 1906), p. vii.

59 A. B. Grant, *The Indian Manual of Hygiene. Being King's Madras Manual of Hygiene revised, rearranged and in great part re-written* (Madras, 1894), pp. xxiii–xxiv.

60 Z. Cope, *Almroth Wright. Founder of Modern Vaccine Therapy* (London, 1966), pp. 21–33. Though there was some uncertainty over the effectiveness of the typhoid vaccine, the Advisory Board's reluctance to carry out trials in order to test the vaccine suggests that other factors lay behind their opposition to Wright. Existing scholarship has tended to view this decision as a 'purely' medical one, ignoring other dimensions of the inoculation controversy, for example Curtin's *Death by Migration*, p. 154.

61 Cope, *Almroth Wright*, pp. 21–2.

62 The shortage of recruits to the British Army – around one-third of which was stationed in India – is considered in Hewlett's *Enteric Fever*, p. 170.

63 Roberts, *Enteric Fever in India*.

64 R. H. Firth, *Military Hygiene: A Manual of Sanitation for Soldiers* (London, 1908).

65 Caldwell, *Military Hygiene*, p. 41.

66 *SCGI* (1870), pp. 48–52.

67 R. Hyam, *Empire and Sexuality: The British Experience* (Manchester, 1990), p. 123.

68 Ballhatchet, *Race, Sex, and Class under the Raj*, pp. 11–19.

69 *Ibid.*, pp. 35–6.

70 *SCGI* (1867), 157; IOR P/674. GOI (Sanitary), no. 204, 1871.

71 IOR P/434/34. GOI (Sanitary), resolution on the new duties of sanitary commissioners, no. 9-681-88, 12 February 1868; *BHO*, 1 (1871), 8; *BHO*, 1 (1872), 7.

72 IOR P/;674. GOI (Sanitary), commissioner of police, Calcutta, to GOBe., submitting report of the superintendent of lock hospitals for 1870.

73 IOR P/1002. GOI (Sanitary), extract from the procs. Govt. of Bengal (Judicial Dept.), 6 August 1873.

74 D. Arnold, *Police Power and Colonial Rule* (Delhi, 1986), p. 64.

75 IOR P/438. GOBo. (Genl. Dept.), no. 41, letter from the municipal commissioner of Bombay to GOBo., 4 June 1871.

76 *BHO*, 3 (1871), 8.

77 IOR P/674. GOI supt. of lock hospitals, Calcutta, to commissioner of police, Calcutta, 1871.
78 Hyam, *Empire and Sexuality*, p. 123.
79 IOR P/1002 GOI (Sanitary), procs. GOBe., 6 August 1873, no. 13.
80 IOR P/1203. GOI (Sanitary), resoln. no. 357, 21 December 1877.
81 *SCGI* (1875), 76.
82 *SCGI* (1876), 31.
83 *SCGI* (1878), 25–8; (1879), 31.
84 IOR P/1664. GOI (Sanitary), no. 1037, sec. to GOBe. to sec. to GOI, 30 August 1881.
85 *SCGI* (1871), 111. Evelyn Baring (later Lord Cromer), legal member of the viceroy's council was one of the staunchest opponents of the CD Acts, but for financial rather than moral reasons. See Lord Zetland, *Lord Cromer* (London, 1932), pp. 77, 165.
86 IOR P/1781. GOI (Medical), resoln. no. 120, 7 June 1881.
87 *Bengalee*, 30 July 1887.
88 *Bengalee*, 2 July 1887.
89 Ballhatchet, *Race, Sex, and Class under the Raj*, pp. 43, 49.
90 *Hindoo Patriot*, 17 May 1875, p. 234.
91 *Bengalee*, 21 August 1886.
92 *Bengalee*, 2 July 1887.
93 IOR P/3195. GOI (Sanitary), no. 24 October 1888, sec. of state to gov.-gen. in council, 14 June 1888.
94 IOR P/4753. GOI (Sanitary), no. 19 May 1895, enclosing copy of Military Cantonments Act 1889.
95 IOR P/4753. GOI (Sanitary), no. 19 May 1895.
96 *Bengalee*, 20 February 1897, p. 89.
97 See chapters 5 and 6.
98 Ballhatchet, *Race, Sex, and Class under the Raj*, p. 95.
99 Nightingale, *Observations*, p. 25.
100 *Gazette of India*, 2 March 1864, pp. 84–6.
101 *SCGI* (1868), 60.
102 *SCGI* (1869), 74–5.
103 *SCGI* (1869), 104–5.
104 IOR P/434/45. GOI (Sanitary), sec. to GOI to sec. to GOBe. (Judicial Dept), 5 February 1870.
105 *Suggestions in Regard to Sanitary Works and Measures required for Improving Indian Stations and their Vicinity, prepared and revised by the Army Sanitary Commission* (London, 1882), p. 43.
106 *SCGI* (1875), 121; (1876), 128–9.
107 *SCGI* (1878), 108–9.
108 *SCGI* (1892), 25.
109 *BHO*, 2 (1869), 4.
110 *Gazette of India*, 1864, pp. 84–6; IOR P/434/34. GOI (Sanitary), nos. 1–18, 'Duties to be performed by sanitary commissioners with the local governments and administrations in the Bengal Presidence', 19 September 1868.
111 *SCGI* (1868), 61, 97.

112	IOR P/434/45. GOI (Sanitary) no. 27a, 'Draft rules for the registration of deaths among the native population in the NWP', 10 February 1870; cf. T. Dyson, 'The historical demography of Berar 1881–1980', in T. Dyson (ed.), *India's Historical Demography: Studies in Famine, Disease and Society* (London, 1989), pp. 150–96.

113	*SCGI* (1870), 104.

114	IOR P/434/45. GOI (Sanitary), no. 23A, sanitary commissioner to NWP to sec. to govt. of NWP, 17 August 1869.

115	IOR P/434/45. GOI (Sanitary), no. 1A, Walker to sec. to govt., NWP, 19 August 1869.

116	IOR P/524. GOI (Sanitary), no. 123, Cuningham to sec. to GOI, 11 March 1871.

117	*SCBo.* (1868), 175.

118	*SCGI* (1874), 41.

119	*SCGI* (1875), 107. The classification of deaths had to be simplified in 1873 to take account of these problems. One of the changes made was a change from the old 5–10 year approximate age categories to the even broader categories of 'infant', 'boy/girl', 'adult' and 'old person'. See IOR P/525. GOI (Sanitary), resoln. no. 5, 31 December 1873.

120	*SCGI* (1875), 111.

121	*BHO* (1877), 6.

122	IOR P/525. GOI (Sanitary), resident of Hyderabad to sec. to GOI, 3 September 1874.

123	IOR P/1003 GOI (Sanitary), no. 46, procs. of GOI (Home Dept.), 23 March 1877.

124	IOR P/1851. GOI (Sanitary) no. 41 resoln. 8-285-96, 10 August 1882. The Famine Commission advocated compulsory registration in the hope that it would give a better impression of the 'condition of the people'.

125	IOR P/1432. GOBo. (Genl.), no. 260, note on the progress of birth and death registration in British India, 10 June 1879.

126	IOR P/4112. GOI (Sanitary), no. 33, Bengal Municipal Dept. resoln. no. 2223, 1 July 1893.

127	*SCGI* (1894), 131.

128	*SCGI* (1896), 101.

129	*SCGI* (1899), 101.

130	See chapter 6.

131	See for example *BHO*, 1 (1899), 1–2.

132	*IPC*, V, pp. 328–34, 408–9.

133	*BHO*, 1 (1901), 1.

134	*BHO*, 2 (1901), 1; 3 (1901), 1.

135	*BHO*, 4 (1901), 3.

136	*BHO*, 1 (1902), 1–2.

137	*Procs. All-India San. Conf.* (1911), 11–12.

138	Arnold, 'Smallpox and colonial medicine', p. 53.

139	S. P. James, *Smallpox and Vaccination in British India* (Calcutta, 1909), p. 21.

140	J. Ranken, *Report on the Malignant Fever called the Pali Plague which has Prevailed in some part of Rajputana since the month of July, 1836* (Calcutta, 1838), p. iv.

141	J. Schoolbred, *Report on the Progress of Vaccine Inoculation in Bengal, 1802–3* (Calcutta, 1804), p. 82.

142 D. Porter and R. Porter, 'The politics of prevention: anti-vaccinationism and public health in nineteenth-century England', *Medical History*, 32 (1988), 231–52.

143 Cowpox was rare, if not non-existent in India, and vaccine was not manufactured from animal lymph in India until after 1860. See James, *Smallpox and Vaccination*, p. 32.

144 *Bengal VR* (1867–8), 13; Arnold, 'Smallpox and colonial medicine', p. 55.

145 James, *Smallpox and Vaccination*, p. vi; Arnold, 'Smallpox and colonial medicine', pp. 48–9.

146 J. Z. Holwell, *An Account of the Manner of Inoculating for the Smallpox in the East Indies* (London, 1767). Inoculation was also practised on slave plantations and on slave ships in order to maximise productivity and profits. See L. Stewart, 'The edge of utility: slaves and smallpox in the early eighteenth century', *Medical History*, 29 (1985), 54–70.

147 For example: Schoolbred, *Smallpox in the East Indies*, pp. 27–8; W. Cameron, 'On vaccination in Bengal', *Procs. Calcutta Medical and Physical Society* (1831), 385–95.

148 James, *Smallpox and Vaccination*, pp. 10–11.

149 Vaccination required a large number of subordinate staff. Even in 1878, a total of 2,559 vaccinators were employed throughout British India, the largest number (591) in the NWP, and the lowest number (139) in the Punjab and the Central Provinces respectively. See *SCGI* (1878), 96.

150 *Report of the Charitable Dispensaries of Bengal* (1870), pp. 64–5.

151 *SCGI* (1868), 50.

152 IOR P/524. GOI (Sanitary), no. 209, sanitary commissioner with the Indian government to sec. to GOI, 21 April 1871.

153 *BHO*, 1 (1869), 9–10. Inoculation had already been banned in Calcutta and surrounding villages. See James, *Smallpox and Vaccination*, p. 14.

154 IOR P/674. GOI (Sanitary), memo no. 400 circulated by sec. to GOI to GOBo., 26 August 1872. The Bill provided for the compulsory vaccination of all children over six months old born, or newly arrived in, the city of Bombay. This was an optimistic, if not unrealistic, objective, given that rapidly industrialising Bombay was attracting large numbers of immigrants from its rural hinterland. See I. Klein, 'Urban development and death: Bombay City, 1870–1914', *Modern Asian Studies*, 20 (1986), 725–54.

155 *SCGI* (1870), pp. 105–6.

156 E. Stokes, *English Utilitarians and India* (Oxford, 1959), pp. 50, 148–50.

157 *SCGI* (1869), 121.

158 IOR P/2510. GOI (Sanitary), no. 4, 25 November 1884. Surg.-capt. Pringle subsequently resigned from the IMS.

159 *Madras VR* (1891–2), 16.

160 *Madras VR* (1893–4), 9.

161 *SCGI* (1877), 101.

162 *SCGI* (1879), 100.

163 *SCBo.* (1887), 55.

164 James, *Smallpox and Vaccination*, pp. 31–3; *SCGI* (1879), 83.

165 *Madras Times*, 3 July 1880, pp. 2–3.

166 *Hindoo Patriot*, 6 May 1878, p. 211.

167 IOR P/1432. GOBo. (Genl.), no. 141, resoln. no. 748, 25 March 1879.

168 *Madras Times*, 30 January 1884, p. 2; 16 March 1885, p. 14.

169 Arnold, 'Smallpox and colonial medicine', p. 60.

170 *SCBo.* (1888), 52.

171 *Bengal VR* (1879–80), 7.

172 *SCGI* (1881), 152.

173 IOR P/2708. GOI (Sanitary), no. 42, sanitary commissioner for Hyderabad to sec. to GOI, 24 June 1886.

174 IOR P/2708. GOI (Sanitary), Simpson to sanitary commissioner for Bengal, 5 July 1886.

175 *Bengal VR* (1877–8), 6–7.

176 IOR P/4346. GOI (Sanitary), no. 13, under sec. to GOI to chief sec. to Punjab govt.

177 IOR P/4346. GOI (Sanitary), no. 16, gov.-gen. in council to sec. of state, September 1893.

178 IOR P/4555. GOI (Sanitary), no. 98, Bengal Municipal Dept. resoln. no. 3391-8, 7 November 1893.

179 IOR P/4753. GOI (Sanitary), no. 33, procs. chief commissioner, CPs, no. 5738, 20 August 1894.

180 IOR P/4753. GOI (Sanitary), no. 41, procs. chief commissioner, Assam, no. 5179, 21 July 1894.

181 Arnold, 'Smallpox and colonial medicine', p. 54.

182 *Madras VR* (1905–6), 18.

183 See *Reports of the Sanitary Commissioner with the Government of India*.

184 IOr P/4753. GOI (Sanitary), no. 310, sec. to GOI to sec. to GOBe., 31 October 1894.

185 *SCGI* for 1892 and 1902.

186 *SCGI* (1899), 143. See also Arnold, 'Touching the body', pp. 68–76 and chapter 6 below.

187 *Amrita Bazar Patrika*, 1 May 1912, p. 9; 2 May 1912, p. 7.

188 *IPHMJ*, February 1909, p. 244.

189 *Moslem Chronicle*, 5 September 1895, p. 379.

190 *Madras VR* (1901–2), 7.

191 *Madras VR* (1897–8), 6–8.

192 IOR P/525. GOI (Sanitary), Cuningham to sec. to GOI, 18 August 1873.

193 *Reports on the Charitable Dispensaries of Bengal* (hereafter, *Bengal Dispensary Reports*), 2.

194 *Ibid.*, 1.

195 *Bengal Dispensary Report* (1869), 37.

196 *Ibid.*, 30.

197 *Bengal Dispensary Report* (1870), xxii.

198 *Bengal Dispensary Report* (1871), xix.

199 *Bengal Dispensary Report* (1867), 5.

200 *Bengal Dispensary Report* (1900), i, xv.

201 *Bengal Dispensary Report* (1869), 55.

202 *Ibid.*, 63.

203 *Bengal Dispensary Report* (1870), ix.

204 *Bengal Dispensary Report* (1869), 41.

205 *Bengal Dispensary Report* (1870), 91.

206 *Bengal Dispensary Report* (1869), xvii.
207 *Bengal Dispensary Report* (1871), ix.
208 *Bengal Dispensary Report* (1900), cv.
209 *Bengal Dispensary Report* (1901), 24. There had been little improvement by 1908, see *Bengal Dispensary Report* (1908), 6.
210 NAI. GOI (Education) (nos. 14–17), 'Introduction of the sanitary primer entitled *The Way to Health* (enclosed)', October 1887.
211 IOR P/1851. GOI (Sanitary), sec. to chief commissioner of Assam to sec. to GOI, 29 June 1882; under-sec. to GOI to chief commissioner, Assam.
212 In 1899 there were 268 missionaries holding British medical qualifications. See G. F. Reynolds, 'Blackwater fever, some cases and notes', *JTM* (January 1899), 151.
213 Madras CVES, *The Way to Health*, p. 5. Like the Ladies Sanitary Association, and other bodies which ministered to the lower classes in Britain, Indian sanitary associations were an outgrowth of Bible mission societies: A. S. Wohl, *Endangered Lives. Public Health in Victorian Britain* (London, 1983), p. 36.
214 M. I. Balfour and R. Young, *The Work of Medical Women in India* (London, 1929), pp. 13–14. The first class for the training of Indian midwives was established in Amritsar in 1866 by the civil surveon, Dr Aitchison.
215 B. Harrison, 'Women's health and the women's movement in Britain: 1840–1940', in C. Webster (ed.), *Biology, Medicine and Society, 1840–1940* (Cambridge, 1981), pp. 15–73.
216 *Ibid.*, pp. 15–18. The society's endeavours met with a limited success, and some Indian women were even induced to undergo medical training in the West. Mrs Anandibai Joshi was the first Indian woman to be trained as a medical practitioner, graduating from the Women's Medical College at Pennsylvania in 1886.
217 *Bombay Gazette*, 2 February 1883, p. 17, and *Bombay Gazette*, 23 February, p. 16.
218 *Bombay Gazette*, 19 June 1883, p. 19.
219 *IMG* (January 1884), 21.
220 Florence Nightingale was among those calling for a service of 'village missioners'; i.e. Indian (especially female) health visitors trained in western hygiene. See *Bombay Times*, 16 January 1897, p. 4.
221 Balfour and Young, *Medical Women in India*, pp. 33–7.
222 *IMG* (January 1886), 15.
223 *Bombay Gazette*, 5 February 1886, p. 16.
224 *Bombay Gazette*, 28 July 1885, p. 6.
225 Balfour and Young, *Medical Women in India*, pp. 39–40.
226 *Bombay Gazette*, 5 February 1886, p. 16.
227 *Hindoo Patriot*, 13 February 1888.
228 *IMG* (February 1891), 42.
229 *IMG* (March 1892), 113.
230 *Bombay Gazette*, 7 July 1886, p. 15.
231 *Moslem Chronicle*, 31 January 1895.
232 *Trans. Ind. Medl. Cong.* (1891), 222.
233 NAI. GOI (Sanitary), no. 171, ASC memo. on the report of the sanitary commissioner for Bengal (1894), February 1897.
234 Sir Henry Holland, *Frontier Doctor. An Autobiography* (London, 1958), pp. 171–2.
235 *Bengalee*, 13 December 1890.

236 *Bengalee*, 28 February 1891.
237 *IMG* (April 1904), 144.
238 Third Report of the Madras Branch of the Dufferin Fund (1888), reproduced in the *Madras Times*, 23 January 1889.
239 Balfour and Young, *Medical Women in India*, pp. 46–9.
240 NAI. GOI (Medical), nos. 124–48, 'Medical education among Indian women', September 1914.
241 Balfour and Young, *Medical Women in India*, pp. 46–8.
242 *Procs. All-India San. Conf.* (1912), 48, 55–6.
243 *IMG* (December 1913), 477–9. Government financial support for voluntary organisations in India mirrored government involvement in the voluntary sphere in Britain, including the areas of maternal and child welfare. See M. Rooff, *Voluntary Societies and Social Policy* (London, 1937), pp. 23, 45–50.
244 Balfour and Young, *Medical Women in India*, pp. 142–3. These efforts appear to have been modelled on milk depots set up in some British towns, as a consequence of concerns over national efficiency and racial degeneration. See D. Dwork, 'The milk option. An aspect of the history of the infant welfare movement in England 1898–1908', *Medical History*, 31 (1987), 51–69.
245 J. A. Turner, *A Plea for Education in Hygiene and Public Health in India* (Bombay, 1919), p. 37.
246 Turner, *Plea for Education*, pp. 25–7.
247 *IPHMJ* (April 1908), 337–9. Similar views had been expressed by British MOsH, see M. Richards, 'The origins of the medical inspection of schools', *Public Health*, 19 (1906–7), 96.
248 C. T. H. Johnson, *A Catechism on Hygiene for use in Elementary Schools* (Madras, 1908).
249 J. A. Turner, *Plea for Education*, pp. 42–5, 60; see also H. Banbury, *School Hygiene for Indian Teachers* (Lucknow, 1909). See also H. B. Collins, 'Health and empire', *Public Health*, 16 (1903–4), pp. 406, 408.
250 Turner, *Plea for Education*, p. 4, and *IPHMJ* (December 1907), 166.

4 Cholera theory and sanitary policy

1 Annesley, *Sketches of the Most Prevalent Diseases of India*, pp. xvii, 4, 9.
2 *Ibid.*, p. 122.
3 This was the most common view of cholera causation in India. See for example: J. Johnson, *Influence of Tropical Climates*, pp. 398–402; Fayrer, *Natural History and Epidemiology of Cholera*; Martin, *Influence of Tropical Climates*, p. 131.
4 Kennedy, *History of the Contagious Cholera*, pp. 241–51.
5 See E. H. Ackerknecht, 'Anticontagionism between 1821 and 1861', *Bull. Hist. Med.*, 22 (1948), 561–93; R. J. Morris, *Cholera 1832: The Social Response to an Epidemic* (London, 1976); Pelling, *Cholera, Fever and English Medicine*; G. P. Parsons, 'The British medical profession and contagion theory: pueperal fever as a case study, 1830–1860', *Medical History*, 22 (1978), 138–50; Durey, *Return of the Plague*; Cooter, 'Anticontagionism and History's medical record'.
6 Crawford, *Roll of the Indian Medical Service*, p. 154, and *Lancet* obituary, 2 (1880), pp. 915–16.

7 Arnold, 'Cholera and colonialism', pp. 121–2.

8 J. L. Bryden, *Cholera Epidemics of Recent Years Viewed in Relation to Former Epidemics. A Record of Cholera in the Bengal Presidency from 1817 to 1872* (Calcutta, 1874), p. 1. See also Bryden's *Epidemic Cholera in Bengal* (Calcutta, 1869), and *Lancet*, 1 (1870), p. 209.

9 L. J. Jordanova, 'Earth science and environmental medicine: the synthesis of the late Enlightenment', in Jordanova and R. Porter (eds.), *Images of the Earth. Essays in the History of the Environmental Sciences* (Oxford, 1979), p. 122, and K. Thomas, *Man and the Natural World. Changing Attitudes in England 1500–1800* (London, 1983), p. 31.

10 Jordanova, 'Earth science and environmental medicine', p. 135.

11 J. L. Bryden, *The Cholera History of 1875 and 1876* (Calcutta, 1878), pp. 308–13.

12 See D. Kumar, 'The evolution of colonial science in India: natural history and the East India Company', in MacKenzie (ed.), *Imperialism and the Natural World*, pp. 51–66.

13 See P. Gay, *The Enlightenment: An Interpretation* (London, 1967); J. M. Eyler, 'The conceptual origins of William Farr's epidemiology: numerical methods and social thought in the 1830s', in A. M. Lilienfeld (ed.), *Times, Places, and Persons. Aspects of the History of Epidemiology* (Baltimore, 1980), pp. 11–13.

14 See Bryden's *Vital Statistics of the Bengal Presidency* (Calcutta, 1866–1879).

15 *Lancet* obituary of Bryden, 2 (1880), 913–16. Farr was somewhat more cautious in making claims about the predictive value of his work than Bryden: Eyler, 'William Farr's epidemiology', pp. 8–9.

16 *BMJ* (15 August 1868), 173.

17 Bryden quoted in *Lancet*, 5 February 1870, p. 209.

18 *Ibid.*, p. 81.

19 *Lancet* (1905), p. 122; Crawford, *Roll of the Indian Medical Service*, p. 138. Cuningham graduated 4 years before Bryden.

20 Klein, 'Cholera: theory and treatment', p. 38.

21 IOR P/674. GOI (Sanitary), DeRenzy to sec. to GOI, 13 September 1871. DeRenzy's emphasis on sanitary measures designed to protect the water supply is clearly stated in *SCP* (1868), pp. 25, 39. DeRenzy advocated a closed-pipe water-supply for towns and military cantonments.

22 Parkes, *Practical Hygiene*, pp. 21–4, 36 and 47–8. However, no causal organism had yet been identified in the case of cholera, and there existed considerable uncertainty in Britain at this time as to the exact nature of the threat posed by impure water. See C. Hamlin, 'Politics and germ theories in Victorian Britain: the metropolitan water commissions of 1867–9 and 1892–3', in R. MacLeod (ed.), *Government and Expertise. Specialists Administrators and Professionals, 1860–1919* (Cambridge, 1988), pp. 110–27.

23 IOR P/674. GOI (Sanitary), DeRenzy to sec. to GOI, 13 September 1871.

24 GOI (Sanitary), DeRenzy to sec. to GOI, 13 September 1871: 'Dr. Bryden's theory is merely the old one professing to rest on a statistical basis and until now there were few Indian Medical Officers who disagreed with or dissented from it.'

25 *BMJ*, 1 (1899), 635–6. MacNamara left India in 1870.

26 GOI (Sanitary), DeRenzy to sec. to GOI, 13 September 1871: citation of Cuningham's sanitary report for 1870.

27 IOR P/674. GOI (Sanitary), sec. to GOI to sec. to Punjab govt., no. 38, 23 January 1872.
28 *Indian Public Opinion and Punjab Times*, 29 March 1870.
29 IOR P/434/45. GOI (Sanitary), sec. to GOB to sec. to GOI, no. 1221, 6 April 1870.
30 IOR P/434/45. GOI (Sanitary), san. comm. to Central Provinces to chief commissioner Central Provinces, 8 October 1869.
31 IOR P/1338. GOI (Sanitary), memo. of ASC on the report of the san. comm. of the NWP and O for 1877, no. 2, November 1879.
32 IOR P/1498. GOI (Sanitary), memo. of ASC on report of san. comm. for Bengal for 1878, no. 17, January 1880.
33 *IMG* (June 1872), 186.
34 *IMG* (October 1873), 265.
35 Ramasubban, 'Imperial health in British India', p. 41.
36 F. Nightingale, *Life or Death in India? A Paper read at the meeting of the National Association for the Promotion of Social Science, Norwich, 1873* (London, 1873), p. 15.
37 *Ibid.*, pp. 15–16. In some respects the issues being debated in India in the 1870s resembled those debated in Britain in the 1830s and 40s: the questions of local autonomy, of 'infringement of individual liberties', of the raising of revenue for sanitary programmes. See for example: W. M. Frazer, *A History of English Public Health, 1834–1939* (London, 1950); R. A. Lewis, *Edwin Chadwick and the Public Health Movement, 1832–1854* (London, 1952); S. E. Finer, *The Life and Times of Sir Edwin Chadwick* (London, 1952).
38 Mersey, Viscount, *The Viceroys and Governors-General of India 1757–1947* (London, 1949), pp. 82–7.
39 R. J. Moore, *Liberalism and Indian Politics 1872–1922* (London, 1966), p. 15. The administration of India had become decentralised in 1861, when local legislatures were set up for the first time in Madras, Bombay, and Bengal. Other legislatures were established subsequently under powers conferred by this Act. See S. V. D. Char, *Centralised Legislation* (Delhi, 1963), p. 327.
40 Ramasubban, *Public Health and Medical Research in India*, pp. 22–3.
41 Crawford, *Roll*, p. 105. Murray's best known works were *Topography of Meerut* (1839) and *Topography of Fatehpur Sikri* (1835). His first treatise on cholera was not published until 1869, 2 years after the epidemic.
42 'Report on the Cholera of 1867', in *SCGI* (1867), 134–5.
43 J. Murray, *Report on the Treatment of Epidemic Cholera* (Calcutta, 1869), p. 7.
44 Ramasubban, *Public Health and Medical Research in India*, p. 22. But, though Murray's plan for 'pilgrim stations' *en route* to religious fairs found little favour with government, sanitary provisions continued to be made at places of pilgrimage themselves. See, for example, I. J. Ranking, *Madras Fairs and Festivals* (Madras, 1868).
45 *Report on the Cholera Epidemic of 1867 in Northern India* (Calcutta, 1867), 17–18.
46 Ramasubban, *Public Health*, p. 22.
47 See Arnold, 'Smallpox and colonial medicine', and 'Cholera and colonialism'.
48 *Hindoo Patriot*, 28 July 1879.
49 IOR P/525. GOI (Sanitary), DeRenzy to sec. to Punjab govt., 5 June 1873. Where sanitary measures impinged on indigenous ways of life, DeRenzy favoured the use of indigenous personnel, even practitioners of indigenous medicine. However, the

employment of *vaids* and *hakims* was stubbornly resisted by other members of the medical profession, and in the Punjab the system was brought to an end in the 1880s. See J. C. Hume, 'Rival traditions: western medicine and Yuna-I Tibb in the Punjab, 1849–1889', in *Bull. Hist. Med.*, 51 (1977), 214–31; and 'Colonialism and sanitary medicine: the development of preventive health policy in the Punjab, 1860–1900', *Mod. Asian Stud.*, 20 (1986), 703–24.

50 The commission which investigated the cholera epidemic of 1861 expressed the view that cholera was communicated by 'human intercourse' and had recommended the isolation of sick troops from their healthy counterparts. The Commission's recommendations appear to have been followed in most cantonments and in some civilian areas like the city of Bombay: *Procs. of the San. Comm. for Bombay* (1866), 2, 43–9. The sanitary commissioner of Bombay also attempted, without success, to persuade railway companies to prohibit persons suffering from cholera from using their trains: *Procs. of the San. Comm. for Bombay* (1867), 238. Cordons sanitaires were also resorted to during the Company era: see Ranken, *Report on the . . . Pali Plague.*

51 *Indian Public Opinion and Punjab Times*, 6 January 1877.

52 *SCGI* (1875), 157–8.

53 *SCGI* (1877), 81. See also J. M. Cuningham, *Cholera. What the State can do to prevent it* (Calcutta, 1864).

54 IOR P/525. GOI (Sanitary), Cuningham to sec. to GOI, 18 August 1873.

55 Different conclusions on the spread of cholera could be drawn from the same epidemiological data: H. Letheby, 'Report on the sanitary condition of the city of London', quoted in *BMJ* (22 February 1868), 173, and William Farr's 'Report on the Cholera Epidemic of 1866', in *BMJ* (15 August 1868), 169.

56 N. Howard-Jones, *The Scientific Background of the International Sanitary Conferences, 1851–1938* (Geneva, 1975), pp. 22–34.

57 Cf. Hamlin, 'Germ theories in Victorian Britain'.

58 IOR P/434/45. GOI (Sanitary), no. 283, san. comm. of Madras to sec. to GOI, 8 March 1870.

59 *SCGI* (1871), 73.

60 *SCGI* (1872), 35.

61 IOR P/525. GOI (Sanitary), Lyall to sec. to GOBe (Judicial Dept.), 22 December 1874.

62 IOR P/535. GOI (Sanitary), DeRenzy to sec. to Punjab govt., 11 May 1875.

63 *IMG* (June 1872), 186.

64 IOR P/1003. GOI (Sanitary), memo. of ASC on report of the san. comm. of Bengal for 1877.

65 *SCGI* (1874), 42–3.

66 T. R. Lewis, 'The microscopic organisms found in the blood of man and animals and their relation to disease', in *SCGI* (1877), 157–8. Lewis quotes Charles Murchison, the renowned British expert on fever, in defence of his views: pp. 185–6.

67 *Lancet*, 1 February 1870, p. 209.

68 *Lancet*, 14 January 1871, p. 52.

69 *Lancet*, 15 November 1873, p. 707.

70 *BMJ* (21 August 1880), 234.

71 *Lancet*, 4 April 1874, p. 482.

72 *Ibid.*, p. 477.

73 Essentially the same technique was used by both Southwood Smith and William Budd with respect to cholera theory in Britain, the former categorically opposing all notions of 'contagion', the latter explaining the behaviour of epidemic disease by reference to smallpox. See Pelling, *Cholera, Fever, and English Medicine*, pp. 50–79, 250–93.

74 W. Coleman, 'Koch's comma bacillus: the first year', *Bull. Hist. Med.*, 61 (1987), 315–42; T. D. Brock, *Robert Koch. A Life in Medicine and Bacteriology* (Madison, 1988), pp. 150–67.

75 Coleman, 'Koch's comma bacillus', pp. 324–5.

76 *SCGI* (1884), 159.

77 *Procs. Madras San. Comm.*, no. 42 1884, memo. of 19 May 1884 to all provincial governments.

78 Coleman, 'Koch's cholera bacillus', p. 327.

79 *Procs. Madras San. Comm.*, no. 42 1884, under sec. of state for India to GOI, 26 July 1884.

80 *SCGI* (1884), 159.

81 *The Times*, 19 November 1884.

82 Coleman, 'Koch's comma bacillus', p. 337.

83 *SCGI* (1884), 160. There had, for some years, been complaints about the Government of India's neglect of medical research: see for example *IMG* (January 1882), 17.

84 IOR P/2708. GOI (Sanitary), sec. to GOBe. to sec. to GOI, 14 February 1885.

85 IOR P/2708. GOI (Sanitary), sec. to GOI to sec. of state for India, 18 May 1886. David Douglas Cunningham (1843–1914) was educated at Edinburgh and Munich, where he worked under Pettenköfer, then professor of hygiene. Cunningham joined the IMS in 1868, rising to the rank of surgeon-major at the time of his appointment to the directorship of the cholera laboratory and retiring, in 1892, as a brigade surgeon lt.-colonel with extra pension. In addition to numerous reports on cholera, he was author, with T. R. Lewis, of 'Fungus disease in India', *Quain's Dictionary of Medicine* (1882), and *Physiological and Pathological Researches* (1888). See Crawford, *Roll*, p. 174.

86 D. D. Cunningham, 'On the relation of cholera to schizomycete organisms', *Sci. Mems.* (1884), 1–16.

87 Cunningham, 'Results of examinations of old specimens of choleraic tissues', *Sci. Mems.* (1887), 1–11.

88 Cunningham, 'Are choleraic bacilli really efficient in determining the diffusion of cholera', *Sci. Mems.* (1889), 1–20.

89 Cunningham, 'The results of continued study of various forms of comma bacillus occurring in Calcutta', *Sci. Mems.* (1894), 1–57.

90 Haffkine's inoculation was tested on a number of occasions in India in 1894: allegedly with a certain amount of success. See for example W. J. Simpson, *Cholera in Calcutta in 1894 and Anti-Choleraic Inoculation* (Calcutta, 1894). Simpson – a critic of the government's non-interventionist stance on matters of public health – claimed that 'the results had been so favourable that I trust that steps will now be taken to make the inoculation a permanent institution in Calcutta' (p. 4). Cunningham was more cautious in his assessment of inoculation, but acknowledged

that it might reduce mortality from, if not the actual incidence of, cholera. He was concerned to avoid direct intervention of the kind advocated by Simpson, and continued to recommend a broad and less intrusive approach to public health. See Cunningham, 'The results on continued study . . . of comma bacilli', p. 57.

91 *IMG* (May 1884), 142.

92 *IMG* (May 1885), 115.

93 Kenneth MacLeod (1840–1922) held the post of professor of surgery and first surgeon at Calcutta Medical College from 1879 to 1896. He was an active propagandist of a more interventionist approach to public health, being chairman of the Calcutta Health Society. See Crawford, *Roll*; *BMJ* obit., 2 (1922), 1246; *Lancet*, 2 (1922), p. 1403; *Plarr's Lives of the Fellows of the Royal College of Surgeons of England* (1930), 2, pp. 8–9.

94 Coleman, 'Koch's comma bacillus', p. 341.

95 R. J. Evans, *Death in Hamburg. Society and politics in the Cholera Years 1830–1910* (Oxford, 1910). Koch's demand for strong state intervention against cholera accorded with the imperial government's desire to impose its authority on the Federal States (p. 270).

96 Klein, 'Cholera: theory and treatment', p. 45. That these developments were followed by at least some medical officers in India is clear from Simpson, *Cholera in Calcutta*, p. 6. However, Pettenköfer had also drunk a culture containing cholera bacilli, apparently without ill effect, in an attempt to refute Koch's claim.

97 *BMJ* (25 February 1893), 429–30. There were, however, exceptions. See *BMJ* (20 January 1894), 120–2; C. Creighton, *A History of Epidemics in Britain*, 2 vols. (London, 1894).

98 *SCGI* (1895), p. 181.

99 D. D. Cunningham, 'Choleraic and other commas; on the influence of certain conditions determining morphological variations in vibrionic organisms', *Sci. Mems.* (1897), 1–29.

100 Klein, 'Cholera: theory and treatment', p. 47.

101 *Ibid.*, pp. 47–50.

102 See, for example, *Procs. All-India Sanitary Conference, 1911* (Calcutta, 1912), especially the presidential address, pp. 1–2.

5 Quarantine, pilgrimage, and colonial trade: India 1866–1900

1 As Beloff points out, 'It was almost inevitable that the Government of India's views would differ from those entertained at home. Its first responsibility was to the defence and security of India, and it naturally regarded these as the first claim on British resources and as the prior consideration in the formation of British policy.' See M. Beloff, *Britain's Liberal Empire 1897–1921*, 2nd edn. (London, 1987), pp. 35–6.

2 A. Basu, *The Growth of Education and Political Development in India 1898–1920* (Delhi, 1974), pp. 147–57; P. Hardy, *The Muslims of British India* (Cambridge, 1972), pp. 116–20; S. R. Mehrotra, *Towards India's Freedom and Partition* (Delhi, 1979), pp. 73–4; A. Seal, *The Emergence of Indian Nationalism. Competition and Collaboration in the later Nineteenth Century* (Cambridge, 1971), pp. 300–39; the

later period is covered in D. Page, *Prelude to Partition: The Indian Muslims and the Imperial System of Control, 1920–32* (Delhi, 1982).

3 N. E. Goodman, *International Health Organizations and their Work* (London, 1952), pp. 52–3; N. Howard-Jones, *The Scientific Background of the International Sanitary Conferences, 1851–1938* (Geneva, 1975), p. 30. With the exception of the British delegate, the conference agreed unanimously that cholera was communicated with the discharges of infected persons mingling with air and water. They did not, however, believe that cholera was directly communicable from person to person in the same sense as smallpox. See Government of India, *Proceedings of the International Sanitary Conference, Constantinople, 1866* (Calcutta, 1868), p. 2.

4 J. Baldry, 'The Ottoman quarantine station on Kamaran Island 1882–1914', *Studies in the History of Medicine*, 2 (Delhi, 1978), 18–19; Howard-Jones, *Sanitary Conferences*, p. 29.

5 Baldry, 'Ottoman quarantine', p. 19.

6 IOR P/434/45. GOI (Sanitary), sec. to GOM (Marine Dept.) to sec. to GOI (Home Dept.), August 1869.

7 The Native Passenger Ships Act was a sanitary, rather than a quarantine, measure, intended to improve conditions on board pilgrim ships. As such, the measure had the support of Muslim leaders, but not necessarily of lower-class Muslims, since such measures tended to make the voyage more expensive.

8 IOR P/434/45. GOI (Sanitary), sec. to GOM (Marine Dept.) to sec. to GOI (Home Dept.), 10 August 1869.

9 Howard-Jones, *Sanitary Conferences*, pp. 35–45.

10 IOR P/1002. GOI (Sanitary), sec. of state to viceroy, encl. letter from Goodeve to sec. of state, 30 December 1870.

11 IOR P/1003. GOI (Sanitary), sec. of state to sec. to Local Government Board, article 9 (encl.), 22 December 1875.

12 IOR P/1002. GOI (Sanitary), sec. to GOI (Home Dept.) to sec. of state, 12 June 1876.

13 IOR P/400. GOBo. (Genl. Dept.), resoln. 2275, 24 July 1875.

14 IOR P/1003. GOI (Sanitary), sec. to GOI (Home Dept.) to sec. to GOB, 21 June 1876.

15 See for example *BHO*, 1 (1871), 1.

16 IOR P/1003. GOI (Sanitary), report of port health officer for Calcutta, 22 June 1876.

17 A. Mayne, '"The dreadful scourge": responses to smallpox in Sydney and Melbourne, 1881–2', in MacLeod and Lewis (eds.), *Medicine and Empire*, 219–41.

18 IOR P/1851. GOI (Sanitary), Mohammed Hali, gov. of Jeddah, to HM consul, Jeddah, 23 June 1881.

19 IOR P/1851. GOI (Sanitary), sec. to GOBo to sec. to GOI (Home Dept.), 31 August 1881.

20 *Bombay Gazette*, 12 July 1881, pp. 16–17.

21 IOR P/1851. GOI (Sanitary), Hon. Mir Husmayum Jah Bahadur to sec. to GOM, 29 September 1881.

22 IOR P/1851. GOI (Sanitary), resoln. 4/198-214, GOI (Home Dept.), 12 January 1882.

23 Baldry, 'Ottoman quarantine', p. 30.

24 *Bombay Gazette*, 19 January 1883, p. 12.

25 Baldry, 'Ottoman quarantine', p. 32.

26 IOR P/2261. GOI (Sanitary), sec. to GOI (Home Dept.) to sec. of state, 24 April 1883.

27 *Bombay Gazette*, 7 August 1883, p. 18.

28 *Bombay Gazette*, 9 February 1882, p. 13.

29 *Bombay Gazette*, 27 October 1881, letter from 'A. Merchant', p. 14.

30 *Bombay Gazette*, 19 January 1882, p. 23.

31 *Bombay Gazette*, 2 March 1882, p. 80.

32 IOR P/1851. GOI (Sanitary), viceroy to sec. of state, February 1882.

33 Quoted in R. Robinson and J. Gallagher, *Africa and the Victorians. The Official Mind of Imperialism* (London, 1961), p. 117.

34 IOR P/1851. GOI (Sanitary), Granville to HM representative in Egypt, 7 March 1882.

35 P. Harnetty, *Imperialism and Free Trade: Lancashire in the Mid-Nineteenth Century* (Columbia, 1972); P. Ray, *India's Foreign Trade Since 1870* (London, 1934), p. 33; I. D. Parshad, *Some Aspects of India's Foreign Trade 1757–1893* (London, 1932), p. 193.

36 B. R. Tomlinson, *Political Economy of the Raj 1914–1947* (London, 1979), p. 17; Ray, *India's Foreign Trade*, p. 30.

37 IOR P/1851. GOI (Sanitary), memo on new Medical Board, Bombay, 5 April 1882.

38 IOR P/1851. GOI (Sanitary), sec. to GOBo (Genl. Dept.) to sec. to GOI (Home Dept.), 16 September 1882.

39 IOR P/2043. GOI (Sanitary), report of the Foreign Office committee on the Red Sea, forwarded by sec. of state to viceroy, 8 February 1883.

40 Sir R. Ensor, *England 1870–1914* (16th edn., Oxford, 1985), pp. 77–80; D. K. Fieldhouse, *Economics and Empire 1830–1914* (2nd edn., London, 1984), pp. 260–8; K. M. Wilson (ed.), *British Foreign Secretaries and Foreign Policy: From Crimean War to First World War* (Beckenham, 1982), p. 96; Robinson and Gallagher, *Africa and the Victorians*, pp. 76–121. The first consul-general of Egypt was Evelyn Baring (later Earl of Cromer), who, as finance member of Ripon's council in 1880–3, was well acquainted with the adverse effects of quarantine upon Indian commerce. See, Stokes, *English Utilitarians*, pp. 312, 315–17, 319–20.

41 *Bombay Gazette*, 3 April 1882, p. 13. Muslim leaders rationalised their 'special relationship' with the British authorities in terms of their history as previous rulers of India, and their shared monotheistic faith. See Metcalfe, 'Nationalist Muslims in British India', p. 3.

42 *Bombay Gazette*, 18 July 1882, p. 13.

43 Hardy, *Muslims of British India*, p. 120; Hindus were generally less concerned about the British invasion of Egypt. The *Hindoo Patriot*, for example, supported the invasion on the grounds that the British force would 'rescue Egypt from anarchy': *Patriot*, 28 January 1884.

44 *Bombay Gazette*, 18 July 1882, pp. 15, 23.

45 IOR P/2043. GOI (Sanitary), sec. to GOBo (Genl. Dept.) to sec. of state, encl. 11, 24 April 1883.

46 IOR P/2261. GOI (Sanitary), sec. to Bombay chamber of commerce, to sec. to GOBo, 22 January 1884.

47 *SCGI* (1883), 115.

48 IOR P/2043. GOI (Sanitary), sec. to GOBo (Genl. Dept.) to sec. of state, encl. 11, 24 April 1883.

49 IOR P/2661. GOI (Sanitary), under sec. of state for India to foreign sec., 23 January 1884.

50 IOR P/2261. GOI (Sanitary), chargé d'affaires to Assim Pasha to sec. to Ottoman govt., 7 March 1885.

51 IOR P/2510. GOI (Sanitary), Wyndham to foreign sec., May 1885.

52 *Bombay Gazette*, 9 February 1882, p. 15; 30 May, p. 11; Fieldhouse, *Economics and Empire*, p. 261.

53 Howard-Jones, *Sanitary Conferences*, p. 21.

54 *Ibid.*, pp. 54–5.

55 One of these – Italy – was committed to a thorough revision of existing regulations at Suez. British delegates were optimistic that with Italian support they would soon be able to effect material changes in arrangements in the Red Sea. See R. Thorne-Thorne, 'On the results of the International Sanitary Conference of Rome, 1885', *Trans. Epid. Soc.*, 5 (1885–6), 135–49.

56 *Ibid.*, p. 56. After securing its proposed reform of the Egyptian (Sanitary, Maritime and Quarantine) board, Britain was still entitled to only one delegate with one vote, along with the other principal European nations and Turkey. But the Egyptian delegation, subject to heavy pressure from Britain, was entitled to 3 votes. This assured Britain of at least 4 out of 12 votes. See M. A. Ruffer, 'Measures taken at Tor and Suez against ships coming from the Red Sea and the Far East', *Trans. Epid. Soc.*, 19 (1899–1900), 25–47.

57 Baldry, 'Ottoman quarantine', pp. 37, 40.

58 *Times of India*, 31 October 1885, p. 2.

59 *Bombay Gazette*, 25 April 1886, pp. 11–12.

60 *Bombay Gazette*, 17 August 1886, pp. 10–11.

61 IOR P/2708 and P/3656. GOI (Sanitary), J. M. Cook to sec. to GOI (Home Dept.), 8 September 1886.

62 *Bombay Gazette*, 29 January 1886, p. 17.

63 *Bombay Gazette*, 31 August 1886, p. 14.

64 IOR P/3195. GOI (Sanitary), E. D. Dickson, British delegate to Ottoman Board of Health to Sir W. A. White, British ambassador to Turkey, 26 December 1887.

65 IOR P/3195. GOI (Sanitary), sec. to GOBo (Genl. Dept.) to sec. to GOI (Home Dept.), 17 December 1888.

66 IOR P/3429. GOI (Sanitary), commissioner of Rohikhund Div. to sec. to govt. of NWP and O, 30 April 1889.

67 IOR P/3656. GOI (Sanitary), J. M. Cook to sec. to GOI (Home Dept.), 9 December 1889.

68 IOR P/3656. GOI (Sanitary), J. M. Cook to sec. to GOI (Home Dept.), 8 February 1890.

69 IOR P/3885. GOI (Sanitary), sec. of state (Viscount Cross) to viceroy (Lansdowne), 14 August 1890; sec. to Bombay Chamber of Commerce to sec. to GOBo (Genl. Dept.), 18 November 1891.

70 Howard-Jones, *Sanitary Conferences*, p. 56.

71 *Ibid.*, p. 48.

72 Howard-Jones, *Sanitary Conferences*, pp. 63–4.

73 Ensor, *England 1870–1914*; Fieldhouse, *Economics and Empire*, pp. 362–73; G. A. Craig, *Germany 1866–1945* (Oxford, 1978), pp. 123–4.

74 Goodman, *Health Organisations*, pp. 63–4.

75 IOR P/4753. GOI (Sanitary), under sec. for foreign affairs to under sec., Colonial Office, 22 March 1895.

76 IOR P/4555. GOI (Sanitary), sec. of state to viceroy, 7 June 1894.

77 IOR P/4555. GOI (Sanitary), sec. to GOI (Home Dept.) to H. H. Fowler, sec. of state, 11 September 1894. It was by no means unprecedented for the secretary of state to overrule the wishes of the Indian government on important policy questions. According to A. Kaminsky, in his study of *The India Office, 1880–1910* (London, 1896), p. 151: 'there is a clearly identifiable pattern of the exercise of authority by the Home Government in long-range planning and the implementation of policy'.

78 There was criticism of this delay in the Indian medical press. See *IMG* (August 1895), 250.

79 *Moslem Chronicle*, 1 August 1895. There was, apparently, strong opposition to the bill among Muslims in Calcutta, Bombay, the Punjab, and Madras.

80 IOR P/4753. GOI (Sanitary), viceroy to sec. of state, 17 September 1895; no. 118, Oomer Jamal Vayani to sec. to GOBo. (Genl. Dept.), 17 August 1895. See also HM Ismail Khan of Aligarh to the editor of the *Moslem Chronicle*, 9 November 1895.

81 *Moslem Chronicle*, 10 October 1895.

82 *Moslem Chronicle*, 19 October 1895.

83 IOR P/4966. GOI (Sanitary), commissioner of police, Calcutta to sec. to GOBe., 6 August 1895.

84 IOR P/4966. GOI (Sanitary), British consul, Jeddah to GOI (Home Dept.), 23 April 1896.

85 IOR P/4966. GOI (Sanitary), port surgeon to first asst. resident, Aden, July 1895.

86 IOR P/4966. GOI, commissioner of customs to sec. GOI (Home Dept.), 30 October 1895.

87 IOR P/4966. GOI (Sanitary), sec. of state to sec. to GOI (Home Dept.), 5 December 1895; no. 93, viceroy to sec. to GOI (Home Dept.), 4 December 1895.

88 Howard-Jones, *Sanitary Conferences*, p. 74.

89 IOR P/4966. GOI (Sanitary), E. D. Dickinson to Sir Phillip Currie, consul, Peira, 15 April 1896.

90 The social and political tensions sharpened by the plague epidemic of 1896 have already received a good deal of attention. See Arnold, 'Touching the body'; Catanach, 'Plague and the tensions of empire'; Klein, 'Plague, policy and popular unrest'. As yet, there has been no examination of the economic impact of the epidemic.

91 *Bombay Gazette*, 26 September 1896, p. 2.

92 *Bombay Gazette*, 3 October 1896, p. 18.

93 R. Nathan, *The Plague in India, 1896–97*, I (Simla, 1898), pp. 406, 408, 417.

94 *Ibid.*, pp. 409–10.

95 Nathan, *The Plague in India*, pp. 417–19. Some European nations had banned the import of tea from Bombay, but this restriction appears to have been lifted following the 1897 Venice convention. See *Accounts and Papers*, viceroy to sec. of state, 2 April 1897.

96 *Bombay Gazette*, 24 October 1896, p. 16; IOR P/4966. GOI (Sanitary), no. 24, sec. to GOBo. (Genl. Dept.) to sec. to GOI (Home Dept.), 8 October 1896.
97 *Bombay Gazette*, 21 November 1896, p. 22; 26 December 1896, p. 13.
98 *Bombay Gazette*, 23 January 1897, pp. 13–14.
99 *Bombay Gazette*, 27 March 1897, p. 7.
100 Nathan, *Plague in India*, I, pp. 417–20.
101 *Ibid*., pp. 412–13.
102 *Bombay Gazette*, 3 October 1896, p. 13.
103 *Bombay Gazette*, 27 March 1897, p. 19.
104 *Bombat Gazette*, 23 January 1897, p. 23.
105 *Bombay Gazette*, 20 February 1897, p. 23.
106 *Bengalee*, 20 February 1897.
107 *Moslem Chronicle*, 13 February 1897.
108 *Accounts and Papers*, sec. of state to viceroy, 14 January 1897; *Madras Times*, 18 February 1897, p. 3.
109 GOI *Accounts and Papers*, sec. of state to viceroy, 12 February 1897.
110 NAI. GOI (Sanitary), no. 69, sec. to GOI to sec. to GOM, 6 February 1897; GOI *Accounts and Papers*, sec. to GOI (Home Dept.) to sec. to GOM, 6 February 1897; viceroy to sec. of state, 17 February 1897.
111 Baldry, 'Ottoman quarantine', pp. 65–6.

6 Professional visions and political realities

1 Grant, *The Indian Manual of Hygiene*, p. xcvi.
2 Stokes, *English Utilitarians*, p. 310.
3 For the notion of India as a 'giant laboratory' see R. M. MacLeod, 'Scientific advice for British India: imperial perception and administrative goals, 1898–1923', *Modern Asian Studies*, 9 (1975), 344; R. A. Stafford, 'The role of Sir Roderick Murchison in promoting the geological development of the British empire and its sphere of influence' (Oxford University, DPhil thesis, 1985), pp. 6, 173; Grove, 'Conservation and colonial expansion', p. 6.
4 Nathan, *The Plague in India, 1896–1897*, I, pp. 82–92.
5 See chapter 4. Similar considerations affected the reporting of cholera in British ports in 1831: Durey, *Return of the Plague*; Morris, *Cholera*; N. Longmate, *King Cholera: The Biography of a Disease* (London, 1966).
6 For an account of preventive measures taken against plague see F. A. Hirst, *The Conquest of Plague. A Study of the Evolution of Epidemiology* (Oxford, 1953).
7 IOR P/4966. GOI (Sanitary), under sec. to GOI to sec. to GOBo., October 1896.
8 M. E. Couchman, *Account of Plague Administration in the Bombay Presidency from September 1896 till May 1897* (Bombay, 1898), pp. 2–9.
9 The bacillus causing plague had been discovered by a Frenchman, Alexandre Yersin in Hong Kong in 1894, though there was no consensus over how the disease spread. Yersin himself suspected that rats played a major role. See H. H. Mollaret and J. Brossollet, *Alexandre Yersin ou le Vainquer de la Peste* (Paris, 1985), pp. 135–45.
10 See J. Cantlie, 'The spread of plague', *Trans. Epid. Soc.*, 16 (1896–7), 15–63.
11 *IPC*, I, pp. 20, 23, 41–9.
12 Durey, *Return of the Plague*, pp. 114–15.

13 See chapter 1, and Watkins, 'Revolution in social medicine', pp. 347–413.

14 Arnold, 'Touching the body', pp. 58, 62–3. In Bombay 1,000 mill-hands attacked the Arthur Rd. plague hospital, while in the city of Poona the plague commissioner W. C. Rand was assassinated.

15 *Bombay Gazette*, 26 December 1896, p. 13; 2 January 1897, p. 6.

16 *Bombay Gazette*, 19 December 1898, p. 10.

17 *Accounts and Papers*, 63 (1897), sec. of state to gov. of Bombay, 6 January 1897; gov. of Bombay to sec. of state, 8 January 1897.

18 *Accounts and Papers*, sec. of state to gov. of Bombay, 3 February 1897.

19 J. A. Lowson, *Report on the Epidemic of Plague from 22nd February to 18th July 1897* (Bombay, 1897), pp. 13–15.

20 Couchman, *Plague Administration*, pp. 25–8, and *Accounts and Papers*, gov. of Bombay to sec. of state, 14 February 1897.

21 Reade to A. Godley, permanent secretary to the India Office, quoted in Catanach, 'Plague and the tensions of empire', p. 154.

22 *IMG* (February 1897), 63.

23 *IPC*, I, p. 160.

24 *Trans. of Bombay Medl. and Physl. Soc.*, 5 March 1897, pp. 7–13.

25 *IPC*, II, p. 26.

26 *Ibid.*, p. 112.

27 *IPC*, II, p. 164.

28 See Simpson, *Cholera in Calcutta*; and 'Anti-choleraic inoculation: a report to the Government of India', *Public Health*, 8 (1895–6), 91–2. The Indian authorities were concerned lest Haffkine's inoculation experiments antagonise the inmates of Indian prisons.

29 R. W. S. Lyons, *Report of the Plague Research Committee* (Bombay, 1897), p. 1. See following section of present chapter for details on the work of the commission and on the scientific aspects of Haffkine's inoculation.

30 *Bombay Gazette*, 27 February 1897, p. 14.

31 *Accounts and Papers*, sec. of state to gov. of Bombay, 2 February 1897.

32 *Further Papers Relating to the Outbreak of Plague in India* (London, 1897), sec. of state to gov. of Bombay, 19 March 1897; sec. of state to Viceroy, 25 March 1897.

33 *IPC*, I, p. 135.

34 *IPC*, II, pp. 91–2.

35 *IPC*, II, p. 119.

36 Catanach, 'Plague and the tensions of empire', p. 160.

37 B. H. F. Leuman, *Report on Plague Inoculation at Hubli* (Bombay, 1898).

38 A. M. Corthorn, *Report on Anti-Plague Inoculation Work in the Dharwar District* (Bombay, 1899), p. 1.

39 *JTM*, September 1898, p. 135.

40 *IPC*, I, p. 21.

41 *IPC*, I, p. 146.

42 *IPC*, I, pp. 153–4.

43 NAI. GOI (Sanitary), sec. to GOI (Home Dept.) to sec. to GOBo. (Genl. Dept.).

44 *IPC*, I, p. 280. Although Harvey was considered by contemporaries to be 'bright', it was also remarked that he was 'lacking in originality', and this may go some way to explaining his distrust of inoculation. See Crawford, p. 168; *BMJ*, 1, (1901), p. 305.

45 *IPC*, I, p. 268.

46 *IPC*, II, p. 133.

47 *IPC*, III, pp. 2, 235.

48 Arnold, 'Touching the body'; K. Done, 'A study of the fight against an endemic disease: smallpox in India' (Physiological Sciences dissertation, Oxford, 1991).

49 NAI. GOI (Sanitary), no, 294, lt.-gov. of NWP and O to sec. to GOI (Home Dept.), 17 April 1900; no. 298 chief sec. to govt. of NWP and O to sec. to GOI (Home Dept.), 25 May 1900.

50 Arnold, 'Touching the body'.

51 Headrick, *Tentacles of Progress*, pp. 159–67.

52 *IPC*, II, p. 178.

53 *IPC*, I, p. 151.

54 *IPC*, II, pp. 136, 212.

55 NAI. GOI (Sanitary), no. 298, encl. B, amendments to plague regulations Cawnpore, June 1900.

56 *IPC*, I, p. 74; *Accounts and Papers*, sec. to GOI (Home Dept.) to sec. of state, 10 February 1897, encl. 20, 'Plague regulations under the Calcutta Municipal Act' (1888).

57 NAI. GOI (Sanitary), encl. B.

58 See second section of the present chapter for an account of the composition, duties, and scientific conclusions of the plague commissions.

59 *IPC*, V, pp. 337–75.

60 *Ibid.*, pp. 267–8.

61 C. J. Sarkies, *Inoculation and Plague Operations in Ahmednagar and District during the Epidemic of 1899* (Bombay, 1899); *Report of the Dharwar Inoculation Investigation Committee* (Bombay, 1901); memo. from Maj.-Genl. C. J. Burnett, chairman of Poona cantonment plague committee, to commissioner, Central Division, Poona, 20 February 1901 (miscellaneous plague documents, Indian Institute Library, Oxford); Corthorn, *Anti-Plague Inoculation*.

62 *IPC*, V, pp. 319–20.

63 NAI. GOI (Sanitary), no. 250, resolution of 16 July 1900.

64 S. Gopal, *British Policy in India 1858–1905* (Cambridge, 1965), p. 200; Catanach, 'Poona politicians and the plague'.

65 Elgin Collection, MSS. Eur. F. 84.72, no. 280, viceroy's private sec. to A. H. T. Martindale, agent, Rajputana, 27b May 1898.

66 NAI. GOI (Sanitary), resoln., p. 32.

67 NAI. GOI (Sanitary), no. 79, K-W No. 2, 19 September 1897.

68 NAI. GOI (Sanitary), no. 190, sec. to GOI (Home Dept.) to sec. of state, 11 January 1900.

69 *IPC*, I, p. 39. This contradicts Klein's statement that 'during plague's worst ravages the relationship between rat epizootics and human epidemics was unknown': Klein, 'Plague, policy and popular unrest', p. 740.

70 *IPC*, V, p. 127.

71 *IPHMJ*, March 1908, p. 321; February 1909, p. 244.

72 *IPHMJ*, June 1907, p. 363; *JTM*, October 1906, p. 300.

73 *IPHMJ*, July 1907, p. 387.

74 *Procs. All-India San. Conf.* (1911), pp. 14, 24.

75 An incident in 1902, in which nineteen villagers in the Punjab died of tetanus as a result of inoculation with contaminated serum, cast a shadow over inoculation for some years. The Indian government was quick to pin blame on Haffkine and procedures taken at his laboratory in Bombay, though the source of contamination was far from certain. An unpopular outsider, and convenient scapegoat, Haffkine was suspended from duty for 3 years. But following an active campaign in the British press, orchestrated by Ross and Simpson, editor of the *BMJ*, and an old friend of Haffkine's, Haffkine was re-employed by the Bombay government, though not in his old position. See Catanach, 'Plague and the tensions of empire', pp. 160–1; S. A. Waksman, *The Brilliant and Tragic Life of W. M. W. Haffkine* (New Brunswick, 1964).

76 *IPHMJ*, November 1910, p. 113.

77 The working definition of a scientific discipline used here is similar to that employed by Keith Vernon in his study of microbiology in Britain; that is, a body of knowledge which had become embodied in distinct institutional structures. See K. Vernon, 'Pus, sewage, beer and milk: microbiology in Britain, 1870–1940', *History of Science*, 28 (1990), 289–325.

78 Address by Manson to the BMA Tropical Diseases Section, July 1898, *JTM* (August 1898), 22.

79 Worboys, 'Science and British colonial imperialism, 1895–1940'; 'The emergence of tropical medicine: a study in the establishment of a scientific speciality'; 'The emergence and early development of parasitology'; 'Manson, Ross and colonial medical policy: tropical medicine in London and Liverpool, 1899–1914'.

80 C. W. Daniels, *Studies in Laboratory Work* (London, 1907).

81 Grant, *Indian Manual of Hygiene*, pp. xviii–xix.

82 Dr A. C. Crombie, IMS, quoted in *Proc. Genl. Malaria Comm.* (1912), p. 6.

83 Once it had accepted the validity of Ross' claims, the British medical press backed Ross to the hilt against foreign competitors. See, for example, *JTM* (August 1898), 21. Ross, however, was equally involved in professional disputes in Britain: E. Chernin, 'Sir Ronald Ross vs. Sir Patrick Manson: a matter of libel', *J. Hist. Med.*, 43, 3 (1888), 262–74.

84 *IMG*, October 1909, p. 382.

85 E. J. Hart, 'An address to the medical profession in India, its position and its work', *BMJ* (1894), 1469–74.

86 Ross, *Memoirs*, p. 17.

87 Sir James Fitzjames Stephen quoted from a letter to *The Times* in 1883, in Stokes, *The English Utilitarians*, p. 288.

88 Lyons, *Report of the Plague Research Committee*, p. 1.

89 *IPC*, II, pp. 243, 311.

90 *IPC*, III, p. 174.

91 Nathan, *Plague in India*, I, pp. 38–40.

92 *Ibid.*, p. 55.

93 *Ibid.*, pp. 26–7, 369.

94 *Ibid.*, pp. 27–30.

95 *Ibid.*, p. 60.

96 *Ibid.*, p. 64.

97 *Ibid.*, pp. 63–4.

98 *Ibid.*, p. 54; Mollaret and Brossollet, *Alexandre Yersin*, pp. 140–50. Among non-medical men in India there was considerable interest in attempts to produce a serum to treat plague, though recognition that any advance – as in the case of the diphtheria serum – would be slow. See *Madras Times*, 8 January 1897, p. 2.

99 Nathan, *Plague in India*, 2, app. 1, Haffkine to sec. to GOI (Home Dept.), 17 February 1897.

100 Nathan, *Plague in India*, 1, p. 58.

101 *IPC*, I, p. 7.

102 *IPC*, V, pp. 68–75.

103 *Ibid.*, pp. 167–70.

104 *Ibid.*, pp. 190–4, 319–20.

105 *DNB*. Marc Armand Ruffer (1859–1916). Born Lyon, son of Baron Alphonse Jacques de Ruffer, and a German mother. Educated Brasenose College Oxford and University College London. Appointed president of International Sanitary, Maritime, and Quarantine Council of Egypt in 1896. After serving on the plague commission, Ruffer actively promoted Haffkine's work in Europe. Ruffer went on to become the first director of the British Institute for Preventive Medicine, and on the outbreak of the First World War was appointed head of the Red Cross in Egypt.

106 *IPC*, V, pp. 409–11. See also: *Annual Reports upon the Work of the Bacteriological Section of the King Institute of Preventive Medicine* (1906–14); *Reports on the Bombay Plague Research Laboratory*. Both these laboratories were engaged primarily in the production of vaccines and sera and in routine bacteriological analysis, though some original research was carried out.

107 The Pasteur Institute at Kasauli was the first of its kind in the British Empire. The number of patients treated at the Institute rose from 321 in 1901 to 4,585 in 1914; its bacteriological work, however, was taken over in 1905 by its neighbour the Central Research Institute. As the Institute gained in stature, it received annual grants from most Indian provincial governments, and, after 1911, the IRFA. See *Annual Reports of the Pasteur Institute* (1901–14), esp. 1901, pp. 1–9.

108 *SCGI* (1899), 242–3.

109 *JTM* (August 1898), 1; June 1900, p. 279.

110 M. Worboys, 'The Imperial Institute: the state and the development of the natural resources of the Colonial Empire, 1887–1923', in J. M. MacKenzie (ed.), *Imperialism and the Natural World*, pp. 164–86; and 'The emergence of tropical medicine'.

111 MacLeod, 'Scientific advice', pp. 344–58.

112 *JTM* (April 1900), 236.

113 *SCGI* (1899), 243.

114 *SCGI* (1905), 153. The CRI opened in 1906. As envisaged by the commission, it combined research and limited teaching functions with the manufacture of vaccines and sera.

115 Ramasubban, 'Public health and medical research', p. 32.

116 The Bombay Plague Research Laboratory – renamed the Haffkine Institute – for example, celebrated its platunum jubilee in 1974: *Haffkine Institute Platinum Jubilee Commemoration Volume, 1899–1974* (Bombay, 1974).

117 Ramasubban, p. 32. There was no systematic official support or direction of medical research in Britain prior to the establishment of the Medical Research

Committee in 1913, and then only in a very limited sense until the formation of its successor the Medical Research Council in 1919: L. Bryder and J. Austoker (eds.), *Historical Perspectives on the Role of the MRC. Essays in the History of the Medical Research Council of the United Kingdom and its Predecessor, the Medical Research Committee, 1913–1953* (Oxford, 1989).

118 Ramasubban, 'Public health', p. 39.

119 Worboys, 'Manson, Ross and colonial medical policy'.

120 Headrick, *Tools of Empire*; Brockway, *Science and Colonial Expansion*, pp. 114–22.

121 NAI. GOI (Medical), nos. 38–9, 'Report of the director of government cinchona plantations, Madras', October 1887. The Nilgiri plantation was in deficit in 1860–76 and 1883–7.

122 Harrison, *Mosquitoes, Malaria and Man*, p. 122.

123 *SCGI* (1900), 131; (1901), 121–3.

124 C. F. Fearnside, 'Inoculation of malaria by Anopheles', *Sci. Mems.* (1901), 19–33.

125 W. J. Buchanan, 'The value of prophylactic issue of cinchona preparations. An experiment in Indian jails', IJTM (March 1899), 21–3.

126 S. R. Christophers, 'Second report of the anti-malarial operations at Mian Mir, 1901–1903', *Sci. Mems.* (1904), 1–13; 'Malaria in the Punjab', *Sci. Mems.* (1911), 1–32. See also S. P. James, 'Malaria in India', *Sci. Mems.* (1902), 1–85; 'First report of the anti-malarial operations at Mian Mir, 1901–3', *Sci. Mems.* (1903), 1–29.

127 L. Rogers, *Fevers in the Tropics. Their Clinical and Microscopical Differentiation, including the Milroy Lectures on Kala-azar* (London, 1908), pp. 237, 239.

128 J. A. Turner, 'Report on malaria in Bombay from 1902–1909', *Paludism*, 4 (1910), 39–40.

129 Lukis quoted in *Paludism*, 4 (1902), 4–5.

130 *Paludism*, 3 (1911), 10-14.

131 *SCGI* (1902), 106.

132 Headrick, *Tentacles of Progress*, pp. 163–4.

133 Though Sambon argued that blackwater fever was a specific disease, and not a form of quinine poisoning, he did believe that quinine was toxic and that its use should be discontinued. See L. W. Sambon, 'The etiology and treatment of blackwater fever', IJTM (May 1899), 295–6.

134 J. W. W. Stephens, *Blackwater Fever. A Historical Survey of Observations made over a Century* (London, 1937); L. W. Sambon, 'Blackwater fever', *JTM* (October 1898), 70–4; 'The etiology and treatment of blackwater fever', *JTM* (June 1899), 293–6; R. Koch (transl. P. Falcke), 'Blackwater fever', *JTM* (August 1899), 333–5; P. Manson, *Tropical Diseases. A Manual of the Diseases of Warm Climates* (London, 1898).

135 A. Beck, 'Medicine and society in Tanganyika 1890–1930. A Historical Inquiry', *Transactions of the American Philosophical Society*, 67 (1977), 1–59.

136 *JTM* (October 1898), 76.

137 *JTM* (September 1908), 283–4.

138 J. W. W. Stephens and S. R. Christophers, *The Practical Study of Malaria* (London, 1904).

139 Rogers, *Fevers in the Tropics*, pp. 229–30; *Recent Advances in Tropical Medicine* (London, 1924), pp. 106–10. Other colonial medical men persisted in quinine

prophylaxis and treatment. See for example: R. K. C. Bose, 'The use of quinine in malarious fevers', *JTM* (September 1900), 27–30; A. H. Hanley, 'Mosquito-screened houses versus quinine', *JTM* (December 1900), 112–13.

140 A. Powell, 'Haemoglobinuric fever in Assam', IJTM (December 1898), 117–19.

141 *Indian Medico-Chirurgical Review* (January 1894), 2. Doubts had been expressed about the safety of administering quinine during pregnancy. See H. P. Dimmock and H. K. Tavaria, 'The effect of quinine on pregnancy', *ibid.*, 92–8.

142 T. W. Jackson, *Tropical Medicine. With Special Reference to the West Indies, Central America, Hawaii, and the Philippines* (London, 1901), pp. 302–3.

143 Rogers, *Recent Advances*, p. 111; Chantemesse and Mosny (eds.), *Traité d'Hygiène*, pp. 361–2.

144 Stephens, *Blackwater Fever*, pp. vii–viii.

145 V. R. Muraleedharan, 'Malady in Madras: the colonial government's response to malaria in the early twentieth century', in D. Kumar (ed.), *Science and Empire*, pp. 101–14; Muraleedharan and D. Veeravagharan, 'Anti-malarial policy in the Madras Presidency: an overview of the early decades of the twentieth century', *Medical History*, 36 (1992), 290–305.

146 *SCGI* (1908), 66–139.

147 *Paludism*, 1 (1910), 4–5, 13–14.

148 *Procs. All-India San. Conf.* (1912), 18.

149 *Procs. Genl. Malaria Comm.* (1912), 21–4.

150 Muraleedharan, 'Malaria in the Madras Presidency'.

151 *SCGI* (1910), 57.

152 *DNB*. Sir Spencer Harcourt Butler (1869–1938). Educated at Harrow and Balliol; entered the ICS in 1902. As deputy commissioner of Lucknow District from 1906–8, he did much to enhance public amenities in the area; was made secretary to the Foreign Department in 1907; appointed to the viceroy's executive council as education member in 1910, where his duties included public health and local government; in 1913 he drafted an important resolution which reconstituted educational policy in India; in 1915 he became lt.-gov. of Burma and in 1918, lt.-gov. of the NWP; in 1927, after retiring from the ICS, he became chairman of the Indian States Committee and in 1931, chairman of the governing body of the School of Oriental and African Studies.

153 *IJMR* (July 1913), 1–2.

154 *SCGI* (1912), 68.

155 *SCGI* (1911), 67–9.

156 *IJMR* (July 1913), 7. For a breakdown of the association's research activities, see *Annual Report of the Board of Scientific Advice for India 1912–13* (Calcutta 1914).

157 NAI. GOI (Medical), no. 10, sec. to GOBe. to sec. to GOI, 27 October 1913.

158 NAI. GOI (Medical), no. 460-c, sec. to GOI to sec. to GOBo. (demi-official), 16 December 1913.

7 Public health and local self-government

1 IOR P/525. GOI (Sanitary), Lyall to sec. to govt. NWP and O, 31 January 1874. Lyall was convinced that government was limited in its capacity to intervene in

matters directly affecting indigenous practices. During his time in the NWP and as commissioner of Berar he had come to believe that government was too distant from the people to be able to predict accurately the effects of its policies on their day-to-day life. For this reason he was committed to local self-government, and local responsibility for public health.

2 R. Basu, 'Colonial municipal policy and Indian response: municipal government and police in Calcutta 1850–1872', *Bengal Past and Present*, 190 (1981), 4.

3 H. R. Tinker, *The Foundations of Local Self-Government in India, Pakistan and Burma* (London, 1954), pp. 43–8, and R. J. Moore, *Liberalism and Indian Politics 1872–1922* (London, 1966), pp. 34–6.

4 *Ibid.*, pp. 74–5.

5 Moore, *Liberalism and Indian Politics*, p. 33.

6 Basu, 'Colonial municipal policy'.

7 Stokes, *English Utilitarians*, p. 288.

8 Tinker, *Foundations of Local Self-Government*, p. 73.

9 Ramasubban, *Public Health and Medical Research in India*, p. 41.

10 Basu, 'Colonial municipal policy'.

11 *Bombay Gazette*, 19 January 1882, p. 15.

12 *Ibid.*, pp. 15–16.

13 *BHO*, 1 (1869), 11.

14 *Ibid.*, 11.

15 *Procs. San. Comm. for Bombay* (1867), 321.

16 See for example: *BHO*, 2 (1877), 1, and *BHO*, 1 (1879), 17.

17 *Madras Times*, 1 July 1880.

18 *Madras Times*, 3 July 1880.

19 *Madras Times*, 22 July 1880.

20 *Madras Times*, 9 September 1880.

21 *Madras Times*, 28 October 1880.

22 *Madras Times*, 23 September 1880.

23 *SCGI* (1881), 164–6.

24 Basu, 'Colonial municipal policy', p. 6.

25 *SCGI* (1881), 167.

26 Tinker, *Self-Government in India*, p. 43.

27 Moore, *Liberalism in Indian Politics*, pp. 34, 41; Stokes, *English Utilitarians*, p. 288.

28 Moore, *Liberalism*, p. 41.

29 Tinker, *Self-Government*, p. 42. In most provinces, the electorate (which comprised local ratepayers) did not exceed 2 per cent of the total population.

30 Towns applied individually to the provincial government for municipal status.

31 Tinker, *Local Self-Government*, p. 74.

32 *SCGI* (1880), 150; and *SCBe.* (1881), 67.

33 In 1894 in Bengal 25 per cent of municipal commissioners were landlords, 22 per cent lawyers, 17 per cent government servants, 4 per cent doctors, 4 per cent schoolmasters, 3 per cent pensioners, and 1 per cent planters. See Tinker, *Local Self-Government*, pp. 50–1.

34 IOR. Bengal Municipal Procs., nos. 9–13, January 1885.

35 IOR. Bengal Municipal Procs., no. 3, February 1885.

36 *SCGI* (1887), 176, and (1890), 186. There are numerous other instances, for example, *SCGI* (1889), 177, and (1891), 162.
37 *SCGI* (1891), 162.
38 *SCGI* (1892), 192.
39 *SCGI* (1893), 185.
40 *SCGI* (1892), 192.
41 Tinker, *Local Self-Government*, p. 58.
42 Tinker, *Local Self-Government*, p. 74.
43 *SCGI* (1884), 157.
44 *SCGI* (1886), 187–8.
45 *Madras Times*, 26 March 1884.
46 *Madras Times*, 1 May 1889.
47 *Madras Times*, 11 July 1890.
48 See chapter 8.
49 It was in Bengal that western science made its greatest impact on indigenous life styles, being actively cultivated by the 'westernised' *bhadralok* community. See Raj, 'Knowledge, power and modern science', in Kumar, *Science and Empire*.
50 Raj, 'Knowledge, power and modern science'.
51 *Madras Times*, 26 March 1884.
52 *Madras Times*, 26 March 1884.
53 *Madras Times*, 26 March 1884; 1 May 1889.
54 *SCM* (1890), 54.
55 *SCGI* (1893), 192.
56 *SCBo* (1879), 93; (1880), 105; (1881), 26.
57 *IPHMJ* (February 1908), 273.
58 *IPHMJ* (June 1909), 455–6.
59 *IPHMJ* (October 1909), 135–6.
60 *Ibid.*, 193.
61 See for example: *SCBo.* (1893), 46, and *SCGI* (1879), 97.
62 *SCBo.* (1888), 59–60.
63 *SCBo.* (1889), 59.
64 *Ibid.*, 65–6.
65 *SCBo.* (1891), 55.
66 *Bombay Gazette*, 2 February 1883, pp. 16–17.
67 *Bombay Gazette*, 8 September 1885, p. 20.
68 *Bombay Gazette*, 3 October 1896, p. 13.
69 S. Arjun, 'Our water supply (chemically and microscopically considered)', *Trans. Medl. and Physl. Soc., Bombay* (1883), 9–31.
70 *SCBo.* (1889), 63.
71 *Ibid.*, 58.
72 *SCBo.* (1891), 68.
73 *SCBo.* (1899), 118.
74 C. Dobbin, *Urban Leadership in Western India. Politics and Communities in Bombay City 1840–1885* (Oxford, 1972); N. Gupta, *Delhi Between Two Empires, 1803–1931. Society, Government and Urban Growth* (Delhi, 1981); and Basu, 'Colonial Municipal Policy'.

75 NAI. GOI (Political), nos. 278–81, July 1897, 'Memorandum on the vernacular and Anglo-Indian press of the North-West provinces and Oudh for 1896'.

76 *SCBo.* (1891), 64.

77 Johnson, *Provincial Politics and Indian Nationalism*, pp. 53–93. See also Catanach, 'Poona politicians and the plague'.

78 *SCBo.* (1894), 83.

79 These figures have been abstracted from the *Reports of the Sanitary Commissioner to the Government of the Punjab* (1880–99) and *Reports on the Working of the Municipalities in the Punjab* (1885–1915).

80 These figures have been abstracted from the *Reports of the Sanitary Commissioner for the Central Provinces* (1878–1904), and *Reviews of Municipal Reports and Statements, Central Provinces* (1905–14).

81 Tinker, *Local Self-Government*, p. 74.

82 IOL P/3429. GOI (Sanitary), sec. to GOBe. to sec. to GOI, 31 October 1889. But these arrangements were reached only after several municipalities objected to their having to finance the new appointment: P/3656. GOI (Sanitary), no. 2, 25 July 1889.

83 *SCGI* (1887), 188–9.

84 Curtin, *Death by Migration*, pp. 119–21.

85 *SCGI* (1890), 178; (1891), 165.

86 *Procs. Madras San. Comm.* (1889), 194.

87 IOR. Bengal Municipal Procs., March 1890, Surg.-Maj. W. H. Gregg to sec. to GOBe., submitting inspection report on Patna municipal commission for 1889.

88 IOR. Bengal Municipal Procs., April 1890, Gregg to sec. to GOBe., submitting inspection report for Howrah municipal commission.

89 *Bengalee*, 7 November 1896.

90 *Accounts and Papers*, gov. of Bombay to sec. of state for India, 1 March 1897; *IPC*, I, p. 44.

91 *IPC*, II, p. 203.

92 *IPC*, II, p. 240.

93 The same was true of other cities: according to Dr Amritaraj, health officer for Bangalore, attention was 'first directed' to problems of congestion and the sanitary environment in his city 'by the perpetual recrudescence of plague from 1898 onwards'. *Trans. All-India San. Conf.* (1912), 14.

94 *Report of the Bombay Improvement Trust* (1898–9), 1–2.

95 *Ibid.*, 1.

96 *Ibid.*, 5–6.

97 *Report of the Bombay Improvement Trust* (1907–8), p. iv.

98 *BHO* (1905), 1, p. 5.

99 *Trans. All-India San. Conf.* (1912), 11.

100 *Trans. All-India San. Conf.* (1912), 107.

101 *Trans. All-India San. Conf.* (1911), 9; Government of Bombay, *Some Recent Sanitary Developments in the Bombay Presidency* (Bombay, 1914), p. 6.

102 *Trans. All-India San. Conf.* (1912), 9.

103 P. Boardman, *The Worlds of Patrick Geddes. Biologist, Town-Planner, Re-educator, Peace Warrior* (London, 1978), p. 263.

104 *SCGI* (1898), 265; see also *SCGI* (1899), 225.

105 *SCGI* (1900), 118.

106 *SCGI* (1898), 267.
107 NAI. GOI (Sanitary), sec. to GOBo. to sec. to GOI, encl., representation from Bombay corporation, 22 September 1904.
108 NAI. GOI (Sanitary), nos. 12–13, endorsement of GOBo., 30 September 1899.
109 Tinker, *Local Self-Government*, pp. 68–9.
110 *Ibid.*, p. 59.
111 *Ibid.*, p. 282. The amount spent on civilian public health by provincial and central government increased from an annual average of 6.2 lakhs in 1870–9 (1.1 per cent of total expenditure) to 23 lakhs (1.6 per cent) in 1910–19; still a small percentage of income, but a substantial increase in total expenditure: Jeffery, *Politics of Health in India*, p. 69.
112 *SCGI* (1911), 55.
113 Tinker, *Local Self-Government*, p. 73.
114 *General Municipal Review, Madras* (1908), p. 8.
115 *SCBe.* (1913), 20.
116 *SCGI* (1903), 111.
117 *SCGI* (1906), 128; (1907), 113; (1914), 105.
118 *SCGI* (1911), 57.
119 *Ibid.*, p. 55.
120 *Trans. Bomb. Medl. and Phyl. Soc.* (1903), 38.
121 *Procs. All-India San. Conf.* (1912), 69.
122 *IPHMJ* (February 1910), 362–3.
123 *SCGI* (1907), 111
124 *SCTI* (1908), 118.
125 *SCGI* (1909), 107.
126 *SCGI* (1911), 57; (1913), 101; (1914), 108.
127 *Amrita Bazar Patrika*, 25 May 1812; 7 February 1913; 10 February 1913; 17 June 1913.
128 *SCM* (1885), 67.
129 *SCGI* 91878), 112.
130 *SCGI* (1880), 149–50. Local fund circles dated from 1863 in the Bombay, Bengal, and Madras presidencies; their powers to raise revenue were legalised in all presidencies in 1870–1. The revenue of district and local (*taluka*) boards was derived from a cess on land revenues, usually amounting to not more than one anna per rupee of revenue. See *Imperial Gazetteers of India* for *Bombay Presidency* (Calcutta, 1909), pp. 112–14; *Madras Presidency* (Calcutta, 1908), pp. 108–11; *Bengal Presidency* (Calcutta, 1909), pp. 138–40.
131 *Report of the Charitable Dispensaries of Bengal* (1869), p. 122.
132 The zemindars of Bengal disliked Ripon's reforms, which conferred substantial powers on the professional classes; they seldom stood for elections to local bodies. See Ripon Papers, Rivers Thompson (lt.-gov. of Bengal) to Ripon, 6 January 1883.
133 *Hindoo Patriot*, 12 April 1875. A massive proportion of annual mortality among the Indian population in most provinces of India was attributable to fevers. In Bengal, in 1879, the total death-rate from all causes was 15.85 per thousand and the death-rate from fevers 10.37. In the NWP the figures were 44.81 and 37.87 per thousand, respectively. See *SCGI* (1879), p. 77.

134 Roy, *The Causes, Symptoms and Treatment of the Burdwan Fever*, p. 1.
135 *Hindoo Patriot*, 4 February 1878.
136 *Hindoo Patriot*, 7 February 1876.
137 *Hindoo Patriot*, 4 February 1878.
138 *Hindoo Patriot*, 5 March 1877.
139 *Hindoo Patriot*, 26 March 1877.
140 *Hindoo Patriot*, 6 August 1877.
141 See J. G. French, *Endemic Fever in Lower Bengal, commonly called 'Burdwan Fever'* (Calcutta, 1875).
142 *SCGI* (1879), 101–2.
143 *SCGI* (1887), 143, and (1890), 131.
144 *Bengalee*, 9 February 1889.
145 *SCGI* (1879), 97–8.
146 *SCGI* (1880), 148.
147 *SCGI* (1883), 155, and (1885), 187.
148 *SCGI* (1880), 151.
149 *SCGI* (1884), 155.
150 *SCM* (1879), 135.
151 *SCGI* (1883), 158.
152 *Hindoo Patriot*, 1 April 1880.
153 Tinker, *Local Self-Government*, pp. 52–4; A. Rogers, 'The progress of the municipal idea in India', *Asiatic Quarterly Review*, 13 (1902), 270–80.
154 *SCGI* (1885), 189; *SCM* (1885), 67.
155 *SCGI* (1886), 189–90.
156 See appendix C.
157 *SCM* (1890), 54.
158 *SCGI* (1886), 186.
159 *Ibid.*, 187.
160 Tinker, *Local Self-Government*, pp. 54, 57.
161 *SCGI* (1888), 188.
162 *Ibid.*, 189.
163 See chapter 3.
164 Davis and Huttenback, *Mammon and the Pursuit of Empire*, pp. 130–2.
165 *SCGI* (1887), 185.
166 H. A. D. Phillips, 'Cheap village sanitation', offprint from *Calcutta Review* (1888), 1–21; WIHM, Crawford Collection.
167 *Ibid.*, pp. 186–8.
168 *Bengalee*, 4 August 1888.
169 *Ibid.*, p. 189. The Bengal Sanitary Board, for example, did not acquire to make even small grants independently of government until 1913. See *Recent Developments in the Bombay Presidency*, p. 21.
170 Davis and Huttenback, *Mammon and the Pursuit of Empire*, pp. 135–6. From 1860 to 1912, the Indian government invested only £0.1 per year in human capital (education, sanitation, etc.), on average (4 per cent of its total expenditure), compared with £0.2 in the Princely States (10 per cent of total expenditure).
171 *SCGI* (1889), 129.
172 *SCGI* (1894), 180.

173 *SCGI* (1890), 186–7.
174 *SCGI* (1897), 227.
175 IOR P/4112. GOI (Sanitary), sec. to GOI to sec. of state, 13 January 1892.
176 *SCGI* (1898), 263.
177 IOR P/4112. GOI (Sanitary), sec. of state to viceroy in council, 14 April 1892.
178 IOR P/4112. GOI (Sanitary), commissioner Fyzabad division to sec. to govt. NWP and O, 8 September 1890.
179 *SCGI* (1895), 173.
180 *Hindoo Patriot*, 28 April 1884.
181 *SCGI* (1894), 259.
182 *SCGI* (1893), 46.
183 *Report on the Working of the District Councils and Local Boards in the Central Provinces* (1899), p. 1.
184 *Trans. Ind. Medl. Cong.* (1894), 220.
185 *Ibid.*, 221.
186 IOR P/4555. GOI (Sanitary), lt.-gov. to sec. to GOI (Home Dept.).
187 *SCGI* 91898), 262.
188 H. Fukazawa, 'Western India: the land and the people', in D. Kumar (ed.), *Cambridge Economic History of India* (Cambridge, 1982), II, pp. 194–7, and I. J. Catanach, *Rural Credit in Western India 1875–1930. Rural Credit and the Co-operative Movement in the Bombay Presidency* (London, 1970), pp. 24–6.
189 M. B. McAlpin, *Subject to Famine: Food Crises and Economic Change in Western India, 1860–1920* (Princeton, 1983). Most critics of McAlpin emphasise the need to understand the revenue burden borne by the smallholder within the broader context of local power structures and indebtedness. See, for example, K. Currie, 'British colonial policy and famines: some effects and implications of "free trade" in Bombay, Bengal and Madras Presidencies, 1860–1900', *South Asia*, 14 (1991), 23–56.
190 R. R. Kumar, *Western India in the Nineteenth Century* (London, 1968), pp. 319–30.
191 Government of India. *Land Revenue Policy of the Indian Government* (Calcutta, 1902), pp. 58–9.
192 *SCGI* (1897), 283.
193 *SCGI* (1899), 223; see also *SCBo.* (1896), 59.
194 *SCGI* (1899), 227.
195 *SCGI* (1900), 116–19.
196 *SCGI* (1902), 98; (1904), 134.
197 R. C. Dutt, *The Economic History of India under British Rule* (Calcutta, 1901).
198 The *Report of the Leprosy Commission in India 1890–1891* (Calcutta, 1892) was one of the first official reports to link explicitly the issues of poverty and ill health. The inability of the government to tackle these problems made it highly vulnerable to critics of colonial rule. See W. Digby, *'Prosperous' British India: A Revelation from Official Records* (Calcutta, 1901); D. Naoroji, *Poverty and Un-British Rule in India* (London, 1901).
199 *SCGI* (1898), 257.
200 *SCGI* (1903), 116.
201 *SCBe.* (1897), app. IV, ccvi–ccxx.
202 *SCGI* (1903), 110; *SCBe.* (1904), 29.

203 *SCGI* (1914), 102.
204 *SCGI* (1902), 95; (1903), 113.
205 *SCGI* (1907), 110.
206 *Ibid.*, 9.
207 *Procs. All-India San. Conf.* (1912), 33.
208 *Ibid.*, ciii.
209 *Procs. All-India San. Conf.* (1912), 95.
210 *Ibid.*, 95.
211 Jeffery, *Politics of Health in India*, p. 71.
212 *Procs. All-India San. Conf.* (1911), 1, 3.
213 *Procs. All-India San. Conf.* (1912), 27.
214 Ramasubban, 'Imperial health in British India', p. 55.

8 The politics of public health in Calcutta, 1876–1899

1 By stressing the role of Indian landed and commercial interests in constraining the development of public health, this study casts further doubt on Radhika Ramasubban's claim that there was considerable enthusiasm for sanitary reform among the Indian élite, and that this was resisted by British officials: Ramasubban, *Public Health and Medical Research in India*.
2 K. Blechynden, *Calcutta, Past and Present* (London, 1975).
3 *Report of the Commissioners of Calcutta* (1867), p. 1.
4 The origins and fortunes of the *bhadralok* are discussed in R. V. M. Baumer (ed.), *Aspects of Bengali History and Society* (New Delhi, 1976); J. H. Broomfield, *Elite Conflict in a Plural Society: Twentieth-Century Bengal* (Oxford, 1968); E. Leach and S. N. Mukherjee (eds.), *Elites in South Asia* (Cambridge, 1970); R. K. Ray, *Social Conflict and Political Unrest in Bengal 1875–1927* (Delhi, 1984); Seal, *The Emergence of Indian Nationalism*; and with respect to medical education in Bala, *Imperialism and Medicine in Bengal*.
5 *Report of the Commissioners for the Improvement of Calcutta*, 1 (1848), 13. For a full account of municipal administration in Calcutta see S. W. Goode, *Municipal Calcutta: Its Institutions and Their Origins* (Edinburgh, 1916).
6 These moves stemmed from the distrust of local management characteristic of the technocratic, centralising, governor-generalship of the Marquess of Dalhousie (1848–56). See Stokes, *English Utilitarians*, pp. 248–51.
7 Basu, 'Colonial municipal policy and Indian response', p. 4.
8 It was often alleged that Indians showed little interest in public health, and that their 'insanitary habits' were responsible for many of the health problems experienced by inhabitants of Calcutta. See for example Martin, *Notes on the Medical Topography of Calcutta*. Such attitudes reflected a more general sense of racial superiority among the British, and increasing racial antagonism which was especially marked in Bengal: Ray, *Social Conflict and Political Unrest in Bengal*, pp. 21–9.
9 D. B. Smith, *Report on the Drainage and Conservancy of Calcutta* (Calcutta, 1869), p. 2.
10 *Ibid.*, p. 16.
11 *Report of the Commissioners for the Improvement of Calcutta*, 2 (1850), 1.
12 *Report of the Commissioners*, 2 (1853), 8.

13 Smith, *Drainage and Conservancy of Calcutta*.
14 *Ibid.*, p. 89.
15 Quoted *ibid.*, p. 14.
16 *Ibid.*, pp. 89–90.
17 *Report of the Commissioners* (1867), 19–20.
18 *Ibid.*, 18.
19 *Report of the Commissioners* (1867), 8–10.
20 Basu, 'Colonial municipal policy', p. 23.
21 Smith, *Drainage and Conservancy of Calcutta*, pp. 93–4.
22 Moore, *Liberalism and Indian Politics*, p. 15.
23 Basu, 'Colonial municipal policy', pp. 5–8; *Hindoo Patriot*, 19 March 1877, p. 114. The British Indian Association was formed by a group of Bengali notables in Calcutta in 1851 to represent the interests of high-caste Hindu landowners. See Gordon, *Bengal: The Nationalist Movement 1876–1940*, p. 27.
24 *Hindoo Patriot*, 7 February 1876.
25 See R. Ray, *Urban Roots of Indian Nationalism: Pressure Groups and Conflict of Interests in Calcutta City Politics 1875–1939* (New Delhi, 1979).
26 *Amritar Bazar Patrika*, 17 February 1876. Within a matter of years, this new group led by Banerjea had wrested power away from the old landowning class, despite quasi-official support. See IOR. Ripon Papers, no. 335, Bayley (member of viceroy's council) to Ripon's private sec.
27 *Report of the Commissioners* (1876), 1–8.
28 *Report of the Commissioners* (1879), 1.
29 *Hindoo Patriot*, 11 January 1875, pp. 18–19.
30 *Report of the Health Officer of Calcutta* (1877), pp. 15, 26. *Bustis* were lines of one-storied huts usually built around a central square containing a water-tank. Over time, these tanks were sometimes filled in, and the square covered with more dwellings. Throughout this period these huts were usually built of wood, but, by the 1890s, an increasing number were built of brick.
31 The corporation's powers were such that if it declared a *busti* injurious to health, it could serve notice upon the owner, specifying the necessary improvements and calling upon him to make them at his own expense. See K. Choudhuri, *Calcutta: Story of its Government* (New Delhi, 1973), pp. 136–7.
32 *Report of the Commissioners* (1879), p. 41.
33 *Hindoo Patriot*, 15 March 1875, pp. 122–3.
34 The *Hindoo Patriot* was traditionally the mouthpiece of the large landowners, or zemindars, but it also defended the interests of the smaller landholders and their agents, who comprised a substantial proportion of the municipal commission.
35 *Hindoo Patriot*, 29 March 1875, p. 148. The absence of suitable alternative accommodation also acted as a brake upon slum clearance in British cities. See A. S. Wohl, *The Eternal Slum: Housing and Social Policy in Victorian London* (London, 1977), pp. 117–19.
36 *Hindoo Patriot*, 3 December 1875, pp. 570–1.
37 *Hindoo Patriot*, 8 October 1877, p. 485.
38 *Hindoo Patriot*, 15 October 1877, p. 499.
39 *Ibid.*, p. 500.
40 *Report of the Commissioners* (1876), 13.

41 *Ibid.*, 11. 36 per cent of revenue came from house rates, 20 per cent from water rates, and 11 per cent from lighting rates, the remainder from various indirect taxes, fines, and charges for municipal services.
42 *Report of the Health Officer for Calcutta* (1881), 7.
43 *SCGI* (1881), 164.
44 *Report of the Commissioners*, 1.
45 *Hindoo Patriot*, 13 July 1886, p. 330.
46 *Englishman*, 7 January 1881, p. 1.
47 *Englishman*, 8 January 1885, p. 4.
48 *IMG* (July 1884), 14.
49 *Englishman*, 10 March 1885, pp. 7–8.
50 See chapter 4.
51 *Report of the Sanitary Commission into the Health of Calcutta*, quoted in *Bengalee*, 21 February 1885.
52 *Bengalee*, 21 February 1885.
53 *Hindoo Patriot*, 9 February 1885, pp. 62–3.
54 *Hindoo Patriot*, 13 April 1885, p. 171.
55 *Hindoo Patriot*, 13 July 1885, p. 330.
56 Letter from 'Vibrio' to the *Englishman*, 13 March, p. 3.
57 *Englishman*, 11 May 1885, p. 4.
58 *Englishman*, 1 July 1885, p. 6.
59 *Englishman*, 2 July 1885, p. 4; *Report of the Commissioners*, 2 (1891), 2–3.
60 *Hindoo Patriot*, 21 December 1885, p. 591.
61 *Bengalee*, 26 September 1885.
62 Hindu voters formed 80.5 per cent of the electorate, but only 56.5 per cent of elected commissioners were Hindus. Muslims, by contrast, formed only 10.4 per cent of the electorate, but 16.7 per cent of elected commissioners. Christians constituted 9.1 per cent of the electorate and 27.1 per cent of elected commissioners. *Bengalee*, 19 December 1885.
63 *Hindoo Patriot*, 5 April 1886, p. 163.
64 *Hindoo Patriot*, 21 December 1885, p. 591.
65 *Hindoo Patriot*, 6 January 1886, p. 40; see *Report of the Commissioners* (1891), p. 7, for the increase in deaths from cholera over these years.
66 *Hindoo Patriot*, 8 March 1886, p. 113.
67 *SCBe.* (1888), 30.
68 *Hindoo Patriot*, 15 April 1889, p. 173.
69 *Hindoo Patriot*, 22 July 1889, p. 340.
70 *Bengalee*, 16 March 1889.
71 *Bengalee*, 20 February 1886.
72 *Bengalee*, 12 May 1888.
73 *Report of the Commissioners* (1888–9), 90.
74 Reported in the *Bengalee*, 12 May 1888.
75 Many of Calcutta's municipal commissioners regarded the Act as a 'retrograde step' which placed the corporation in a position of greater subordination to government. Under the terms of the new Act, the lieutenant-governor now had the power to appoint agents to perform duties which had been neglected by the municipality. *Bengalee*, 7 April 1888.

76 *Report of the Health Officer for Calcutta* (1887–8), 26.
77 *Report of the Commissioners* (1888–9), 91.
78 *Ibid.*, 93.
79 *Bengalee*, 22 March 1890.
80 *Report of the Commissioners* (1893), 5.
81 *Report of the Commissioners* (1893), 132.
82 *Report of the Commissioners* (1894), 130.
83 *Trans. Indian Medl. Congress* (1895), 224.
84 *Report of the Commissioners* (1886), 8.
85 *Moslem Chronicle*, 20 June 1895, p. 259.
86 *Report of the Commissioners* (1895), 3.
87 *Moslem Chronicle*, 12 June 1895, p. 246.
88 *Moslem Chronicle*, 25 April 1895, p. 174.
89 *Ibid.*, p. 174.
90 *Bengal Times*, 8 February 1897, p. 4.
91 Reported in the *Bengalee*, 11 July 1890.
92 *Bengalee*, 14 June 1888.
93 *Report of the Health Officer for Calcutta* (1888–9), 24.
94 *Report of the Commissioners* (1981), 3.
95 *Report of Mr. Baldwin Latham on the Drainage of Calcutta* (1891), 2–3.
96 *Report of the Health Officer for Calcutta* (1894), 119-20.
97 *IPC*, I, p. 52.
98 *Report of the Commissioners* (1897), p. 25; IOR P/5171 – Bengal Municipal Proceedings, no. 270, sec. to GOBe. (Municip. Dept.) to sec. to GOI (Home Dept.), 25 February 1897.
99 *The Bengalee*, 10 October 1896, pp. 485–6.
100 *Bengalee*, 4 January 1897, p. 51.
101 *Englishman*, 27 January 1897, p. 13.
102 *Englishman*, 27 January 1897, p. 13.
103 IOR P/5171 – Bengal Municipal Procs., nos. 129–30, sec. to Bengal Medical Board to sec. to GOBe. Municip. Dept.
104 *Report of the Commissioners* (1898), 117.
105 *Bengalee*, 30 April 1898, p. 209.
106 *Report of the Health Officer for Calcutta* (1898), 163.
107 *IPC*, I, p. 275.
108 *Bengalee*, 30 April 1898, p. 209.
109 *IPC*, I, p. 280.
110 *Bengalee*, 28 May 1898, pp. 255–6.
111 *Bengalee*, 22 October 1898, p. 508, and 4 March 1899, p. 99.
112 *Bengalee*, 28 May 1898, p. 256.
113 *Report of the Health Officer for Calcutta* (1897), 265.
114 *Englishman*, 17 February 1897, pp. 10–11.
115 *Bengal Times*, 16 January 1897, p. 4.
116 IOR P/5171 – Bengal Municip. Procs., no. 13, sec. to Medical Board to sec. to GOB. Municip. Dept., forwarding report of the sanitary inspection committee, 30 November 1896; *Accounts and Papers relating to the Plague Epidemic in India* (London, 1897), 1, encl. 12 – sec. to GOI to sec. of state, 27 January 1897.

117 IOR P/5171 – Bengal Municip. Procs., no. 13. For a comparison with housing conditions in nineteenth-century London see Wohl, *Eternal Slum*.

118 *Englishman*, 10 August 1898.

119 *Ibid*.

120 *IPC*, I, pp. 233, 268. The removal of insanitary dwellings was sanctioned under the emergency provisions of the 1888 Municipal Act.

121 *Englishman*, 10 August 1898.

122 Choudhuri, *Calcutta*, pp. 168–9.

123 *Report of the Bombay Improvement Trust* (1898–99), pp. 5–7.

124 Under section 8 of the Calcutta Municipal Bill, the general committee was to be comprised of 4 members elected by the commissioners, 2 by the Chamber of Commerce, 1 by the Calcutta Trades Association, 1 by the Port Commissioners, and 4 to be appointed by the Bengal government.

125 *Englishman*, 24 August 1898.

126 *Englishman*, 13 October 1898.

127 *Englishman*, 30 March 1899.

128 *Bengalee*, 16 April 1898.

129 *Basumati*, 6 October; *Bengalee*, 16 April.

130 IOR P/5629. Bengal Municip. Procs., May 1900.

131 *Bengalee*, 16 April 1898.

132 *Bengalee*, 25 March 1899.

133 Letter from a retired Anglo-Indian reprinted in *Bengalee*, 25 February 1899.

134 *Bengalee*, 4 March 1899.

135 *Bengalee*, 16 April 1898.

136 *Englishman*, 23 March 1899.

137 *Bengalee*, 3 December 1898.

138 *Bengalee*, 25 March 1899.

139 *Englishman*, 1 December 1898.

140 Curzon quoted in the *Englishman*, 19 January 1899.

141 *Englishman*, 5 October 1899.

142 Choudhuri, *Calcutta*, p. 201.

143 *Mihir o Sudhahar*, 14 September.

144 Ray, *Urban Roots of Indian Nationalism*, p. 65.

145 An improvement trust was established in Allahabad in the United Provinces in 1909. See J. B. Harrison, 'Allahabad: a sanitary history', in K. Ballhatchet and J. B. Harrison (eds.), *The City in South Asia* (London, 1980), pp. 167–96.

146 *Report on the Operations of the Calcutta Improvement Trust* (1912–13), 6–8.

147 *Amrita Bazar Patrika*, 5 February 1911.

148 *Bengalee*, 1 March 1911.

149 *Bengalee*, 7 March 1911.

150 *Amrita Bazar Patrika*, 3 September 1912, p. 8.

151 *Ibid*., pp. 25–7.

152 *Amrita Bazar Patrika*, 3 September 1912, p. 8.

153 *Report on the Operations of the Calcutta Improvement Trust* (1912–13), 27.

154 *Report of the Bombay Improvement Trust* (1898–9), 5–7.

155 *Report of the Bombay Improvement Trust* (1907–8), iv.

156 *Report on the Operations of the Calcutta Improvement Trust* (1912–13), 11.

157 *Report of the Calcutta Improvement Trust* (1913–14), 4–5.
158 *Report of the Municipal Administration of Calcutta* (1912–13), 65.

Conclusion

1 PRO. WO 30/114: minutes of procs. of the Army Medical Re-organisation Committee, 13 December 1901; statement by Surgeon-General Taylor.
2 For example, D. G. Crawford, 'What the Indian Medical Service has done for India', reprinted from *IMG*, June 1912. WIHM, Crawford Collection.
3 T. Dyson, 'The historical demography of Berar', p. 159.
4 Jeffery, *Politics of Health*, pp. 40-1.
5 Arnold, 'The Indian Ocean as a disease zone'; 'Cholera mortality in British India'.
6 Ramasubban, *Public Health and Medical Research in India*.
7 With the exception of Arnold, 'Touching the body' and 'Smallpox and colonial medicine'; Harrison, 'Quarantine, pilgrimage and colonial trade'.
8 With the exception of Catanach, 'Plague and the tensions of empire'; Harrison, 'Towards a sanitary utopia'.
9 With the exception of Jeffery, *The Politics of Health in India*.
10 A. Ghosh, *History of the Armed Forces Medical Services* (Hyderabad, 1988), p. 105.
11 Turner and Goldsmith, *Sanitation in India*, pp. 913–34; Balfour and Young, *The Work of Medical Women in India*, pp. 145–9.
12 V. R. Muraleedharan, 'Rural health care in Madras Presidency: 1919–39', *Indian Economic and Social History Review*, 24 (1987), 324-34.
13 Balfour and Scott, *Health Problems of Empire*, p. 134.
14 R. P. Dutt, *India Today* (London, 1940), p. 79.
15 Ramasubban, *Public Health and Medical Research in India*.
16 Arnold, 'Medical priorities', p. 172.
17 Jeffery, *Politics of Health in India*, p. 102.

Select bibliography

Unpublished official sources

National Archives of India, New Delhi

Government of India   Home (Sanitary)
                                     Home (Medical)
                                     Home (Political)
Government of Bombay   General

India Office Library, London

Government of India   Home (Sanitary)
                                     Home (Medical)
                                     Home (Political)
                                     Military
Government of Bengal   Municipal
Government of Bombay   General

Public Record Office, London

War Office

Wellcome Institute for the History of Medicine

Crawford Collection
RAMC Collection

Indian Institute Library, Oxford

Miscellaneous papers relating to sanitation and plague.

Published official sources

Accounts and Papers Relating to the Plague Epidemic in India (London, 1897), 2 vols.
Annual Reports of the Board of Scientific Advice (Calcutta, 1911–14).

Annual Reports of the Pasteur Institute of India (Calcutta, 1901–14).

Annual Reports upon the Work of the Bacteriological Section of the King Institute of Preventive Medicine, Madras (Madras, 1909–14).

General Local Fund Review, Madras (Madras, 1900–15).

General Municipal Review, Madras (Madras, 1900–15).

Government of India, *Memorandum on Measures Adopted for Sanitary Improvements in India up to the End of 1867* (London, 1868).

　Land Revenue Policy of the Indian Government (Calcutta, 1902).

　Improvements in India up till the end of 1867 (London, 1868).

HM Government, *Qualifications and Examinations of Candidates for Commissions in the Medical Services of the British and Indian Armies* (London, 1860).

　Principles of Construction for Barracks for Single and Married Men: Remarks of the Army Sanitary Commission (London, 1864).

Imperial Gazetteer of India, Bengal Presidency (Calcutta, 1909).

Imperial Gazetteer of India, Bombay Presidency (Calcutta, 1909).

Imperial Gazetteer of India, Madras Presidency (Calcutta, 1908).

Leprosy in India: Report of the Leprosy Commission in India 1890–91 (Calcutta, 1892).

Proceedings of the General Malaria Committee (Simla, 1911–14).

Proceedings of the Sanitary Commission for Bengal (Calcutta, 1864–70).

Proceedings of the Sanitary Commission for Bombay (Bombay, 1865–70).

Proceedings of the Sanitary Commission for Madras (Madras, 1865–70).

Quarterly Reports of the Health Officer for Bombay (Bombay, 1869–1914).

Report of the Dharwar Plague Inoculation Investigation Committee (Bombay, 1901).

Report on the Cholera Epidemic of 1867 in Northern India (Calcutta, 1867).

Report of the Commissioners Appointed to Enquire into the Sanitary State of the Army in India, Parliamentary Papers, I and II (1868).

Report on the Working of the District Councils and Local Boards in the Central Provinces (Nagpur, 1898–1915).

Reports of the Indian Plague Commission, 5 vols. (London, 1900).

Reports on the Charitable Dispensaries of Bengal (Calcutta, 1869–1908).

Reports of the Sanitary Commissioner for the Government of Assam (Shillong, 1876–1915).

Reports of the Sanitary Commissioner for the Government of Bengal (Calcutta, 1868–1915).

Reports of the Sanitary Commissioner for the Government of Bombay (Bombay, 1868–1915).

Reports of the Sanitary Commissioner for the Government of the Central Provinces (Nagpur, 1868–1915).

Reports of the Sanitary Commissioner with the Government of India (Calcutta, 1868–1915).

Reports of the Sanitary Commissioner for the Government of Madras (Madras, 1868–1915).

Reports on Vaccination in the Madras Presidency (Madras, 1891–1906).

Reports of the Sanitary Commissioner for the Government of the North West Provinces and Oudh (Allahabad, 1868–1915).

Reports of the Sanitary Commissioner for the Government of Punjab (Lahore, 1868–1915).

Reports on the Administration of Municipalities in the Bombay Presidency (Bombay, 1889–1915).
Reports of the Bombay Improvement Trust (Bombay, 1898–1914).
Reports on the Administration of Local Boards in the Bombay Presidency (Bombay, 1889–1915).
Reports on the Bombay Plague Research Laboratory (Bombay, 1896–1914).
Reports on Vaccination in the Province of Bengal (Calcutta, 1867–81).
Reports on the Working of District Boards in Bengal (Calcutta, 1889–1915).
Reports on the Working of Municipalities in Bengal (Calcutta, 1889–1915).
Report of the Commissioners for the Improvement of Calcutta (Calcutta, 1848–53).
Reports of the Commissioners for Calcutta (Calcutta, 1875–1914).
Reports of the Health Officer of Calcutta (Calcutta, 1875–1914).
Reports of the Calcutta Improvement Trust (Calcutta, 1911–14).
Reviews of Municipal Reports and Statements, Central Provinces (Nagpur, 1889–1915).
Some Recent Sanitary Developments in the Bombay Presidency (Bombay, 1914).
Transactions of the All-India Sanitary Conferences (Calcutta, 1911–14).

Newspapers and journals

Amrita Bazar Patrika
Bengalee
Bengal Times
Bombay Gazette
British Medical Journal
Englishman
Gazette of India
Hindoo Patriot
Indian Journal of Medical Research
Indian Medical Gazette
Indian Medico-Chirurgical Review
Indian Public Health and Municipal Journal
Journal of Tropical Medicine
Lancet
Madras Quarterly Medical Review
Madras Times
Moslem Chronicle and Mohamedan Observer
Pioneer
Public Health
Punjab Times
Scientific Memoirs of Medical Officers of the Army of India
Times of India
Transactions of the Bombay Medical and Physical Society
Transactions of the Calcutta Medical and Physical Society
Transactions of the Epidemiological Society
Transactions of the Indian Medical Congress
Transactions of the International Congresses of Hygiene and Demography

Published primary sources

Annesley, C. A., *Researches into the Causes, Nature, and Treatment of the More Prevalent Diseases of India* (Calcutta, 1828).

Annesley, J., *Sketches of the Most Prevalent Diseases of India* (London, 1831).

Arjun, S., 'Our water supply (chemically and microscopically considered)', *Trans. Medl. Soc. Bombay* (1883), 9–31.

Baetson, W. B., 'Indian Medical Service: past and present', *Asiatic Quarterly Review*, 4, 14 (1902), 272–320.

Balfour, A. and H. H. Scott, *Health Problems of the Empire* (London, 1924).

Balfour, F., *Treatise on the Influence of the Moon in Fevers* (Calcutta, 1784).

Balfour, M. I. and R. Young, *The Work of Medical Women in India* (London, 1929).

Ballingall, G., *Practical Observations on Fever, Dysentery, and Liver Complaints, as they Occur amongst the European Troops in India* (Edinburgh, 1818).

Banbury, H., *School Hygiene for Indian Teachers* (Lucknow, 1909).

Bellew, H. H., *The Nature, Causes and Treatment of Cholera* (London, 1887).

Blackham, R. J., *Scalpel, Sword and Stretcher: Forty Years of Work and Play* (London, 1931).

Bose, R. K. C., 'The use of quinine in malarious fevers', *JTM*, September 1900, 27–30.

Bryden, J. L., *Vital Statistics of the Bengal Presidency* (Calcutta, 1866–79).

  Epidemic Cholera in Bengal (Calcutta, 1869).

  Cholera Epidemics of Recent Years Viewed in Relation to Former Epidemics. A Record of Cholera in the Bengal Presidency from 1817 to 1872 (Calcutta, 1874).

  The Cholera History of 1875 and 1876 (Calcutta, 1878).

Buchanan, W. J., 'The value of prophylactic issues of cinchona preparations. An experiment in Indian jails', *JTM* (March 1899), 21–3.

Burt, A., *A Tract on the Biliary Complaints of Europeans in Hot Climates; founded on Observations in Bengal; and Consequently Designed to be Particularly Useful to those in that Country* (Calcutta, 1785).

Caldwell, R., *Military Hygiene* (London, 1905).

Cameron, W., 'On vaccination in Bengal', *Trans. Calcutta Medical and Physical Soc.* (1831), 385–95.

Cantlie, J., 'The spread of plague', *Trans. Epid. Soc.*, 16 (1896–7), 15–63.

  'Tropical life as it affects life insurance', *JTM* (January 1911), 35–41.

Chambers, C. A., 'Enteric fever in Indians, with special reference to its occurrence in the Indian Army', *JTM* (September 1913), 280–2.

Chantemesse, A. and E. Mosny (eds.), *Traité d'Hygiène. Etiologie et Prophylaxie des Maladies Transmissibles par la Peau et les Muqueses Externes* (Paris, 1911).

Chesson, J., *Report on the Hill-Station of Panchgunny, near Mahableshwar* (Bombay, 1862).

Christophers, S. R., 'Second report of the anti-malarial operations at Mian Mir, 1901–1903', *Sci. Mems.* (1904), 1–13.

  'Malaria in the Punjab', *Sci. Mems.* (1911), 1–132.

Clark, J., *Observations of the Diseases which Prevail in Long Voyages to Hot Countries, Particularly those in the East Indies; and on the same Diseases as they Appear in Britain* (London, 1809).

Cole, J., *Notes on Hygiene With Hints on Self-Discipline for Young Soldiers in India* (London, 1882).

Collins, H. B., 'Health and empire', *Public Health*, 16 (1903–4), 406–8.

Cornish, W. R., *Reports on the Nature of Food of the Inhabitants of the Madras Presidency and the Dietaries of Prisoners in Zillah Jails* (Madras, 1863).

Corthorn, A. M., *Report on Anti-Plague Inoculation Work in the Dharwar District* (Bombay, 1899).

Couchman, M. E., *Account of Plague Administration in the Bombay Presidency from September 1896 till May 1897* (Bombay, 1898).

Crawford, D. G., 'What the Indian Medical Service has done for India', reprinted from *IMG*, June 1912; WIHM, Crawford Collection.

'The Medical Services in 1905', reprinted from *IMG*, March 1906; WIHM, Crawford Collection.

Creighton, C., *A History of Epidemics in Britain*, 2 vols. (London, 1894).

Cuningham, J. M., *Cholera. What the State Can do to Prevent it* (Calcutta, 1864).

Cunningham, D. D., 'On the relation of cholera to schizomycete organisms', *Sci. Mems.* (1884), 1–16.

'Results of examinations of old specimens of choleraic tissues', *Sci. Mems.* (1887), 1–11.

'Are choleraic bacilli really efficient in determining the diffusion of cholera', *Sci. Mems.* (1889), 1–20.

'The results of continued study of various forms of comma bacillus occurring in Calcutta', *Sci. Mems.* (1894), 1–57.

'Choleraic and other commas; on the influence of certain conditions determining morphological variations in vibrionic organisms', *Sci. Mems.* (1897), 1–29.

Curtis, C., *An Account of the Diseases in India, as they Appeared in the English Fleet, and in the Naval Hospital at Madras, in 1782 and 1783; with Observations on Ulcers, and the Hospital Sores of that Country* (Edinburgh, 1807).

Daniels, C. W., *Studies in Laboratory Work* (London, 1907).

DeRenzy, A. C. C., 'The prevention of heat apoplexy', *Trans. Epid. Soc.*, 4 (1884–5), 63–71.

Digby, W., *'Prosperous' British India: A Revelation from Official Records* (Calcutta, 1901).

Dimmock, H. P. and H. K. Tavaria, 'The effect of quinine on pregnancy', *Indian Medico-Chirurgical Review* (January 1894), 92–8.

Duvivier, Général, *Solution de la Quèstion de l'Algérie* (Paris, 1841).

Eames, W. J., 'Chill and malaria', *BMJ*, 23 (January 1875), 109.

Ewart, J., 'On the colonisation of the sub-Himalayahs and Neilgherries, with remarks on the management of European children in India', *Trans. Epid. Soc.*, 3 (1883–4), 96–117.

Farr, W., 'Report on the cholera epidemic of 1866', *BMJ* (15 August 1868), 169.

Fayrer, J., *European Child Life in Bengal* (London, 1873).

On the Climate and Fevers of India (London, 1882).

The Natural History and Epidemiology of Cholera (London, 1888).

Recollections of My Life (Edinburgh, 1890).

The Preservation of Health in India (London, 1894).

'Enteric fever among British soldiers in India', *JTM* (September 1898), 29-31.

Fearnside, C. F., 'Inoculation of malaria by Anopheles', *Sci. Mems.* (1901), 19–33.

Fink, G. H., 'Food of the natives of India', *JTM* (October 1906), 310–12.

Goldsmith, D. K. and J. A. Turner, *Sanitation in India* (Bombay, 1922).

Gordon, G. A., *Army Hygiene* (London, 1866).

'Experiences in relation to cholera in India from 1842 to 1879', in *Trans. Epid. Soc.*, 15 (1895–6), 48–67.

Grierson, J., 'On the endemic fever of Arracan, with a sketch of the medical topography of that country', *Trans. Calcutta Medical and Physical Soc.*, 2, 5 (March 1825), 201–19.

Guyer-Hunter, W., 'The origin of the cholera epidemic of 1883 in Egypt', *Trans. Epid. Soc.*, 3 (1883–4), 43–64.

Hall, J., *Observations on the Report of the Sanitary Commissioners in the Crimea, during the Years 1855 and 1856* (London, 1857).

Hanley, A. H., 'Mosquito-screened houses versus quinine', *JTM* (December 1900), 112–13.

Harvey, W., 'The Indian Medical Services as a career', reprinted from *Dollar Magazine*; WIHM, Crawford Collection.

Hewlett, T. G., *Report on Enteric Fever* (Bombay, 1883).

Holwell, J. Z., *An Account of the Manner of Inoculating for the Smallpox in the East Indies* (London, 1767).

Jackson, T., 'General and medical topography of Meerut', *Trans. Calcutta Medical and Physical Soc.*, 1, 4 (September 1824), 292–8.

Jackson, T. W., *Tropical Medicine with Special Reference to the West Indies, Central America, Hawaii, and the Philippines* (London, 1901).

James, S. P., 'Malaria in India', *Sci. Mems.* (1902), 1–85.

'First report of the anti-malarial operations at Mian Mir, 1901–3', *Sci. Mems.* (1903), 1–29.

Jeffreys, J., *The British Army in India: Its Preservation by an Appropriate Clothing, Housing, Locating, Recreative Employment, and Hopeful Encouragement of the Troops* (London, 1858).

Johnson, C. T. H., *A Catechism on Hygiene for use in Elementary Schools* (Madras, 1908).

Johnson, J., *The Influence of Tropical Climates, More Especially of the Climate of India, On European Constitutions; and the Principal Effects and Diseases Thereby Induced, their Prevention and Removal, and the Means of Preserving Health in Hot Climates Rendered Obvious to Europeans of Every Capacity*, 2nd edn. (London, 1815).

A Practical Treatise on Derangements of the Liver, Digestive Organs and Nervous System to Which is Added an Essay on the Prolongation of Life and Conservation of Health (London, 1918).

The Economy of Health or the Stream of Human Life from the Cradle to the Grave, with Reflections Moral, Physical, and Philosophical on the Successive Stages of Human Existence, the Maladies to which they are Subjected and the Dangers that may be Averted (London, 1837).

Kennedy, J., *The History of the Contagious Cholera; with Facts Explanatory of its Origin and Laws, and of a Rational Method of Cure* (London, 1831).

Koch, R., 'Blackwater fever', transl. P. Falcke, *JTM* (August 1899), 333–5.

Letheby, H., 'Report on the sanitary condition of the city of London', *BMJ* (22 February 1868), 173.

Leuman, B. H. F., *Report on Plague Inoculation at Hubli* (Bombay, 1898).

Lewis, T. R., 'The microscopic organisms found in the blood of man and animals and their relation to disease', *SCGI* (1877), 157–8.

Lind, J., *Essay on the Diseases Incidental to Europeans in Hot Climates*, 1st edn. (London, 1768).

Lowson, J. A., *Report on the Epidemic of Plague from 22nd February to 18th July 1897* (Bombay, 1897).

Lyons, R. W. S., *Report of the Plague Research Committee* (Bombay, 1897).

MacDonald, D., *Surgeons Twoe and a Barber: Being Some Account of the Life and Work of the Indian Medical Service (1600–1947)* (London, 1950).

Maclean, C., *Results of an Investigation Respecting Epidemic Fevers and Pestilential Diseases; Including Researches in the Levant Concerning the Plague* (London, 1817).

Madras Christian Vernacular Education Society, *The Way to Health* (Madras, 1887).

Mair, R. S., *Medical Guide for Anglo-Indians* (London, 1874).

Manson, P., *Tropical Diseases. A Manual of the Diseases of Warm Climates* (London, 1898).

Martin, J. R., *Notes on the Medical Topography of Calcutta* (Calcutta, 1837).

   The Influence of Tropical Climates on European Constitutions, Including Practical Observations on the Nature and Treatment of the Diseases of Europeans on their Return from Tropical Climates (London, 1856).

McCoy, D., 'Investigations on Bengali jail dietaries with some observations on the physical development and well-being of the people of Bengal', *Sci. Mems.*, 37 (1910), 1–226.

Montesquieu, Baron, *The Spirit of the Laws*, transl. T. Nugent, ed. F. Neumann (New York, 1949).

Moore, W., 'The constitutional requirements for tropical climates, with special reference to temperaments', *Trans. Epid. Soc.*, 4 (1884–5), 32–51.

   'Is the colonisation of tropical Africa by Europeans possible', *Trans. Epid. Soc.*, 10 (1890–1), 27–45.

Murchison, C., *Treatise on the Continued Fevers of Great Britain*, 1st edn. (London, 1862).

Murray, J., *Report on the Treatment of Epidemic Cholera* (Calcutta, 1869).

Nathan, R., *The Plague in India, 1896, 1897*, 2 vols. (Simla, 1898).

Naoroji, D., *Poverty and Un-British Rule in India* (London, 1901).

Newsholme, A., 'Tuberculosis in relation to milk supply', *Public Health*, 54 (1900–1), 637–43.

Nightingale, F., *Observations on the Evidence Contained in the Stational Reports Submitted to her by the Royal Commission on the Sanitary State of the Army in India* (London, 1863).

   Life or Death in India (London, 1873).

Parkes, E. A., *Manual of Practical Hygiene. Prepared Especially for Use in the Medical Service of the British Army* (London, 1864).

Pearse, F., 'Prickly heat', *JTM* (June 1899), 297–8.

Perier, J. A. N., *De l'Hygiène en Algèrie* (Paris, 1847).

Playfair, G., *Taleef Shereef* (Calcutta, 1832).

Powell, A., 'Haemoglobinuric fever in Assam', *JTM* (December 1898), 117–19.

Pringle, R., 'Enteric fever in India: its increase, causes, remedies, and probable consequences', *Trans. Epid. Soc.*, 9 (1889–90), 111–32.

Ranken, J., 'On public health in India', *Trans. Calcutta Medl. and Physical Society* (Calcutta, 1836), 300–50.

Report on the Malignant Fever called the Pali Plague Which has Prevailed in some part of Rajputana since the month of July, 1836 (Calcutta, 1838).

Ranking, I. J., *Report on the Military Sanitation in the Presidency of Madras* (Madras, 1868).

Reynolds, G. F., 'Blackwater fever, some cases and notes', *JTM* (January 1899), 146–55.

Richards, M., 'The origins of the medical inspection of schools', *Public Health*, 19 (1906–7).

Roberts, E., *Enteric Fever in India, and other Tropical and Sub-Tropical Regions: A Study in Epidemiology and Military Hygiene* (London, 1906).

Rogers, A., 'The progress of the municipal idea in India', *Asiatic Quarterly Review*, 13 (1902), 270–80.

Rogers, L., *Fevers in the Tropics. Their Clinical and Microscopical Differentiation, Including the Milroy Lectures on Kala-Azar* (London, 1908).

Ross, R., *Memoirs* (London, 1923).

Roy, G. C., *The Causes, Symptoms, and Treatment of Burdwan Fever, or the Epidemic Fever of Lower Bengal* (London, 1876).

Ruffer, M. A., 'Measures taken at Tor and Suez against ships coming from the Red Sea and the Far East', *Trans. Epid. Soc.*, 19 (1899–1900), 25–47.

Sambon, L. W., 'Blackwater fever', *JTM* (October 1988), 70–4.

'The etiology and treatment of blackwater fever', *JTM* (May 1899), 295–6.

Sarkies, C. J., *Reports on Plague Operations in Ahmednagar and District during the year of 1899* (Bombay, 1899).

Schoolbred, J., *Report on the Progress of Vaccine Inoculation in Bengal, 1802–3* (Calcutta, 1804).

Sergent, E. and L. Parrot, *La Découverte de Laveran* (Paris, 1931).

Simpson, W. J., *Cholera in Calcutta in 1894 and Anti-Choleraic Inoculation* (Calcutta, 1894).

'Anti-choleraic inoculation: a report to the Government of India', *Public Health*, 8 (1895–6), 91–2.

Skey-Muir, H., 'On the cause of enteric fever in India', *Trans. Epid. Soc.*, 10 (1890–1), 222–6.

Smith, D. B., *Report on the Drainage and Conservancy of Calcutta* (Calcutta, 1869).

Snow, J., *On Continuous Molecular Changes, More Particularly in their Relation to Epidemic Disease* (London, 1853).

On the Mode of Communication of Cholera, 2nd edn. (London, 1855).

Stephens, J. W. W., *Blackwater Fever. A Historical Survey of Observations Made over a Century* (London, 1937).

Stephens, J. W. W. and S. R. Christophers, *The Practical Study of Malaria* (London, 1904).

Stewart, A. P. and E. Jenkins, *The Medical and Legal Aspects of Sanitary Reform, 1866–69* (London, 1869).

Strachey, J., *India: Its Administration and Progress*, 3rd edn. (London, 1903).

Thompson, A. S., 'On the doctrine of acclimatization', *Madras Quarterly Medical Review*, 2 (1840), 69–76.

Thorne-Thorne, R., 'On the results of the International Sanitary Conference of Rome', *Trans. Epid. Soc.*, 5 (1885–6), 135–49.

Thornton, J. H., *Memories of Seven Campaigns. A Record of Thirty-Five Years' Service in the Indian Medical Department in India, China, Egypt, and the Sudan* (London, 1895).

Tilt, E. J., *Health in India for British Women* (London, 1875).

Turner, J. A., 'Report on malaria in Bombay from 1902–1909', *Paludism*, 4 (1910), 39–40.

A Plea for Education in Hygiene and Public Health in India (Bombay, 1919).

Turner, J. A. and D. K. Goldsmith, *Sanitation in India* (Bombay, 1922).

Twining, W., *Clinical Illustrations of the More Important Diseases of Bengal with the Results of an Enquiry into their Pathology and Treatment* (Calcutta, 1835).

Wilson, H. H., 'Kushta, or leprosy; as known to the Hindus', *Trans. Medical and Physical Soc. of Calcutta*, 1, 3 (May 1823), 1-44.

Young, D. S., 'An account of the general and medical topography of the Neelgerries', *Trans. Calcutta Medical and Physical Soc.*, 4, 7 (July 1827), 36–78.

Published and unpublished secondary sources

Ackerknecht, E. H., 'Anticontagionism between 1821 and 1861', *Bull. Hist. Med.*, 22 (1948), 561–93.

Anderson, W., 'Climates of opinion: acclimatization in nineteenth-century France and England', *Victorian Studies*, 35 (1992), 135–57.

Arnold, D., 'Medical priorities and practice in nineteenth-century British India', *South Asia Research*, 5 (1985), 167–83.

Police Power and Colonial Rule. Madras 1859–1947 (Delhi, 1986).

'Cholera and colonialism in British India', *Past and Present*, 113 (1986), 118–51.

'Touching the body: perspectives on the Indian plague, 1896–1900', in R. Guha (ed.), *Subaltern Studies V* (Delhi, 1987), pp. 55–90.

(ed.), *Imperial Medicine and Indigenous Societies* (Manchester, 1988).

'Smallpox and colonial medicine in nineteenth-century India', in Arnold (ed.), *Imperial Medicine*, pp. 45–65.

Austoker, J. and L. Bryder (eds.), *Historical Perspectives on the Role of the MRC. Essays in the History of the Medical Research Council of the United Kingdom and its Predecessor, the Medical Research Committee, 1913–1953* (Oxford, 1989).

Bala, P., 'State and indigenous medicine in nineteenth- and twentieth-century Bengal: 1800–1947' (Edinburgh University Ph.D. thesis, 1987).

Imperialism and Medicine in Bengal. A Socio-Historical Perspective (Delhi, 1991).

Baldry, J., 'The Ottoman quarantine station on Kamaran Island 1882–1914', *Studies in the History of Medicine*, 2 (Delhi, 1978).

Ballhatchet, K., *Race, Sex and Class under the Raj. Imperial Attitudes and Policies and their Critics* (London, 1980).

Basalla, G., 'The spread of western science', *Science*, 156 (1967), 611-22.

Basu, A., *The Growth of Education and Political Development in India 1898–1920* (Delhi, 1974).

'The Indian response to scientific and technical education in the colonial era, 1820–1920', in Kumar (ed.), *Science and Empire* (1991), pp. 126–38.

Basu, R., 'Colonial municipal policy and Indian response: municipal government and police in Calcutta 1850–1872', *Bengal Past and Present*, 190, 1 (1981), 1–47.

Baumer, R. V. M. (ed.), *Aspects of Bengali History and Society* (New Delhi, 1976).

Bearce, G. D., *British Attitudes Towards India, 1784–1858* (London, 1982).

Beck, A., 'Problems of British medical administration in East Africa between 1900 and 1930', *Bull. Hist. Med.*, 36 (1962), 275–83.

'Medicine and society in Tanganyika 1890–1930. A Historical Inquiry', *Trans. American Philosophical Society*, 67, 3 (1977), 1–59.

Beloff, M., *Britain's Liberal Empire 1897–1921* (London, 1987).

Bilson, G., 'Public health and the medical profession in nineteenth-century Canada', in MacLeod and Lewis (eds.), *Disease, Medicine, and Empire*, pp. 156–75.

Blechynden, K., *Calcutta, Past and Present* (London, 1975).

Blunt, E., *The Indian Civil Service* (London, 1937).

Boardman, P., *The Worlds of Patrick Geddes. Biologist, Town Planner, Re-educator, Peace Warrior* (London, 1978).

Brand, J. L., *Doctors and the State: The Medical Profession and Government Action in Public Health* (Baltimore, 1965).

Brock, T. D., *Robert Koch. A Life in Medicine and Bacteriology* (Madison, 1988).

Broomfield, J. H., *Elite Conflict in a Plural Society: Twentieth-Century Bengal* (Oxford, 1968).

Buchanan, L., 'The introduction and spread of western medical science in India', *Calcutta Review* (1914), 419–30.

Bulloch, W., *The History of Bacteriology* (London, 1938).

Bynum, W. and V. Nutton (eds.), *Theories of Fever from Antiquity to the Enlightenment. Medical History Supplement* (London, 1981).

Bynum, W. and R. Porter (eds.), *Medical Fringe and Medical Orthodoxy 1750–1850* (London, 1987).

Calcutta Medical College, *Centenary of the Medical College of Bengal* (Calcutta, 1935).

Cantlie, N., *A History of the Army Medical Department*, 2 vols. (London, 1974).

Catanach, I. J., *Rural Credit in Western India 1875–1930. Rural Credit and the Co-operative Movement in the Bombay Presidency* (London, 1970).

'Plague and the Indian village, 1896–1914', in P. Robb (ed.), *Rural India: Land, Power and Society Under British Rule* (London, 1983), pp. 216–43.

'Poona politicians and the plague', *South Asia*, 7 (1984), 1–18.

'Plague and the tensions of empire: India, 1896–1918', in D. Arnold (ed.), *Imperial Medicine and Indigenous Societies*, pp. 149–71.

Char, S. V. D., *Centralised Legislation. A History of the Legislative System of British India from 1834–1881* (Delhi, 1963).

Chernin, E., 'Sir Ronald Ross vs. Sir Patrick Manson: a matter of libel', *J. Hist. Med.*, 43 (1988), 262–74.

Chitnis, A. C., *The Scottish Enlightenment: A Social History* (London, 1976).

Cohn, B. S., 'The command of language and the language of command', in R. Guha (ed.), *Subaltern Studies IV* (New Delhi, 1985), pp. 276–329.

Coleman, W., 'Koch's comma bacillus: the first year', *Bull. Hist. Med.*, 61 (1987), 315–42.

Cooter, R., 'Anticontagionism and history's medical record', in P. Wright and A. Treacher (eds.), *The Problem of Medical Knowledge.*

The Cultural Meaning of Popular Science. Phrenology and the Organisation of Consent in Nineteenth-Century Britain (Cambridge, 1984), pp. 87–108.

Cope, Z., *Almroth Wright. Founder of Modern Vaccine Therapy* (London, 1966).

Crawford, D. G., *A History of the Indian Medical Service, 1600-1913*, 2 vols. (London, 1914).

Roll of the Indian Medical Service (London, 1930).

Crosby, A. W., *The Columbian Exchange: The Biological and Cultural Consequences of 1492* (Westport, Conn., 1974).

Ecological Imperialism. The Biological Expansion of Europe, 900–1900 (Cambridge, 1986).

Crowther, M. A., 'Paupers or patients? Obstacles to professionalization in the Poor Law Medical Services before 1914', *J. Hist. Med.*, 29 (1984), 33–54.

Curson, P. and K. McCracken, *Plague in Sydney. The Anatomy of an Epidemic* (Kensington, New South Wales, 1989).

Curtin, P. D., '"The White Man's Grave": image and reality, 1750–1850', *J. Brit. Stud.*, 1 (1961), 94–110.

'Medical knowledge and urban planning in tropical Africa', *American Historical Review*, 90 (1985), 594–613.

The Image of Africa. British Ideas and Action, 1780–1850 (Madison, Wisc., 1964).

Death by Migration. Europe's Encounter with the Tropical World in the Nineteenth Century (Cambridge, 1989).

Darby, P., *Three Faces of Imperialism. British and American Approaches to Asia and Africa 1870–1970* (New Haven, 1987).

Das, M. N., *India Under Morley and Minto. Politics Behind Revolution, Repression and Reforms* (London, 1964).

Davis, L. E. and R. A. Huttenback, *Mammon and the Pursuit of Empire. The Political Economy of British Imperialism 1860–1912* (Cambridge, 1986).

Dilks, D., *Curzon in India*, 2 vols. (London, 1969).

Dingwall, R. and P. Lewis (eds.), *The Sociology of the Professions. Lawyers, Doctors and Others* (London, 1983).

Dobbin, C., *Urban Leadership in Western India. Politics and Communities in Bombay City 1840–1855* (Oxford, 1972).

Done, K., 'A study of the fight against an endemic disease: smallpox in India' (University of Oxford Physiological Sciences dissertation, 1991).

dos Santos Pereira, R., *Piso e a Medicine Indigena* (Pernambuco, 1980).

Douglas, M., *Purity and Danger. An Analysis of Concepts of Purity and Taboo* (London, 1966).

Durand, M., *Life of the Honourable Sir Alfred Comyn Lyall* (Edinburgh, 1913).

Durey, M., *Return of the Plague: British Society and the Cholera 1831–2* (Dublin, 1979).

Dutt, R. P., *India Today* (London, 1940).

Dwork, D., 'The milk option. An aspect of the history of the infant welfare movement in England 1898–1908', *Medical History*, 31 (1987), 51–69.

Dyason, D., 'The medical profession in colonial Victoria, 1834–1901', in R. M. MacLeod and M. Lewis (eds.), *Disease, Medicine, and Empire*, pp. 194–216.

Dyson, T. (ed.), *India's Historical Demography: Studies in Famine, Disease and Society* (London, 1989).

Edwardes, M., *High Noon of Empire: India Under Lord Curzon* (London, 1965).

Ernst, W., 'The European insane in British India, 1800–1858: a case study in psychiatry and colonial rule', in D. Arnold (ed.), *Imperial Medicine and Indigenous Societies*, pp. 27–44.

　　'Doctor-patient relationship in colonial India: a case of "intellectual insanity"', *History of Psychiatry*, 1 (1990), 207–22.

Evans, R. J., *Death in Hamburg. Society and Politics in the Cholera Years 1830–1910* (Oxford, 1987).

Eyler, J. M., 'The conceptual origins of William Farr's epidemiology: numerical methods and social thought in the 1830s', in A. M. Lilienfeld (ed.), *Times, Places, and Persons. Aspects of the History of Epidemiology* (Baltimore, 1980), pp. 1-24.

Feierman, S., 'Struggles for control: the social roots of health and healing in modern Africa', *African Studies Review*, 28, 2/3 (1985), 73–147.

Fermor, L., 'The development of scientific research in India to the end of the nineteenth century', *Asiatic Society of Bengal Yearbook*, 1 (1935), 9–22.

Fieldhouse, D. K., *Economic and Empire 1830–1914*, 2nd edn. (London, 1984).

Finer, S. E., *The Life and Times of Sir Edwin Chadwick* (London, 1952).

Foucault, M., *The Order of Things. An Archaeology of the Human Sciences* (London, 1970).

Fraser, W. M., *A History of English Public Health, 1834–1939* (London, 1950).

Freeden, M., *The New Liberalism. An Ideology of Social Reform* (Oxford, 1978).

Freidson, E., *Profession of Medicine. A Study in the Sociology of Applied Knowledge* (New York, 1970).

Fukazawa, H., 'Western India: the land and the people', in Kumar (ed.), *The Cambridge Economic History of India*, II (Cambridge, 1982), pp. 177–206.

Gaitonde, P. D., *Portuguese Pioneers in India: Spotlight on Medicine* (London, 1983).

Geggus, D., 'Yellow fever in the 1790s: the British Army in occupied Saint Dominique', *Medical History*, 23 (1979), 38–58.

Ghosh, A., *History of the Armed Forces Medical Services* (Hyderabad, 1988).

Glacken, C. J., *Traces on the Rhodian Shore. Nature and Culture in Western Thought from Ancient Times to the End of the Century* (Berkeley, 1973).

Goodman, N. E., *International Health Organizations and their Work* (London, 1952).

Gopal, S., *British Policy in India 1858–1905* (Cambridge, 1965).

Gordon, L. A., *Bengal: The Nationalist Movement 1876–1949* (New York, 1974).

Goubert, J. P., *The Conquest of Water. The Advent of Health in the Industrial Age* (Oxford, 1989).

Grove, R., 'Conservation and colonial expansion: a study of the evolution of environmental attitudes and conservation policies on St. Helena, Mauritius, and in India, 1660–1860' (Cambridge University Ph.D. thesis, 1988).

Gupta, N., *Delhi Between Two Empires, 1803–1831. Society, Government and Urban Growth* (Delhi, 1981).

Haffkine Institute, *Haffkine Institute Platinum Jubilee Commemoration Volume, 1899–1974* (Bombay, 1974).

Hamlin, C., 'Politics and germ theories in Victorian Britain: the metropolitan water commissions of 1867–9 and 1892–3', in R. M. MacLeod (ed.), *Government and Expertise. Specialists, Administrators and Professionals, 1860–1919* (Cambridge, 1988), pp. 110-27.

'Providence and putrefaction: Victorian sanitarians and the natural theology of health and disease', in P. Brantlinger (ed.), *Energy and Entropy. Science and Culture in Victorian Britain* (Bloomington, Ind., 1990), pp. 93–123.

Harnetty, P., *Imperialism and Free Trade: Lancashire in the Mid-Nineteenth Century* (Columbia, 1972).

Hardy, P., *The Muslims of British India* (Cambridge, 1972).

Harrison, G., *Mosquitoes, Malaria, and Man* (London, 1978).

Harrison, J. B., 'Allahabad. A sanitary history', in K. Ballhatchet and J. B. Harrison (eds.), *The City in South Asia* (London, 1980), pp. 167–96.

Harrison, M., 'Towards a sanitary Utopia? Professional visions and public health in India, 1880–1914', *South Asia Research*, 10, 1 (1990), 19–41.

'Quarantine, pilgrimage, and colonial trade: India 1866–1900', *Indian Econ. and Soc. Hist. Rev.*, 29 (1992), 117–44.

'Tropical medicine in nineteenth-century India', *British J. for the Hist. of Science*, 25 (1992), 299–318.

Headrick, D. R., *The Tools of Empire. Technology and European Imperialism in the Nineteenth Century* (Oxford, 1981).

The Tentacles of Progress: Technology Transfer in the Age of Imperialism (Oxford, 1988).

Heathcote, T. A., *The Indian Army: The Garrison of British Imperial India, 1822–1922* (London, 1974).

Hibbert, C., *The Great Mutiny: India 1857* (London, 1978).

Hirst, F. A., *The Conquest of Plague. A Study of the Evolution of Epidemiology* (Oxford, 1953).

Holland, Sir Henry, *Frontier Doctor. An Autobiography* (London, 1958).

Hume, J. C., 'Rival traditions: western medicine and Yuna-i Tibb in the Punjab, 1849–1889', *Bull. Hist. Med.*, 51 (1977), 214–31.

'Colonialism and sanitary medicine: the development of preventive health policy in the Punjab, 1860-1900', *Mod. Asian Stud.*, 20 (1986), 703–24.

Hutchins, F. G., *The Illusion of Permanence. British Imperialism in India* (Princeton, 1967).

Hyam, R., *Empire and Sexuality. The British Experience* (Manchester, 1991).

Ileto, R. C., 'Cholera and the origins of the American sanitary order in the Philippines', in Arnold (ed.), *Imperial Medicine and Indigenous Societies*, pp. 125–48.

Illich, I. D., *Medical Nemesis. The Expropriation of Health* (London, 1975).

Inkster, I., 'Marginal men: aspects of the social role of the medical community in Sheffield, 1790–1850', in D. Richards and J. Woodward (eds.), *Health Care and Popular Medicine in Nineteenth century England* (London, 1977).

Irfan Habib, S., 'Promoting science and its world-view in mid-nineteenth century India', in Kumar (ed.), *Science and Empire*, pp. 139–51.

Jaggi, O. P., *Indian System of Medicine* (Delhi, 1973).

Jeffery, R., 'Recognising India's doctors: the establishment of medical dependency, 1918–39', *Mod. Asian Stud.*, 13 (1979), 301–26.

'Doctors and Congress: the role of medical men and medical politics in Indian nationalism', in M. Shepperdson and C. Simmons (eds.), *The Indian National Congress and the Political Economy of India, 1885–1985* (London, 1987), pp. 160–73.

The Politics of Health in India (Berkeley, 1988).

Johnson, G., *Provincial Politics and Indian Nationalism: Bombay and the Indian National Congress, 1880–1915* (Cambridge, 1973).

Johnson, T., *Professions and Power* (London, 1972).

Jordanova, L. J., 'Earth science and environmental medicine: the synthesis of the late Enlightenment', in Jordanova and R. Porter (eds.), *Images of the Earth. Essays in the History of Environmental Sciences* (Oxford, 1979).

Kaminsky, A., *The India Office, 1880–1910* (London, 1986).

Kaye, M. M. (ed.), *The Golden Calm. An English Lady's Life in Mogul Delhi* (Exeter, 1980).

Kennedy, D., 'The perils of the midday sun: climatic anxieties in the colonial tropics', in MacKenzie (ed.), *Imperialism and the Natural World*, pp. 118–40.

Klein, I., 'Death in India, 1871–1921', *J. Asian Stud.*, 22, 4 (1973), 639–59.

'Cholera: theory and treatment in nineteenth century India', *J. Indian Hist.*, 58 (1980), 35–51.

'Urban development and death: Bombay city, 1870–1914', *Mod. Asian Stud.*, 20 (1986), 725–54.

'Plague, policy and popular unrest in British India', *Mod. Asian Stud.*, 22 (1988), 723–55.

Kopf, D., *British Orientalism and the Bengal Renaissance* (Berkeley, 1969).

Kumar, D., 'Racial discrimination and science in nineteenth-century India', *Indian Econ. and Soc. Hist. Rev.*, 19 (1982), 63–82.

'Science, resources and the Raj', *Indian Hist. Rev.*, 10 (1983), 66–89.

'The evolution of colonial science in India: natural history and the East India Company', in MacKenzie (ed.), *Imperialism and the Natural World*, 51–66.

(ed.), *Science and Empire. Essays in Indian Context (1700–1947)* (Delhi, 1991).

Kumar, R. R., *Western India in the Nineteenth Century* (London, 1968).

Laissus, Y., 'Les voyageurs naturalistes du Jardin du Roi et du Museum d'Histoire Naturelle: essai de portrait-robot', *Rev. Hist. Sci.*, 36 (1981), 259–317.

Lambert, R., *Sir John Simon (1816–1904) and English Social Administration* (London, 1963).

Lange, R., 'Plagues and pestilences in Polynesia: the nineteenth-century Cook Islands experience', *Bull. Hist. Med.*, 58 (1984), 325–46.

Lankford, N. D., 'The Victorian medical profession and military practice: army doctors and national origins', *Bull. Hist. Med.*, 54 (1980), 511–28.

Larson, M. S., *The Rise of Professionalism: A Sociological Analysis* (Berkeley, 1977).

Leach, E. and S. N. Mukherjee (eds.), *Elites in South Asia* (Cambridge, 1980).

Leslie, C. (ed.), *Asian Medical Systems: A Comparative Study* (Berkeley, 1976).

Lewis, R. A., *Edwin Chadwick and the Public Health Movement, 1832–54* (London, 1952).

Livingstone, D. N., 'Human acclimatization: perspectives on a contested field of inquiry in science, medicine and geography', *History of Science*, 25 (1982), 359–94.

Longmate, N., *King Cholera: The Biography of a Disease* (London, 1966).

Loudon, I., *Medical Care and the General Practitioner, 1750–1850* (Oxford, 1986).

Lyons, M., *The Colonial Disease. A Social History of Sleeping Sickness in Northern Zaire, 1900–1940* (Cambridge, 1992).

MacKenzie, J. M. (ed.), *Imperialism and the Natural World* (Manchester, 1990).

MacLeod, R. M., 'Scientific advice for British India: imperial perception and administrative goals, 1898–1923', *Mod. Asian Stud.*, 9, 3 (1975), 343–84.

MacLeod, R. M. and M. Lewis (eds.), *Disease, Medicine, and Empire. Perspectives on Western Medicine and the Experience of European Expansion* (London, 1988).

Marcovich, A., 'French colonial medicine and colonial rule: Algeria and Indochina', in R. M. MacLeod and M. Lewis (eds.), *Disease, Medicine, and Empire*, pp. 103–18.

Marks, S. and N Anderson, 'Typhus and social control: South Africa: 1917–1950', in R. M. MacLeod and M. Lewis (eds.), *Disease, Medicine, and Empire*, pp. 257–83.

Marland, H., *Medicine and Society in Wakefield and Huddersfield 1780–1870* (Cambridge, 1987).

Marshall, P. J. (ed.), *The Discovery of Hinduism in the Eighteenth Century* (Cambridge, 1970).

Mayne, A., '"The dreadful scourge": responses to smallpox in Sydney and Melbourne, 1881-2', in R. M. MacLeod and M. Lewis (eds.), *Disease, Medicine, and Empire*, pp. 219–41.

McAlpin, M. B., *Subject to Famine: Food Crises and Economic Change in Western India, 1860–1920* (Princeton, 1983).

McNeill, W. H., *Plagues and Peoples* (Harmondsworth, 1979).

Meek, R. L., *Social Science and the Ignoble Savage* (Cambridge, 1976).

Mehrotra, S. R., *Towards India's Freedom and Partition* (Delhi, 1979).

Mersey, Viscount, *The Viceroys and Governors-General of India 1757–1947* (London, 1949).

Metcalfe, B. D., 'Nationalist Muslims in British India: the case of Hakim Ajmal Khan', *Mod. Asian Stud.*, 19 (1985), 1–28.

Misra, B. B., *The Indian Middle Classes. Their Growth in Modern Times* (London, 1961).

Mollaret, H. H. and J. Brossollet, *Alexandre Yersin ou le Vainquer de la Peste* (Paris, 1985).

Moore, R. J., *Liberalism and Indian Politics 1872–1922* (London, 1966).

Morrell, J. B., 'The chemist breeders: the research schools of Liebig and Thomas Thompson', *Ambix*, 19 (1972), 1–46.

Morris, R. J., *Cholera 1832: The Social Response to an Epidemic* (London, 1976).

Mukherjee, S. N., *Sir William Jones* (London, 1968).

Muraleedharan, V. R., 'Malady in Madras: the colonial government's response to malaria in the early twentieth century', in D. Kumar (ed.), *Science and Empire*, pp. 101–14.
   'Rural health care in Madras Presidency: 1919–39', *Indian Social and Economic History Review*, 24 (1987), 324–34.

Nicolson, M., 'Medicine and racial politics: changing images of the New Zealand Maori in the nineteenth century', in D. Arnold (ed.), *Imperial Medicine*, pp. 66–104.

O'Brien, P. K., 'The costs and benefits of British imperialism 1846–1914', *Past and Present*, 120 (1988), 163–200.

Page, D., *Prelude to Partition: The Indian Muslims and the Imperial System of Control, 1920–32* (Delhi, 1982).

Parry, J. and N. Parry, *The Rise of the Medical Profession. A Study of Collective Social Mobility* (London, 1976).

Parshad, I. D., *Some Aspects of India's Foreign Trade 1757–1893* (London, 1932).

Patterson, T. J. S., 'Science and medicine in India', in P. Corsi and P. Weindling (eds.), *Information Sources in the History of Science and Medicine* (London, 1983), pp. 457–75.

'The relationship of Indian and European practitioners of medicine from the sixteenth century', in G. J. Meulenbeld and d. D. Wujastyk (eds.), *Studies in Indian Medical History* (Groningen, 1987), pp. 119–29.

Pelling, M., *Cholera, Fever and English Medicine 1825–1865* (Oxford, 1978).

Peterson, M. J., *The Medical Profession in Mid-Victorian London* (Berkeley, 1978).

'Gentlemen and medical men: the problem of professional recruitment', *Bull. Hist. Med.*, 58 (1984), 457–73.

Porter, R., 'Lay medical knowledge in the eighteenth century: the evidence of the Gentleman's Magazine', *Medical History*, 29 (1985), 138–68.

Porter, R. and D. Porter, 'The politics of prevention: anti-vaccinationism and public health in nineteenth-century England', *Medical History*, 32 (1988), 231–52.

Raj, K., 'Knowledge, power and modern science: the Brahmins strike back', in Kumar (ed.), *Science and Empire*, pp. 115–25.

Ramasubban, R., *Public Health and Medical Research in India: Their Origins and Development Under the Impact of British Colonial Policy* (Stockholm, 1982).

'Imperial health in British India, 1857–1900', in MacLeod, R. M. and M. Lewis (eds.), *Disease, Medicine, and Empire*, pp. 38–60.

Ray, R. K., *Social Conflict and Political Unrest in Bengal 1875–1927* (New Delhi, 1984).

Ray, R., *Urban Roots of Indian Nationalism: Pressure Groups and Conflict of Interests in Calcutta City Politics 1875–1939* (New Delhi, 1979).

Raychaudhuri, T., 'Europe in India's xenology: the nineteenth-century record', Past and Present, 137 (1992), 156–82.

Riley, J. C., 'The medicine of the environment in eighteenth-century Germany', *Clio Medica*, 18 (1983), 167–78.

Rooff, M., *Voluntary Societies and Social Policy* (London, 1937).

Sangwan, S., 'Indian response to European science and technology 1757–1857', *British J. for the Hist. of Sci.*, 21 (1988), 211–32.

Scott, H. H., *A History of Tropical Medicine*, 2 vols. (London, 1939–42).

Seal, A., *The Emergence of Indian Nationalism. Competition and Collaboration in the Later Nineteenth Century* (Cambridge, 1971).

Shapin, S. and A. Thackray, 'Prosopography as a research tool in the history of science: the British scientific community 1700–1900', *History of Science*, 12 (1974), 1–24.

Sheridan, R. B., *Doctors and Slaves: A Medical and Demographic History of Slavery in the British West Indies 1680–1834* (Cambridge, 1985).

Sinha, J. N., 'Science and the Indian National Congress', in Kumar (ed.), *Science and Empire*, 161–81.

Skelley, A. R., *The Victorian Army at Home: The Recruitment and Terms and Conditions of the British Regular, 1859–1988* (London, 1977).

Spangenberg, B., *British Bureaucracy in India. Status, Policy and the ICS in the late 19th Century* (Delhi, 1976).

Stafford, R. A., 'The role of Sir Roderick Murchison in promoting the geological development of the British empire and its sphere of influence' (Oxford University D.Phil. thesis, 1985).

Stewart, L., 'The edge of utility: slaves and smallpox in the early eighteenth century', *Medical History*, 29 (1985), 54–70.

Stokes, E., *The English Utilitarians and India* (Oxford, 1959).

Sullivan, R., 'Cholera and colonialism in the Philippines, 1899–1903', in MacLeod and Lewis (eds.), *Disease, Medicine, and Empire*, pp. 284–300.

Summers, A., *Angels and Citizens: British Women as Military Nurses 1854–1914* (London, 1988).

Swanson, M. W., 'The sanitation syndrome: bubonic plague and urban native policy in the Cape Colony, 1900–1909', *J. African Hist.*, 18 (1977), 387–410.

Thomas, K., *Man and the Natural World. Changing Attitudes in England 1500–1800* (London, 1983).

Tinker, H. R., *The Foundations of Local Self-Government in India, Pakistan and Burma* (London, 1954).

Tomlinson, B. R., *Political Economy of the Raj 1914–1947* (London, 1979).

van Heteren, G., et al. (eds.), *Dutch Medicine in the Malay Archipelago 1816–1942* (Amsterdam, 1989).

Vaughan, M., *Curing Their Ills. Colonial Power and African Illness* (Cambridge and Oxford, 1991).

Vernon, K., 'Pus, sewage, beer and milk: microbiology in Britain, 1870–1940', *History of Science*, 28 (1990), 289–325.

Waddington, I., 'General practitioners and consultants in early-nineteenth-century England: the sociology of an intra-professional conflict', in J. Woodward and R. Woods (eds.), *Urban Disease and Mortality in NIneteenth-Century England* (London, 1984), pp. 164–88.

Waksman, S. A., *The Brilliant and Tragic Life of W. M. W. Haffkine* (New Brunswick, 1964).

Watkins, D. E., 'The English revolution in social medicine, 1889–1911' (University of London Ph.D. thesis, 1985).

Weber, G., 'Science and society in nineteenth-century anthropology', *History of Science*, 12 (1974), 260–83.

Wilson, K. M. (ed.), *British Foreign Secretaries and Foreign Policy: From Crimean War to First World War* (Beckenham, 1982).

Wohl, A. S., *Endangered Lives: Public Health in Victorian Britain* (London, 1983).

Worboys, M., 'The emergence of tropical medicine: a study in the establishment of a scientific speciality', in G. Lemaine et al. (eds.), *Perspectives on the Emergence of Scientific Disciplines* (The Hague, 1977), pp. 76–98.

'Science and British colonial imperialism, 1895–1940' (University of Sussex D.Phil. thesis, 1979).

'Manson, Ross, and colonial medical policy: tropical medicine in London and Liverpool, 1899–1914', in MacLeod and Lewis (eds.), *Disease, Medicine and Empire*, pp. 21–37.

'The Imperial Institute: the state and the development of the natural resources of the Colonial Empire, 1887–1823', in MacKenzie (ed.), *Imperialism and the Natural World*, pp. 164–86.

Wright, P. and R. Treacher (eds.), *The Problem of Medical Knowledge* (Edinburgh, 1982).

Zetland, Lord, *Lord Cromer* (London, 1932).

Index

Abdul Kadir, S.S., 133
abhijatas, 203, 207
acclimatisation, 37–9, 43–51
Aden, 125, 137
Afghanistan campaign (1877–80), 68
Agra Medical School, 95
Ahmed, Hon. M. N., 18
Ahmed, Hon. Sayyed, 84
Ahmedabad, 147, 182, 184
Ainslie, Whitelaw, 41
Alban, Sir Arthur, 132–3
alcoholism, 62–3
Alexandria, bombardment of, 126
Alikhan, Muhammed Yakub, 129
All-India Sanitary Conferences, 1911, 81, 95;
    1912, 185, 199
Allahabad, 148
American Army Sanitary Commission, 62, 78,
    109
Amrita Bazar Patrika, Calcutta health officer;
    municipal representation, 207; vaccination,
    87
Amritsar, 104, 163
Arabi, Colonel, 125, 126, 127
Araud, T., 46
Arbuthnot, John, 36
Army Hospital Corps, 14
Army Medical Department, 8, 19, 30–1, 42,
    110, 143, 164, 227
Army Medical Service, see Army Medical
    Department
Army Sanitary Commission, 66, 76–7, 109,
    208, 231
Arnold, David, 2, 229, 233–4
Arracan, 46
Asiatic Society of Bengal, 15
Assam, government of, 90; medical treatment,
    162; sanitation, 169, 195, 198; vaccination,
    86
Association of Medical Women, 95
asylums, 78

Australia, 121
Austro-Hungary, 126, 130, 133, 136
ayurveda, 40–1, 42, 88

Bainbridge, George, 140–1, 145
Ballhatchet, Kenneth, 33, 76
Ballingall, George, 37–9
Banatlava, H. M., 34
Banerjea, M., 172
Banerjea, Surendranath, 207, 213, 218, 222,
    224, 232
Bangalore, 144
Bardwan fever, 189–90
Baring, E., 265n, 277n
barracks, 63–6
Batchman Sirusker, S.S., 119
Beck, Ann, 161
Belgaum Vaccine Institute, 86
Bellary, 143, 147
Bellew, Henry, 56
Benares, 174
Bengal Medical Service, 7, 14, 23, 24–5
Bengal Times, 270
Bengal National Chamber of Commerce, 224
Bengal Coal Company, 88
Bengal Presidency, 44, 47; CD Acts, 73, 76,
    77; Chamber of Commerce, 221; cholera,
    104; dispensaries, 88–90; Drainage Act
    (1880), 190; Local Government Loans Act
    (1879), 172; local self-government, 170,
    221–4; malaria, 160; Medical Board, 218;
    Municipal Acts (1848), 204, (1871), 167,
    206–7, (1884), 172; sanitation, 170, 171–4,
    182–8, 192, 196, 198; vaccination, 83, 84,
    86; vital statistics, 79, 81
Bentinck, William, 47, 48
Bengalee, Calcutta Corporation, 183, 210–11,
    212, 213–14, 216, 217, 222–3; CD Acts, 33,
    75–6; Dufferin Fund, 94; municipal
    representation, 207; plague in Calcutta, 218,
    219; quarantine, 136; sanitary boards, 194

317

Cambridge history of medicine